Selected Heritable Disorders of Connective Tissue and Disability

Paul A. Volberding, Carol Mason Spicer, Tom Cartaxo, and Roberta A. Wedge, *Editors*

Committee on Selected Heritable Disorders of Connective Tissue and Disability

Board on Health Care Services

Health and Medicine Division

A Consensus Study Report of

The National Academies of
SCIENCES · ENGINEERING · MEDICINE

THE NATIONAL ACADEMIES PRESS
Washington, DC
www.nap.edu

THE NATIONAL ACADEMIES PRESS   500 Fifth Street, NW   Washington, DC 20001

This activity was supported by Contract/Task Order No. 28321318D00060015/00003 between the National Academy of Sciences and the U.S. Social Security Administration. Any opinions, findings, conclusions, or recommendations expressed in this publication do not necessarily reflect the views of any organization or agency that provided support for the project.

International Standard Book Number-13: 978-0-309-27553-8
International Standard Book Number-10: 0-309-27553-9
Digital Object Identifier: https://doi.org/10.17226/26431
Library of Congress Control Number: 2022943401

Additional copies of this publication are available from the National Academies Press, 500 Fifth Street, NW, Keck 360, Washington, DC 20001; (800) 624-6242 or (202) 334-3313; http://www.nap.edu.

Copyright 2022 by the National Academy of Sciences. All rights reserved.

Printed in the United States of America

Suggested citation: National Academies of Sciences, Engineering, and Medicine. 2022. *Selected heritable disorders of connective tissue and disability*. Washington, DC: The National Academies Press. https://doi.org/10.17226/26431.

The National Academies of
SCIENCES · ENGINEERING · MEDICINE

The **National Academy of Sciences** was established in 1863 by an Act of Congress, signed by President Lincoln, as a private, nongovernmental institution to advise the nation on issues related to science and technology. Members are elected by their peers for outstanding contributions to research. Dr. Marcia McNutt is president.

The **National Academy of Engineering** was established in 1964 under the charter of the National Academy of Sciences to bring the practices of engineering to advising the nation. Members are elected by their peers for extraordinary contributions to engineering. Dr. John L. Anderson is president.

The **National Academy of Medicine** (formerly the Institute of Medicine) was established in 1970 under the charter of the National Academy of Sciences to advise the nation on medical and health issues. Members are elected by their peers for distinguished contributions to medicine and health. Dr. Victor J. Dzau is president.

The three Academies work together as the **National Academies of Sciences, Engineering, and Medicine** to provide independent, objective analysis and advice to the nation and conduct other activities to solve complex problems and inform public policy decisions. The National Academies also encourage education and research, recognize outstanding contributions to knowledge, and increase public understanding in matters of science, engineering, and medicine.

Learn more about the National Academies of Sciences, Engineering, and Medicine at **www.nationalacademies.org**.

The National Academies of
SCIENCES • ENGINEERING • MEDICINE

Consensus Study Reports published by the National Academies of Sciences, Engineering, and Medicine document the evidence-based consensus on the study's statement of task by an authoring committee of experts. Reports typically include findings, conclusions, and recommendations based on information gathered by the committee and the committee's deliberations. Each report has been subjected to a rigorous and independent peer-review process and it represents the position of the National Academies on the statement of task.

Proceedings published by the National Academies of Sciences, Engineering, and Medicine chronicle the presentations and discussions at a workshop, symposium, or other event convened by the National Academies. The statements and opinions contained in proceedings are those of the participants and are not endorsed by other participants, the planning committee, or the National Academies.

For information about other products and activities of the National Academies, please visit www.nationalacademies.org/about/whatwedo.

COMMITTEE ON SELECTED HERITABLE DISORDERS OF CONNECTIVE TISSUE AND DISABILITY

PAUL A. VOLBERDING (*Chair*), Professor Emeritus, Department of Epidemiology and Biostatistics, University of California, San Francisco

REBECCA BASCOM, Professor, Department of Medicine and Department of Public Health Sciences, Penn State College of Medicine

ADAM D. BITTERMAN, Assistant Professor of Orthopaedic Surgery, Zucker School of Medicine at Hofstra/Northwell

ANTONIO BULBENA-VILARRASA, Distinguished Professor of Psychiatry and Chair, Department of Psychiatry and Forensic Medicine, Universitat Autònoma de Barcelona

PRADEEP CHOPRA, Assistant Professor (Clinical), Department of Medicine, Warren Alpert Medical School of Brown University; Director, Center for Complex Conditions, Rhode Island

HARRY C. DIETZ, III (through July 2021), Victor A. McKusick Professor of Medicine and Genetics; Investigator, Howard Hughes Medical Institute, Johns Hopkins University School of Medicine

CLAIR A. FRANCOMANO, Professor of Medical and Molecular Genetics, Indiana University School of Medicine; Director, Ehlers-Danlos Society Center for the Ehlers-Danlos Syndromes, Indiana University Health Center

WALTER R. FRONTERA, Professor, Department of Physical Medicine, Rehabilitation, and Sports Medicine, and Department of Physiology, University of Puerto Rico School of Medicine

PETRA M. KLINGE, Director, Pediatric Neurosurgery Division; Director, Center for CSF Disorders of the Brain and Spine; Professor, Department of Neurosurgery, Warren Alpert Medical School of Brown University

BARBARA L. KORNBLAU, Executive Director, Coalition for Disability Health Equity; Professor and Director, Occupational Therapy Program, Idaho State University

DEBORAH KRAKOW, Professor and Chair, Department of Obstetrics and Gynecology; Professor of Human Genetics, Pediatrics, and Orthopedic Surgery, David Geffen School of Medicine at the University of California, Los Angeles

CHERYL L. MAIER, Medical Director, Emory Special Coagulation Laboratory; Assistant Professor, Department of Pathology and Laboratory Medicine, Emory University School of Medicine

ANNE L. MAITLAND, Assistant Professor, Department of Medicine, Icahn School of Medicine at Mount Sinai; Attending Physician, Mount Sinai South Nassau Chiari EDS Center Program; Medical Director, Comprehensive Allergy & Asthma Care and 3 Pillars Therapeutics

REED E. PYERITZ, William Smilow Professor of Medicine Emeritus, and Professor of Genetics Emeritus, University of Pennsylvania Perelman School of Medicine

LESLIE N. RUSSEK, Professor Emeritus, Department of Physical Therapy, Clarkson University

ERIC L. SINGMAN, Professor, Department of Ophthalmology and Visual Sciences, University of Maryland School of Medicine

Study Staff

CAROL MASON SPICER, Study Director
TOM CARTAXO, Associate Program Officer (through December 2021)
ROBERTA A. WEDGE, Senior Program Officer (from December 2021)
AUSTEN APPLEGATE, Research Associate (from May 2022)
VICTORIA BROWN, Senior Program Assistant
SHARYL NASS, Senior Director, Board on Health Care Services

Reviewers

This Consensus Study Report was reviewed in draft form by individuals chosen for their diverse perspectives and technical expertise. The purpose of this independent review is to provide candid and critical comments that will assist the National Academies of Sciences, Engineering, and Medicine in making each published report as sound as possible and to ensure that it meets the institutional standards for quality, objectivity, evidence, and responsiveness to the study charge. The review comments and draft manuscript remain confidential to protect the integrity of the deliberative process.

We thank the following individuals for their review of this report:

JAMES H. BLACK, III, Johns Hopkins Hospital
ANN BURKHARDT, Independent Consultant
JEFFERSON J. DOYLE, Johns Hopkins Hospital
HOWARD H. GOLDMAN, University of Maryland School of Medicine
DAVID LEVINE, University of Tennessee at Chattanooga
MARC A. NORMAN, University of California, San Diego
LAURA A. PACE, Metrodora Institute
JONATHAN RODIS, Marfan Foundation, Massachusetts Chapter
JOHNATHAN G. SEIDMAN, Harvard Medical School
MAXWELL SLEPIAN, University Health Network Canada
JOYCE SO, University of California, San Francisco School of Medicine
PAUL DAVID SPONSELLER, Kennedy Krieger Institute
WENDY WAGNER, Wendy 4 Therapy
JESSICA J. WANG, University of California, Los Angeles

Although the reviewers listed above provided many constructive comments and suggestions, they were not asked to endorse the conclusions or recommendations of this report, nor did they see the final draft before its release. The review of this report was overseen by **ALAN JETTE**, MGH Institute of Health Professions, and **ROBERT S. LAWRENCE**, Johns Hopkins Bloomberg School of Public Health. They were responsible for making certain that an independent examination of this report was carried out in accordance with the standards of the National Academies and that all review comments were carefully considered. Responsibility for the final content rests entirely with the authoring committee and the National Academies.

Preface

The U.S. Social Security Administration (SSA) provides support for individuals—adults and children—who are unable to function in employment or school due to chronic disabling medical conditions. While some conditions are straightforward, for example, a disease affecting a single organ, others are more complex, such as disorders that involve multiple organs and body systems. In these, impairments may reflect a summation of dysfunction from an array of sources. Also, while many disabling conditions can be diagnosed easily, others cannot be confirmed with a single biologic test. For these complex disorders affecting multiple organs and body systems determining disability can be challenging.

An example of such complex and difficult-to-diagnose disorders leading to impaired occupational and school function are those termed hereditary disorders of connective tissue (HDCTs). HDCTs, including Marfan syndrome and the Ehlers-Danlos syndromes, can disrupt the structure and function of many organs. Most are inherited with known genetic causes, while some demonstrate involvement of genetic factors with unknown genetic causes. Although often considered uncommon, HDCTs frequently go undiagnosed or are only detected after prolonged delays. Disability in HDCTs varies by the organs affected and the severity of resulting dysfunction. Additionally, many people with these conditions experience pain, fatigue, impaired cognition, and other neurological and immunological disorders. The constellation of clinical manifestations and severity in each person often varies over time. Functional disability in HDCTs can be linked to a single or multiple comorbidities potentially affecting multiple organ systems. HDCTs are not curable, and treatment is directed at preventing or mitigating specific consequences, often termed secondary impairments.

SSA, appreciating the difficulty in disability determinations for HDCTs, asked the Health and Medicine Division (HMD) of the National Academies of Sciences, Engineering, and Medicine to convene a committee of experts to review these disorders. SSA sought clarification on the epidemiology and diagnosis of HDCTs, on the ways in which these conditions affect the individual and insights into the disability determination process. To this end, the HMD convened a committee who carefully considered evidence in the literature and from invited discussants with both professional and personal experience in this area. The committee collected their findings and conclusions to assist SSA in its consideration of this group of medical conditions.

On behalf of the committee and the HMD project staff, I extend my sincere thanks to the many individuals who shared their time and expertise to support the committee's work and inform its deliberations. The study was sponsored by the SSA, and we thank Andrea Bento, Megan Butson, Gina Clemons, Alayna Ness, Vincent Nibali, and Steven Rollins for their guidance and support. The committee also acknowledges SSA for verifying relevant technical content pertaining to the disability determination process for accuracy. The committee benefited greatly from discussions with individuals who presented at the committee's open sessions: Andrea Bento, Maggie Buckley, Antonio Bulbena-Vilarrasa, Laura Pace, Jon Rodis, Peter Rowe, and Alissa Zingman. The committee is grateful to these presenters for volunteering to share their expertise, knowledge, data, and opinions with the committee and SSA. We also thank Peter Rowe for preparing a commissioned paper based on his presentation. Our appreciation goes to the reviewers for their invaluable feedback on an earlier draft of the report and to the monitor and coordinator who oversaw the report review.

The committee acknowledges the many staff within HMD who provided support in various ways to this project, including Carol Mason Spicer (study director), Tom Cartaxo (associate program officer), Victoria Brown (senior program assistant), Roberta Wedge (senior program officer), Austen Applegate (research associate), Karen Helsing (senior program officer), Micah Winograd (senior finance business partner), and Ron Brown (deputy director program finance). The committee extends great thanks and appreciation to Sharyl Nass, senior board director of the Board on Health Care Services, who oversaw the project. Rebecca Morgan (senior librarian) provided research assistance, and the report review, production, and communications staff all provided valuable guidance to ensure the success of the final product. Rona Brière and her staff are to be credited for the superb editorial assistance they provided in preparing the final report.

PREFACE

Finally, I would like to deeply thank the committee of experts who volunteered their invaluable service in this review. The field of HDCTs is extremely broad, involving experts on a wide variety of affected body systems and the diagnosis and management of persons with HDCTs. The committee worked selflessly to ensure that the final report could be most effective in assisting SSA address their crucial efforts to guide the disability determination process in an accurate and efficient manner.

Paul A. Volberding, *Chair*
Committee on Selected Heritable Disorders
of Connective Tissue and Disability

Contents

ACRONYMS AND ABBREVIATIONS   xxi

SUMMARY   1
    Study Approach and Scope, 2
    Overall Conclusions, 6

1 INTRODUCTION   13
    Context for This Study, 13
    Study Charge and Scope, 15
    Study Approach, 15
    Report Organization, 22
    References, 22

2 OVERVIEW OF HERITABLE DISORDERS OF
    CONNECTIVE TISSUE   25
    History of the Hereditary Disorders of Connective Tissue, 25
    Epidemiology, 26
    Genetics, 27
    Connective Tissue, 28
    Diagnosis, 32
    Clinical Course, 35
    Disease State Management, 37
    Findings and Conclusions, 38
    References, 39

3 MARFAN SYNDROME AND RELATED HEREDITARY AORTOPATHIES 47
History of Marfan Syndrome and Related Hereditary Aortopathies, 47
Diagnosis of Marfan Syndrome and Related Hereditary Aortopathies, 48
Characteristics of Marfan Syndrome and Related Hereditary Aortopathies, 49
Treatment and Management, 58
Emerging Treatments, 61
Findings and Conclusions, 61
References, 63
Annex Table, 70

4 EHLERS-DANLOS SYNDROMES AND HYPERMOBILITY SPECTRUM DISORDERS 73
History of Ehlers-Danlos Syndromes and Hypermobility Spectrum Disorders, 73
Diagnosis of Ehlers-Danlos Syndromes and Hypermobility Spectrum Disorders, 77
Characteristics of Ehlers-Danlos Syndromes and Hypermobility Spectrum Disorders, 81
Treatment and Management, 88
Prognosis, 95
Emerging Treatments, 96
Findings and Conclusions, 97
References, 99
Annex Table, 114

5 HERITABLE DISORDERS OF CONNECTIVE TISSUE AND EFFECTS ON FUNCTION 125
Secondary Impairments, 126
Environmental Factors and Functioning, 128
Global Functioning, 129
Physical Functioning, 145
Vision, Hearing, and Speech Functioning, 149
Mental Functioning, 152
Heritable Disorders of Connective Tissue and the U.S. Social Security Administration's Listing of Impairments, 155
Findings and Conclusions, 158
References, 161
Annex Tables, 195

6 OVERALL CONCLUSIONS   291
   Overall Conclusions, 291
   Selected Findings and Conclusions in Support of the
      Committee's Overall Conclusions, 299

APPENDIXES
A Public Session Agendas   313
B Commissioned Paper   317
C Selected Resources   357
D Biographical Sketches of Committee Members   363

Boxes, Figures, and Tables

BOXES

1-1 Statement of Task, 16

3-1 Revised Ghent Criteria for Diagnosis of Marfan Syndrome and Related Conditions, 50
3-2 Ghent II Criteria for Scoring of Systemic Measures, 52

6-1 Overall Conclusions and Selected Chapter-Specific Findings and Conclusions, 300

B-1 Methods and Reporting Form for the Passive Standing Test, 326

FIGURES

1-1 ICF model of functioning and disability, 18

2-1 Connective tissue, 29

B-1 Pathophysiologic factors in orthostatic intolerance, 320
B-2 Changes in cerebral blood flow during 30 minutes of head-up tilt compared to supine values in 44 healthy controls and 429 adults with ME/CFS, 331
B-3 Reductions in cerebral blood flow (CBF) from supine values after 30 minutes of head-up tilt in 100 hypermobile and 100 nonhypermobile

adults with myalgic encephalomyelitis/chronic fatigue syndrome (ME/CFS), 334

TABLES

4-1 Clinical Classification of the Ehlers-Danlos Syndromes, Inheritance Pattern, and Genetic Basis, 75
4-2 Selected Hypermobility Assessment Scales, 78
4-3 Surgical and Anesthetic Recommendations for Joint Hypermobility Syndrome/Ehlers-Danlos Syndrome Hypermobility Type (JHS/EDS-HT), 94

B-1 Symptoms of Orthostatic Intolerance, 319
B-2 Medications for Orthostatic Intolerance, 338
B-3 Response to Ivabradine in a Young Adult with Joint Hypermobility and Inappropriate Sinus Tachycardia, 341

ANNEX TABLES

Annex Table 3-1 Overview of Marfan Syndrome and Related Hereditary Aortopathies, 70

Annex Table 4-1 Overview of Ehlers-Danlos Syndromes and Hypermobility Spectrum Disorders, 114

Annex Table 5-1 Levels of Work Based on Physical Exertion Requirements, 195
Annex Table 5-2 Physical; Vision, Hearing, and Speech; and Mental Activities, 197
Annex Table 5-3 Selected Musculoskeletal Manifestations Associated with Heritable Disorders of Connective Tissue, 201
Annex Table 5-4 Selected Neurologic Manifestations Associated with Heritable Disorders of Connective Tissue, 213
Annex Table 5-5 Selected Cardiovascular and Hematologic Manifestations Associated with Heritable Disorders of Connective Tissue, 222
Annex Table 5-6 Selected Respiratory Manifestations Associated with Heritable Disorders of Connective Tissue, 225
Annex Table 5-7 Selected Immunologic Manifestations Associated with Heritable Disorders of Connective Tissue, 231
Annex Table 5-8 Selected Gastrointestinal Manifestations Associated with Heritable Disorders of Connective Tissue, 241

Annex Table 5-9	Selected Cutaneous Manifestations Associated with Heritable Disorders of Connective Tissue, 244
Annex Table 5-10	Selected Genitourinary Manifestations Associated with Heritable Disorders of Connective Tissue, 248
Annex Table 5-11	Selected Vision, Hearing, and Speech Manifestations Associated with Heritable Disorders of Connective Tissue, 252
Annex Table 5-12	Selected Neuropsychiatric Conditions Potentially Connected with Heritable Disorders of Connective Tissue, 260
Annex Table 5-13	Global Functioning Associated with Heritable Disorders of Connective Tissue, 265
Annex Table 5-14	Functional Implications for Physical Activities of Conditions Associated with Heritable Disorders of Connective Tissue, 270
Annex Table 5-15	Functional Implications for Vision, Hearing, and Speaking Activities of Conditions Associated with Heritable Disorders of Connective Tissue, 279
Annex Table 5-16	Functional Implications for Mental Activities of Conditions Associated with Heritable Disorders of Connective Tissue, 282
Annex Table 5-17	Examples of Social Security Administration Listings that May Apply to Individuals with Heritable Disorders of Connective Tissue, 288

Acronyms and Abbreviations

6MWD	six minute walk distance
ABC Scale	Activities-specific Balance Confidence Scale
ACTH	adrenocorticotropic hormone
ADA	Americans with Disabilities Act
ADHD	attention-deficit/hyperactivity disorder
ADL	activity of daily living
aEDS	arthrochalasia-type Ehlers-Danlos syndrome
ANA	antinuclear antibody
ANCA	antineutrophil cytoplasmic antibody
ASHA	American Speech-Language-Hearing Association
BAI	Beck Anxiety Inventory
BCS	brittle cornea syndrome
BDI	Beck Depression Inventory
BFI	Brief Fatigue Inventory
BHS	Birt-Hogg-Dubé syndrome
BiPAP	bilevel positive airway pressure
BLS	U.S. Bureau of Labor Statistics
BMAT	Bruininks Motor Ability Test
BOT-2	Bruininks-Oseretsky Test of Motor Proficiency, 2nd Edition
CBC	complete blood count
CBT	cognitive behavioral therapy

CCA	congenital contractural arachnodactyly
CDC	Centers for Disease Control and Prevention
cEDS	classical Ehlers-Danlos syndrome
CFS	chronic fatigue syndrome, also myalgic encephalomyelitis
clEDS	classical-like Ehlers-Danlos syndrome
CNS	central nervous system
COMPASS 31	Composite Autonomic Symptom Score
CPAP	continuous positive airway pressure
CRP	C-reactive protein
CSF	cerebrospinal fluid
CT	computed tomography
CTA	computed tomography angiography
cvEDS	cardiac-valvular Ehlers-Danlos syndrome
DASH	Disabilities of the Arm, Shoulder and Hand questionnaire
dEDS	dermatosparaxis Ehlers-Danlos syndrome
DTH	delayed-type hypersensitivity
ECM	extracellular matrix
EDS	Ehlers-Danlos syndromes
EGD	esophagogastroduodenoscopy
EMG	electromyogram
ESR	erythrocyte sedimentation rate
FAMM	Foot and Ankle Ability Measure
FCE	Functional Capacity Evaluation
FSS	Fatigue Severity Scale
GAF	Global Assessment of Functioning scale
GERD	gastroesophageal reflux disease
G-HSD	generalized (joint) hypermobility spectrum disorder
GI	gastrointestinal
HAT	hereditary alpha tryptasemia
HDCT	heritable disorder of connective tissue
hEDS	hypermobile Ehlers-Danlos syndrome
HRQoL	health-related quality of life
HSCT	haematopoietic stem cell transplantation
HSD	hypermobility spectrum disorder
JAN	Job Accommodations Network
JH	joint hypermobility

IADL	instrumental activity of daily living
ICF	*International Classification of Functioning, Disability and Health*
ICP	intracranial pressure
IOM	Institute of Medicine
IOP	intraocular pressure
IPEX	immune dysregulation, polyendocrinopathy, enteropathy, X-linked
ISTH	International Society on Thrombosis and Haemostasis
kEDS	kyphoscoliotic Ehlers-Danlos syndrome
KOOS	Knee Injury and Osteoarthritis Outcome Score
LDS	Loeys-Dietz syndrome
LE	lower extremity
LEFS	Lower Extremity Functional Scale
LPR	laryngopharyngeal reflux
M-BESS	Modified Balance Error Scoring System
MCAD	mast cell activation disease
mcEDS	musculocontractural Ehlers-Danlos syndrome
ME	myalgic encephalomyelitis, also chronic fatigue syndrome
MET	metabolic equivalent of task
MFI	Mutidimensional Fatigue Inventory
MFS	Marfan syndrome
MHQ	Michigan Hand Outcomes Questionnaire
MINI	mini international neuropsychiatric interview
MIRECC	Mental Illness Research, Education, and Clinical Center
MRA	magnetic resonance angiography
MRI	magnetic resonance imaging
MRV	magnetic resonance venography
NASEM	National Academies of Sciences, Engineering, and Medicine
NDI	Neck Disability Index
NLM	U.S. National Library of Medicine
NMDAR	N-methyl-D-aspartate receptors
NMH	neurally mediated hypotension
NORD	National Organization for Rare Disorders
NRS	Numeric Rating Scale
OCT	optical coherence tomography
ODI	Oswestry Disability Index

OI	osteogenesis imperfecta
ORS	Occupational Requirements Survey
PCORI	Patient-Centered Outcomes Research Institute
PedsQL	Functional Disability Inventory of Pediatric Quality of Life
PEM	postexertional malaise
PID	primary immunodeficiency
PIDD	primary immunodeficiency disease
POTS	postural orthostatic tachycardia syndrome
PREE	Patient-Rated Elbow Evaluation
PROMIS	Patient-Reported Outcomes Measurement Information System
PRWE	Patient-Rated Wrist Evaluation
RAST	radioallergosorbent test
RFC	residual functional capacity
RMDQ	Roland-Morris Disability Questionnaire
SCID	severe combined immunodeficiency
SCID	structured clinical interview for DSM
SDS	Sheehan Disability Scale
SFN-SIQ	small fiber neuropathy Symptom Inventory Questionnaire
SGA	substantial gainful activity
SGS	Shprintzen-Goldberg syndrome
SLE	systemic lupus erythematosus
SNAP	sensory nerve action potential
SODA	Sequential Occupational Dexterity Assessment
SOFAS	Social and Occupational Functioning Assessment Scale
spEDS	spondylodysplastic Ehlers-Danlos syndrome
SSA	U.S. Social Security Administration
SSDI	Social Security Disability Insurance
SSI	Supplemental Security Income
TENS	transcutaneous electric nerve stimulation
UBM	ultrasound biomicroscopy
UE	upper extremity
VAS	Visual Analog Scale
vEDS	vascular Ehlers-Danlos syndrome
VUS	variants of uncertain significance
vWF	von Willebrand Factor

WAI	Work Ability Index
WD-FAB	Work Disability Functional Assessment Battery
WHO	World Health Organization
WOMAC	Western Ontario and McMaster Universities Osteoarthritis Index
WOSI	Western Ontario Shoulder Instability Index

Summary[1]

Heritable disorders of connective tissue (HDCTs) are a diverse group of many inherited (genetic) disorders and subtypes. Connective tissue is an integral component of all organ systems and plays a crucial role in their function. Hence, the physical and mental impairments associated with HDCTs manifest throughout the body and affect functioning in every body system. These impairments may develop and vary in severity (wax and wane) throughout an affected individual's lifetime.

The natural history of HDCTs as a general group demonstrates several commonalities, including their multisystem nature and the impairments they may cause. Nevertheless, the clinical course of individuals with an HDCT is highly variable with respect not only to the disease-specific manifestations of each disorder but also to the ways in which the disorders manifest in each affected individual, as well as the effects of environmental factors and physical and psychological demands to which the person is exposed.

The severity of HDCTs cannot be measured by a single genetic or laboratory test. Rather, their severity is determined by the severity of the physical and mental manifestations experienced by affected individuals, which may be measurable with existing clinical and function testing. The impact of HDCTs on functioning results from the combined effects of the multiple impairments with which they are associated in different body systems, which may be severe collectively even if "less severe" individually. In some cases, the impairments experienced by individuals with an HDCT are

---

[1] With the exception of direct quotations, this summary does not include references. Citations to support the text and conclusions herein are provided in the body of the report.

severe enough to qualify them for disability benefits from the U.S. Social Security Administration (SSA).

SSA provides financial assistance to people with disabilities through two programs: Social Security Disability Insurance (SSDI) (Title II of the Social Security Act) and Supplemental Security Income (SSI) (Title XVI of the Social Security Act). The SSDI program, established in 1956, provides benefits to eligible adults with disabilities who have paid into the Disability Insurance Trust Fund, as well as to certain family members. The SSI program, created in 1972, is a means-tested program based on income and financial resources that pays benefits to eligible adults and children with disabilities, individuals who are blind, and adults aged 65 and older.

In 2020, SSA requested that the Health and Medicine Division of the National Academies of Sciences, Engineering, and Medicine convene a committee of relevant experts to review current information and provide findings and conclusions regarding the diagnosis, treatment, and prognosis of selected HDCTs, including Marfan syndrome (MFS) and the Ehlers-Danlos syndromes (EDS), in adults and children. In the statement of task for the study, SSA also asked the committee to provide information on the relative levels of functional limitation typically associated with the disorders and their common treatments, and to identify any "non-exertional physical… and mental limitations (e.g., cognitive or behavioral) that are equivalent in severity to the standard represented in [SSA's] listings (i.e., that would prevent any gainful activity) but are not captured by currently existing listings and are not currently reflected in SSA's disability grid rules."[2] The committee was tasked as well with providing a summary of selected treatments currently being studied in clinical trials.

STUDY APPROACH AND SCOPE

The committee conducted an extensive review of the literature pertaining to HDCTs and work-related functioning. In addition, this review included websites maintained by such organizations as the International Consortium on Ehlers-Danlos Syndromes & Hypermobility Spectrum Disorders, the EDS & HSD Community Coalition (formerly "the EDS Comorbidity Coalition"), The Ehlers-Danlos Society, The Marfan Foundation, and SSA. Committee members and project staff identified additional salient literature and information using traditional academic research methods and online searches throughout the course of the study. The committee also drew on

---

[2] SSA's grid rules reflect functional and vocational patterns and in certain cases, incorporate into disability determinations analysis of vocational factors (i.e., age, education, previous work experience) in combination with the individual's residual functional capacity (https://www.ssa.gov/OP_Home/cfr20/404/404-app-p02.htm [accessed February 24, 2022]).

a variety of additional resources, including invited speakers with expertise in HDCT-associated gastrointestinal conditions, mental health conditions, and orthostatic intolerance (a condition in which individuals develop symptoms upon assuming and maintaining upright posture), as well as a panel discussion with patient advocates. The committee's work was informed further by a commissioned paper on the functional impact of orthostatic intolerance in EDS.

Definition of Disability

The concept of disability has evolved over the past several decades from a medical to a biopsychosocial model. The latter model, exemplified by the World Health Organization's International Classification of Functioning, Disability and Health (ICF), portrays disability as "the interaction between an individual (with a health condition) and that individual's contextual factors (environmental and personal factors)."[3] The ICF model recognizes functioning in three domains: (1) body function and structure, which encompass physiological functions of the body, including psychological functions, as well as the functioning of body structures (e.g., movement of limbs, cardiac function); (2) activities, which are actions or tasks (e.g., running, problem solving); and (3) participation, which is the performance of tasks in a societal context (e.g., participation in school or organized sports). The model refers to deficits in body function and structure as impairments, deficits in completing activities as limitations, and reductions in participation as restrictions. Accommodations, such as assistive technologies and environmental modifications, are environmental contextual factors that act on the ICF domains to enhance an individual's activity and participation.

SSA employs different definitions of disability for adults and children. For adults, the definition is "inability to engage in any SGA [substantial gainful activity] by reason of any medically determinable physical or mental impairment which can be expected to result in death or which has lasted or can be expected to last for a continuous period of not less than 12 months."[4] SGA is work activity that "involves doing significant and productive physical or mental duties" or activity that "is done (or intended) for pay or profit," regardless of whether a profit is realized.[5] In the SSA context, "disability" in adults refers to work disability—an inability to participate in work "in an ordinary work setting, on a regular and continuing basis,

---

[3]WHO (World Health Organization). 2001. *International classification of functioning, disability and health*. Geneva, Switzerland: WHO. https://apps.who.int/iris/handle/10665/ (accessed July 22, 2022).
[4]42 U.S.C. 423(d)(1); see also 20 CFR 404.1505; 20 CFR 416.905.
[5]20 CFR 404.1510; 20 CFR 404.1572.

and for 8 hours per day, 5 days per week, or an equivalent work schedule."[6] SSA incorporates assessment of function into its definition of disability for children (i.e., those less than 18 years of age). It considers children who are not engaged in SGA to be disabled if they have a "medically determinable physical or mental impairment or combination of impairments that causes marked and severe functional limitations, and that can be expected to cause death or that has lasted or can be expected to last for a continuous period of not less than 12 months."[7]

In its consideration of functioning among individuals affected by HDCTs, this report focuses on those physical; vision, hearing, and speech; and mental activities the committee determined to be most relevant to SSA. The committee made this determination based on the information SSA collects about disability applicants and the information the U.S. Bureau of Labor Statistics collects about the physical and mental demands of jobs for inclusion in the Occupational Information System.

Selection of Heritable Disorders of Connective Tissue for This Study

The committee's statement of task requests information about "selected [HDCTs], including but not necessarily limited to Ehlers-Danlos syndrome[s] and Marfan syndrome." As directed in the statement of task, this report focuses primarily on MFS and EDS because of their relative prevalence. MFS is an autosomal-dominant disorder that affects multiple organ systems, especially the ocular, cardiovascular, and skeletal systems. Thirteen types of EDS have been identified, all of which share common elements of joint hypermobility and skin and soft tissue involvement; hypermobile EDS (hEDS) is by far the most prevalent EDS type. In addition to MFS and EDS, the committee identified for inclusion in the report several other hereditary aortopathies (Loeys-Dietz syndrome, congenital contracture arachnodactyly [also known as Beals-Hecht syndrome], and Shprintzen-Goldberg syndrome) and hypermobility spectrum disorders (HSD) because of the features they share with MFS and hEDS, respectively.

Terminology

Secondary Impairments

The committee was tasked with describing, to the extent possible, "secondary impairments" that result from the HDCTs or their treatments.

---

[6] SSA. 2021. *DI 24510.057 sustainability and the residual functional capacity (RFC) assessment* https://secure.ssa.gov/poms.nsf/lnx/0424510057 (accessed May 23, 2022).
[7] 20 CFR 416.906; see also 42 U.S.C. 1382(c).

Because there is not always a known or clear causal link between the disorder and all of its manifestations, the committee understands "secondary impairments" to mean physical and mental manifestations (medical diagnoses, syndromes, or comorbid and other health conditions) that are either associated with or may result from an HDCT. Many of these are not specific to HDCTs and can also occur in other individuals. Use of this term thus defined does not mean that any of the physical or mental manifestations seen in individuals with HDCTs are not core elements of the disorders. Rather, the primary impairment is the underlying genetic disorder (e.g., EDS, MFS), while the secondary impairments encompass all of the physical and mental manifestations of that disorder. The committee considered the number, types, and severity of the secondary impairments experienced by individuals with an HDCT to be of particular importance with regard to the functional implications of these disorders.

Treatment and Management

The committee was tasked with addressing several issues related to the "types of treatments available" for HDCTs. For the purposes of this report, the committee distinguishes between "treatment" and "management": whereas treatment focuses on curing or mitigating a specific disease (in this case an HDCT), management focuses on caring for the person as a whole, which requires a multidisciplinary team and extends throughout the life course. Although no curative treatments currently are available for MFS or EDS, these disorders can be managed. Management involves supportive care, early diagnosis of the multisystem manifestations, treatment of associated physical and mental secondary impairments, and strategies for reducing or preventing problems that may present over time.

Severity

The committee was tasked with identifying possible indicators of "the clinical or medical severity" of HDCTs, and was asked to indicate in this report when the terms "severity" and "severe" are being used as they would be in "clinical or medical care settings" versus in "SSA's work-related program definition (i.e., an impairment of such severity as to be the basis of a finding of an inability to engage in any substantial gainful activity)." For the purposes of this report, the terms "severe" and "severity" are used as they typically would be in clinical or medical care settings. When the terms reflect SSA's program definition, their usage is specified as such.

OVERALL CONCLUSIONS

The committee formulated eight overall conclusions in seven areas: (1) nature of heritable disorders of connective tissue, (2) heritable disorders of connective tissue and disability, (3) diagnosis, (4) management, (5) barriers to access to care, (6) education, and (7) research gaps. In addition, at the end of several chapters, the report contains findings and conclusions specific to the evidence presented in those chapters.

Nature of Heritable Disorders of Connective Tissue

As described above, HDCTs affect connective tissues, which are present in and affect the functioning of all organ systems throughout the body. For this reason, HDCTs manifest in secondary impairments throughout the body that may develop and fluctuate in severity over time, and can have widespread and varied effects on physical and mental functioning. The severity of HDCTs relates to the severity of the physical and mental secondary impairments experienced by affected individuals, including the combined effects of multiple impairments, as well as the frequency, severity, and predictability of their fluctuations. Secondary impairments in any of the body systems can be severe and adversely affect an individual's functioning; limitations associated with pain, fatigue, and anxiety may be particularly pronounced. The functional limitations experienced by individuals with HDCTs are also affected by environmental factors (e.g., extreme heat and cold, noise and vibration, smells, wetness and humidity, other atmospheric conditions, irritants). In addition, physical and mental demands related to school or work may precipitate or exacerbate these limitations.

For these reasons, the committee drew the following overall conclusion:

1. Heritable disorders of connective tissue (HDCTs) comprise a large and varied group of disorders in children and adults that share the common feature of pronounced involvement of connective tissues, usually in multiple organ systems. HDCTs can lead to a variety of physical and mental secondary impairments (i.e., manifestations, medical diagnoses, syndromes, comorbidities, or other health conditions) and associated functional limitations. Impairments can range from minor to severe and even life-threatening and may fluctuate in severity over time in an individual. Functional limitations may be sufficiently severe to interfere with participation in work and school, as well as social and recreational activities, and may include precautions and restrictions on activities to avoid aggravating the condition.

Heritable Disorders of Connective Tissue and Disability

A challenge in assessment of functioning in individuals with HDCTs is capturing the full effect of their impairment(s) on their daily activities, including participation in work and school. This is particularly true when a person has multiple impairments. Individuals with HDCTs may experience significant variability in their physical and/or mental secondary impairments from day to day or even within a single day. This variability is often unpredictable and may limit the ability to sustain gainful employment.

The committee reviewed SSA's Listing of Impairments-Adult Listings and found that some of the listings include severity criteria for some of the secondary impairments that may be experienced by individuals with MFS, EDS, and other HDCTs. The committee also concluded that other listings, with some modification, could apply to certain secondary impairments experienced by individuals with HDCTs. The committee found further that the combined effects of an individual's secondary impairments may limit function with a degree of severity sufficient to preclude the individual's participation in work on a "regular and continuing basis" (i.e., 8 hours per day, 5 days per week, or an equivalent work schedule) or, for children, to cause "marked and severe functional limitations." The concept of functional equivalence used by SSA in some disability determinations in children is particularly well suited to evaluating the combined effects on an applicant's functioning of the many and varied impairments that often manifest in HDCTs and other multisystem disorders.

For these reasons, the committee drew the following overall conclusion:

2. Some of SSA's Adult Listings apply directly to secondary impairments experienced by individuals with HDCTs and could be used to evaluate disability in those individuals. Other listings, with some modification, could apply to certain secondary impairments experienced by individuals with HDCTs.

Diagnosis

Early diagnosis of HDCTs is important to reduce physical injury, reduce psychological harm to the affected individual and family members, and prevent the risks associated with inappropriate or fragmented medical care. HDCTs are diagnosed through a combination of clinical findings and established clinical criteria, followed by confirmatory molecular genetic testing when specific genes have been identified for the suspected disorder. Some HDCTs, such as hEDS, do not yet have a known genetic marker or test, and the absence of molecular genetic testing should not necessarily rule out the diagnosis if the clinical suspicion remains based on clinical findings.

An HDCT diagnosis should be considered for individuals who present with previously undiagnosed complex multisystem disorders; however, diagnosis of some HDCTs, in particular EDS, is often delayed, in some cases for a decade or more. One reason for delayed diagnosis is that because HDCTs can cause a wide variety of physical and mental secondary impairments involving multiple organ systems, patients often are referred to a succession of different specialists. Other factors may contribute to delayed diagnosis, including minimal training in and knowledge about the disorders among health care providers and a corresponding shortage of clinicians with expertise in diagnosing and managing them. Delayed diagnosis may exacerbate manifestations of HDCTs or have life-threatening consequences.

For these reasons, the committee drew the following overall conclusion:

3. **Early diagnosis of HDCTs is important to reduce physical injury, reduce psychological harm to the individual and family members, and prevent the risks associated with inappropriate or fragmented medical care.**
    - Diagnosis of HDCTs is often delayed because of
        - the multisystem, complex, and phenotypically variable nature of the disorders;
        - lack of knowledge about HDCTs among health care providers, patients and family members, and other stakeholders;
        - lack of experience with using the syndromic approach to diagnosis, in which diagnosis is based on characteristic groups of symptoms and signs;
        - lack of access to comprehensive, multidisciplinary care teams with expertise in HDCTs (due to a shortage of clinicians, especially in some geographic areas);
        - historical bias and denial among health care providers, patients, and family members about the reality of the lived experience of manifestations of the disorders; and
        - inaccurate expectations that there will be a diagnostic genetic test for every HDCT.
    - Delayed or misdiagnosis of individuals with HDCTs can result in
        - inappropriate medical interventions;
        - inability to accurately assess the risks and benefits associated with medical procedures;
        - inability to access necessary reasonable accommodations at work or school;
        - family stress and dysfunction;
        - stress associated with unexplained and repeated evidence of trauma, leading to inappropriate suspicion of child abuse;
        - inappropriate assessments and incorrect diagnoses; and

- mistrust of health care providers and negative expectations for future health care encounters.
- Timely diagnosis and recognition of the many physical and mental secondary impairments with which HDCTs can present and action to address them, even if in the absence of a specific molecular diagnosis, can dramatically improve individuals' quality of life and functional status, including the ability to participate in work and school.

Management

As noted, there are currently no curative treatments for HDCTs, but appropriate management can reduce the frequency and severity of the disorders' manifestations and resulting functional limitations. Management of the HDCTs involves supportive care, early diagnosis and treatment of associated physical and mental secondary impairments, and preventive strategies to lessen or prevent problems that may occur over time. Because of the complex, multisystem nature of HDCTs, high-quality care for individuals with these disorders relies on effective coordination among a team of health care providers across a broad range of disciplines with expertise in the disorders.

For these reasons, the committee drew the following overall conclusion:

4. Although curative treatments for HDCTs do not exist at this time, appropriate understanding and management of the disorders can reduce the frequency and severity of their manifestations and resulting functional consequences. High-quality care for individuals with HDCTs relies on effective coordination among a team of clinicians across a broad range of physical and mental health care disciplines who are knowledgeable about these disorders.

Barriers to Access to Care

Given the general lack of knowledge about HDCTs among clinicians, individuals with these disorders often have difficulty obtaining appropriate and integrated multidisciplinary care to address the wide range of associated impairments. Insufficient training in and knowledge about the disorders among health care providers contribute to a shortage of clinicians with expertise in diagnosing and managing them. In addition, access to multidisciplinary teams and relevant specialists is limited or nonexistent in rural areas; even many university centers lack multidisciplinary teams with expertise in HDCTs.

For these reasons, the committee drew the following overall conclusion:

5. Access to comprehensive, multidisciplinary care for the diagnosis and management of HDCTs can be limited by geography and other factors, including the availability of care teams with expertise in the disorders.

Education

Education about HDCTs, including their multisystem manifestations, diagnosis, and management, is important for all health care providers to help increase recognition and earlier diagnosis of the disorders. With appropriate education, a variety of health care providers, including, for example, physicians, nurses, psychologists, neuropsychologists, rehabilitation specialists (e.g., physiatrists; physical, occupational, and speech therapists), nutritionists, and others, should be able to recognize HDCTs and direct affected individuals to the appropriate care providers for management. Clinicians performing procedures or providing anesthesia and periprocedures management need to be aware of the altered procedural and postprocedural risks associated with HDCTs and to have a screening strategy for these disorders. It is also important for individuals with HDCTs and their family members to learn about strategies for preventing or mitigating symptoms, as well as the risks associated with certain activities that may result in physical trauma, such as physically demanding activities or pregnancy and childbirth. Relevant support groups provide valuable education regarding the manifestations and lived experience of the disorders.

For these reasons, the committee drew the following overall conclusions:

6. Education about HDCTs, including their multisystem manifestations, diagnosis, and management, is important for all clinicians to help increase recognition and earlier diagnosis of the disorders and enable the provision of appropriate care.
   - A variety of health care providers should be able to recognize HDCTs and direct affected individuals to the appropriate clinicians for management.
   - Individuals with HDCTs and relevant support groups can provide valuable insight regarding the manifestations and lived experience of the disorders.
   - Increased recognition of the breadth and scope of HDCTs by health care professional education programs, professional organizations, and publishers of quality biomedical research is needed.

7. Education of individuals with the disorders and their families, as well as employers and school staff, is important to improve the quality of life for affected individuals and their families, to facilitate appropriate accommodations at work and school, and to help inform the disability assessment and determination process.

Research Gaps

HDCTs can be difficult to diagnose, and the true prevalence of many of these disorders is unknown. As noted above, HDCTs are diagnosed through a combination of clinical findings and established clinical criteria, followed by confirmatory molecular genetic testing when specific genes have been identified for the suspected disorder. However, diagnosis of hEDS and HSD is based solely on clinical criteria, since currently no associated causative genes have been identified for either disorder. Understanding of and diagnostic criteria for these disorders continue to evolve.

There currently are no curative treatments for MFS and related hereditary aortopathies, EDS, or HSD, making this an important area for research. In addition, more research is needed to improve recognition, management, and outcomes of the many secondary impairments associated with these disorders.

The clinical course of HDCTs and their effects on functioning vary greatly among affected individuals. Longitudinal studies of individuals with different HDCTs would increase understanding of the clinical course of the disorders; associated functional limitations; and potentially the impact of interventions, including reasonable accommodations, on participation in work and school.

While the severity of HDCTs is linked to the severity of the affected individual's physical and mental secondary impairments, including the combined effects of multiple impairments, improved understanding and measurement of the effects of impairments and multiple impairments on functioning could advance management of the disorders and improve functional status and quality of life for patients.

For these reasons, the committee drew the following overall conclusion:

8. Ongoing research on HDCTs is important to advance understanding of the disorders and their effects. In particular, research on care services and interventions for HDCTs and secondary impairments is needed, including
    - more specific diagnostic criteria and biomarkers;
    - functional and biomeasures of severity;

- effective treatment for HDCTs and management of their physical and mental manifestations, including comparative treatment trials;
- the clinical course of the disorders throughout the lifetime of affected individuals;
- the impact of relevant reasonable accommodations on affected individuals' ability to participate in work and school; and
- benefits versus risks of participation in common childhood activities (e.g., contact sports, gymnastics, dance).

1

Introduction

The U.S. Social Security Administration (SSA) provides financial assistance to people with disabilities through the Social Security Disability Insurance (SSDI) (Title II of the Social Security Act) and Supplemental Security Income (SSI) (Title XVI of the Social Security Act) programs. The SSDI program, established in 1956, provides benefits to eligible adults with disabilities who have paid into the Disability Insurance Trust Fund, as well as to certain family members. The SSI program, created in 1972, is a means-tested program based on income and financial resources that pays benefits to eligible adults and children with disabilities, individuals who are blind, and adults aged 65 and older. In December 2020, approximately 9.54 million individuals were receiving SSDI benefits as "disabled workers" (85.5 percent), "disabled widow(er)s" (2.5 percent), or "disabled adult children" (12.1 percent), and about 6.8 million individuals classified as blind or disabled were receiving SSI benefits (SSA, 2021a, pp. 11, 21; 2021b).

CONTEXT FOR THIS STUDY

To receive SSDI or SSI disability benefits, an individual must meet the statutory definition of disability. For adults, disability is defined as an "inability to engage in any substantial gainful activity [SGA] by reason of any medically determinable physical or mental impairment which can be expected to result in death or which has lasted or can be expected to last for a continuous period of not less than 12 months."[1] Children under the age of 18 who are not engaged in SGA are considered disabled if they have "a medically determinable physical or mental impairment or combination of impairments that causes marked and severe functional limitations, and that can be expected to cause death or that has lasted or can be expected to last for a continuous period of not less than 12 months."[2]

SSA uses a five-step process based on medical–vocational evaluations to determine whether an adult meets the definition of disability. After SSA determines an applicant's administrative eligibility and the presence of a medical impairment of sufficient duration and severity in steps 1 and 2 of this process, it assesses, in step 3, whether the applicant's impairment meets or medically equals the criteria listed for a condition in SSA's Listing of Impairments-Adult Listings (listings) (SSA, n.d.-a). The Adult Listings are organized by major body system and describe impairments that SSA considers to be sufficiently severe to prevent an applicant from performing any gainful activity, regardless of age, education, or work experience. Step 3 is used as a "screen-in" step. If an impairment is severe but does not meet or medically equal any listing, SSA assesses in step 4 whether the applicant's physical or mental residual functional capacity (RFC) allows the person to perform past relevant work. Applicants who are able to perform past relevant work are denied benefits, while those who are unable to do so proceed to step 5. At step 5, SSA considers, in combination with the applicant's RFC, such vocational factors as age, education, and work experience, including transferable skills, in determining whether the individual can perform other work in the national economy. Applicants determined to be unable to adjust to performing other work are allowed benefits, while those determined able to adjust are denied.

Disability determinations in children follow a three-step sequential evaluation process. After determining administrative eligibility and the presence of a medical impairment of sufficient duration and severity, SSA assesses in step 3 whether the impairment(s) meets, medically equals (is equivalent in severity to), or functionally equals (i.e., the impairment[s] results in functional limitations equivalent in severity to) the criteria in SSA's Child Listings (SSA, n.d.-b).[3] If a child's impairment or combination of impairments "does not meet or medically equal any listing, [SSA] will

---

[1] 42 U.S.C. 423(d)(1); 42 U.S.C. 416(i); see also 20 CFR 404.1505; 20 CFR 416.905; "Substantial gainful activity" is work activity involving significant physical or mental activities for pay or profit (20 CFR 416.972). Someone earning more than a specified monthly amount ($1,310 after deduction of impairment-related work expenses for a nonblind individual in 2021) ordinarily is considered to be engaging in SGA (SSA, 2022).
[2] 20 CFR 416.906; see also 42 U.S.C. 1382(c).
[3] 20 CFR 416.926; 20 CFR 416.926a.

decide whether it results in limitations that functionally equal the listings."[4] Functional equivalence refers to functionally equaling the listings: SSA's technique for determining functional equivalence is a "whole child" approach that "accounts for all of the effects of a child's impairments singly and in combination—the interactive and cumulative effects of the impairments—because it starts with a consideration of actual functioning in all settings" (SSA, 2009).

For both adults and children, disability claims related to heritable disorders of connective tissue (HDCTs) are evaluated under listings for the affected body systems. With the exception of Marfan syndrome (MFS), which is identified under the cardiovascular listing 4.10 (aneurysm of aorta or major branches), HDCTs are not specified in the listings.

STUDY CHARGE AND SCOPE

In 2020, SSA requested that the Health and Medicine Division of the National Academies of Sciences, Engineering, and Medicine convene a committee of relevant experts to review the current state of medical knowledge and practice regarding selected HDCTs. The Committee on Selected Heritable Disorders of Connective Tissue was charged with determining the latest standards of care, technology for understanding disease processes, treatment modalities, and science demonstrating the effect of these disorders on the health and functional capacity of adults and children (see Box 1-1 for the committee's statement of task). The 16-member committee comprised experts in general medicine, immunology, orthopedics, neurology, cardiology, hematology, ophthalmology, psychiatry, rehabilitation, pain management, and genetics.

STUDY APPROACH

Definition of Disability

The concept of disability has evolved over the past several decades from a medical to a biopsychosocial model. In the medical model, disability is viewed as a feature of a person that is caused by injury, disease, or other health condition and managed through medical treatment or modification of an individual's behavior (IOM, 1991; Kaplan, 2000; WHO, 2001, 2002). In contrast, the biopsychosocial model, exemplified by the World Health Organization's International Classification of Functioning, Disability and Health (ICF), portrays disability as "the interaction between an individual (with a health condition) and that individual's contextual factors

---
[4] 20 CFR 416.926a.

BOX 1-1
Statement of Task

An ad hoc committee of the National Academies of Sciences, Engineering, and Medicine will review selected heritable conditions related to connective tissues and produce a report addressing the current status of the diagnosis, treatment, and prognosis of those conditions in adults and children based on published evidence (to the extent possible) and professional judgement (where evidence is lacking):

1. Provide an overview of the current status of the diagnosis, treatment, and prognosis of selected heritable connective tissue disorders, including but not necessarily limited to Ehlers-Danlos syndrome and Marfan syndrome, in the U.S. population and the relative levels of functional limitation typically associated with the disorders and their common treatments.
2. For the connective tissue disorders identified in task 1, describe to the degree possible:
   a. The average age of onset and gender distributions;
   b. The professionally accepted diagnostic techniques used in identifying the disorders (e.g., laboratory test results and clinical findings) and how the techniques differ for adults and children (if applicable);
   c. The methods in common use for differentiating clinical or medical severity (e.g., classifiers such as "moderate" or "severe"), what the method entails (e.g., a specific laboratory test) and what the findings from these methods mean in terms of treatment, prognosis, and functional limitation;
   d. The usual clinical course of the disorders, including any differences in the clinical course of the disorders for adults and children (if applicable);
   e. The likelihood, frequency, and duration of changes in the clinical or medical severity of symptoms, such as flare-ups or remissions (if applicable);
   f. The possibility and likelihood of reducing the work-related severity of symptoms (if applicable), and the treatments or circumstances that may lead to vocationally relevant improvement; and
   g. Secondary impairments that result from either the disorders or their treatments (if applicable).
3. For the connective tissue disorders identified in task 1, identify the types of treatments available and describe to the degree possible:
   a. The clinical practice guidelines for receiving the treatments;
   b. The settings in which the treatments are provided;

    c. What receipt of the treatments indicates about the clinical or medical severity of the medical condition;
    d. The likelihood of improvement when receiving the treatments and the period over which the improvement would be expected; and
    e. Any limitations on the availability of the treatments (other than due to financial circumstances or the patient's preferences), such as whether treatments are considered experimental, remain in the trial phase, or are limited to certain geographic areas.
4. For the connective tissue disorders identified in task 1, provide a summary of selected treatments currently being studied in clinical trials.
5. For the connective tissue disorders identified in task 1, identify to the degree possible the functional limitations associated with each disorder, including physical functioning limitations, mental functioning limitations, limitations resulting from common treatments, and variations in functioning (e.g., during flare-ups vs. remission), and how such limitations would present in a typical medical record.
6. For the connective tissue disorders identified in task 1, identify nonexertional physical limitations (e.g., balancing or using the upper extremities for fine or gross movements) and mental limitations (e.g., cognitive or behavioral) that are equivalent in severity to the standard represented in the listings (i.e., that would prevent any gainful activity) but are not captured by currently existing listings and are not currently reflected in SSA's disability grid rules.

The report will include consensus conclusions but not recommendations.

    In the report, when terms such as "severity" or "severe" are used, the committee shall identify to the degree possible whether the term is being used with SSA's work-related program definition (i.e., an impairment of such severity as to be the basis of a finding of an inability to engage in any substantial gainful activity) or as it is used in the clinical or medical care settings, and, if necessary, will specify the pertinent differences between the two definitions.

    The committee shall not describe issues with respect to access to treatments due to financial circumstances, including insurance limitations. While SSA recognizes some patients may have difficulty accessing care or particular forms of treatment due to financial circumstances, others do successfully access those treatments. SSA may receive information about those treatments in the medical records SSA considers when making disability determinations and conducting continuing disability reviews (CDRs). SSA understands improvement is not certain in all cases. SSA makes individual decisions on each case based on all the evidence they receive.

(environmental and personal factors)" (WHO, 2001). The ICF model recognizes functioning in three domains (middle tier of Figure 1-1): (1) body functions and structures, which encompass physiological functions of the body, including psychological functions, as well as the functioning of body structures (e.g., movement of limbs, cardiac function); (2) activities, which are actions or tasks (e.g., running, problem solving); and (3) participation, which is the performance of tasks in a societal context (e.g., participation in school or organized sports). The ICF model refers to deficits in body functions and structures as impairments, deficits in completing activities as limitations, and reductions in participation as restrictions. It should be noted that such accommodations as assistive technologies and environmental modifications are environmental contextual factors that act on the ICF domains to enhance an individual's activity and participation.

As noted above, SSA's definition of disability in adults is "inability to engage in any SGA by reason of any medically determinable physical or mental impairment which can be expected to result in death or which has lasted or can be expected to last for a continuous period of not less than 12 months."[5] SGA is work activity that "involves doing significant and productive physical or mental duties" or activity that "is done (or intended) for

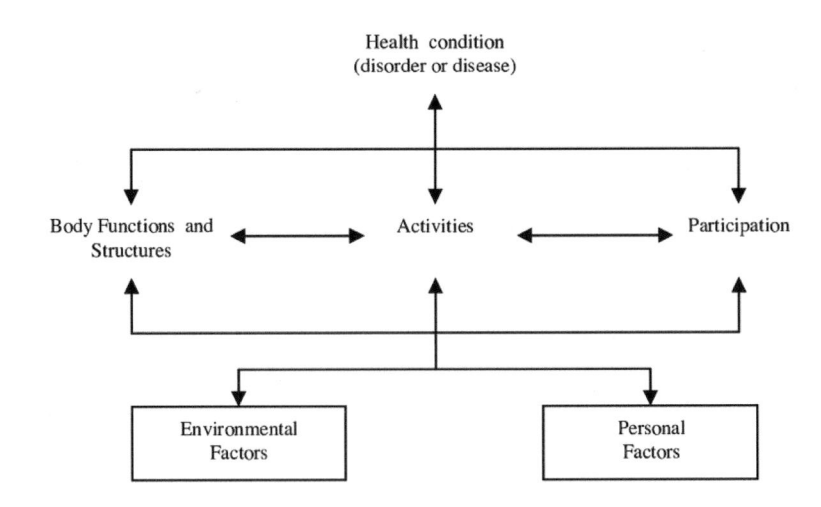

FIGURE 1-1 ICF model of functioning and disability.
SOURCE: WHO, 2001. Reproduced from *International Classification of Functioning, Disability and Health*, World Health Organization, Introduction: 5. Model of Functioning and Disability, p. 18, copyright 2001.

---

[5] 42 U.S.C. 423(d)(1); 42 U.S.C. 416(i); see also 20 CFR 404.1505; 20 CFR 416.905.

pay or profit," regardless of whether a profit is realized.[6] In the SSA context, "disability" in adults refers to work disability—an inability to participate in work "in an ordinary work setting, on a regular and continuing basis, and for 8 hours per day, 5 days per week, or an equivalent work schedule" (SSA, 2021c).

This report focuses on those physical; vision, hearing, and speech; and mental activities the committee determined to be most relevant to SSA based on the information SSA collects about applicants and the information the U.S. Bureau of Labor Statistics collects about the physical and mental demands of jobs for inclusion in the Occupational Information System. SSA classifies jobs as sedentary, light, medium, heavy, and very heavy based on the level of physical exertion required for the work.[7] SSA distinguishes between two types of limitations: exertional and nonexertional. Exertional limitations relate to the strength demands of jobs (sitting, standing, walking, lifting, carrying, pushing, and pulling) and are classified by level (sedentary, light, medium, heavy, and very heavy). All other limitations (e.g., mental limitations, sensory limitations, environmental intolerance) are considered nonexertional (SSA, 1999).

SSA incorporates function into its definition of disability for children, stating that a child's qualifying impairment(s) must cause "marked and severe functional limitations."[8] SSA considers a number of factors when evaluating the effects of an impairment or combination of impairments on a child's functioning.[9] These factors include but are not limited to

- how well the child can initiate and sustain activities, how much extra help he or she needs, and the effects of structured or supportive settings (see § 416.924a(b)(5));
- how the child functions in school (see § 416.924a(b)(7)); and
- the effects of the child's medications or other treatment (see § 416.924a(b)(9)).[10]

SSA considers "how appropriately, effectively, and independently" the child performs their activities (everything they do at home, at school, and in the community) "compared to the performance of other children [their] age who do not have impairments."[11] In particular, SSA considers functioning in six domains:

---

[6] 20 CFR 404.1510; 20 CFR 404.1572.
[7] 20 CFR 416.967.
[8] 20 CFR 416.906.
[9] 20 CFR 416.924a.
[10] See 20 CFR 416.926a.
[11] 20 CFR 416.926a.

- acquiring and using information,
- attending and completing tasks,
- interacting and relating with others,
- moving about and manipulating objects,
- caring for [oneself], and
- health and physical well-being.[12]

Selection of Heritable Disorders of Connective Tissue

HDCTs are a heterogeneous group of inherited disorders that affect the body's connective tissue. As directed in its statement of task, the committee addressed in particular the Ehlers-Danlos syndromes (EDS) and MFS, two of the most prevalent HDCTs. The EDS are a group of 13 disorders characterized by joint hypermobility and tissue fragility (Malfait et al., 2017). MFS is an autosomal-dominant disorder that affects multiple organ systems, with cardiovascular, ocular, and skeletal features being most prominent (Loeys et al., 2010). In addition, the committee identified for inclusion in this report hypermobility spectrum disorders (HSD) and several other hereditary aortopathies (Loeys-Dietz syndrome, congenital contractural arachnodactyly [also known as Beals-Hecht syndrome], and Shprintzen-Goldberg syndrome) because of the features they share with hypermobile EDS (hEDS, the most prevalent EDS type) and MFS, respectively.

Terminology

Secondary Impairments

The committee was tasked with describing, to the extent possible, secondary impairments that result from the HDCTs or their treatments. Because there is not always a known or clear causal link between the disorder and all of its manifestations, the committee understands "secondary impairments" to mean physical and mental manifestations (medical diagnoses, syndromes, or comorbid and other health conditions) that are either associated with or may result from an HDCT. Many of these are not specific to HDCTs and can also occur in other individuals. Use of this term thus defined does not mean that any of the physical or mental manifestations seen in individuals with HDCTs are not core elements of the disorders. Rather, the primary impairment is the underlying genetic disorder (e.g., EDS, MFS), and the secondary impairments encompass all of the physical and mental manifestations of that disorder.

---

[12] 20 CFR 416.926a.

Because connective tissues are found throughout the body, HDCTs manifest in multiple body systems. The symptoms and secondary impairments associated with HDCTs vary widely, as do the severity of the manifestations experienced by different individuals and the timing of their appearance. The committee considers the number, types, and severity of the physical and mental secondary impairments experienced by individuals—which may develop and vary in severity (wax and wane) over time—to be of particular importance with regard to the functional implications of HDCTs.

Treatment and Management

The committee was tasked with addressing several issues related to the treatment of HDCTs. For the purposes of this report, the committee distinguishes between "treatment" and "management": whereas treatment focuses on curing or mitigating a specific disease, in this case an HDCT, management focuses on caring for the person as a whole, which requires a multidisciplinary team and extends throughout the life course. Although no curative treatments currently are available for EDS and MFS, these disorders can be managed through surveillance and treatment of associated secondary impairments.

Severity

The committee was tasked with describing the severity of HDCTs. For the purposes of this report, the terms "severe" and "severity" are used as they typically would be in clinical or medical care settings. When the terms reflect SSA's program definition (i.e., an impairment of such severity as to be the basis of a finding of an inability to engage in any SGA), their usage is specified as such.

Information Gathering

The committee conducted an extensive review of the literature pertaining to heritable disorders of connective tissue and work-related functioning. This review began with a search of online databases for U.S. and international English- and Spanish-language literature from 2006 through 2021. This search encompassed PubMed and Scopus, as well as websites including those of the International Consortium on Ehlers-Danlos Syndromes & Hypermobility Spectrum Disorders, the EDS & HSD Community Coalition (formerly "the EDS Comorbidity Coalition"), The Ehlers-Danlos Society, The Marfan Foundation, and SSA. Committee members and project staff identified additional salient literature and information using traditional academic research methods and online searches throughout the course of the study.

The committee used a variety of resources to supplement its review of the literature. Meeting virtually six times, the committee held two public workshops to hear from invited experts in areas pertinent to its charge (see Appendix A). Speakers at the workshops included experts in HDCT-associated gastrointestinal conditions, mental health conditions, and orthostatic intolerance. Additionally, the committee participated in a panel discussion with patient advocates and commissioned a paper on the functional impact of orthostatic intolerance in EDS (Appendix B). The committee's work was further informed by several previous reports of the National Academies: *Cardiovascular Disability: Updating the Social Security Listings* (IOM, 2010), *The Promise of Assistive Technology to Enhance Activity and Work Participation* (NASEM, 2017), *Functional Assessment for Adults with Disabilities* (NASEM, 2019), and *Childhood Cancer and Functional Impacts across the Care Continuum* (NASEM, 2021).

REPORT ORGANIZATION

Chapter 2 provides an overview of the history, etiology, diagnosis, and management considerations common to all HDCTs. Chapter 3 addresses the diagnosis and management of MFS and several other hereditary aortopathies and the secondary impairments associated with these disorders. Chapter 4 does the same for EDS and HSD. Chapter 5 includes more information on physical and mental secondary impairments associated with the selected HDCTs and their potential effects on functioning, with particular focus on activities of interest to SSA (e.g., for adults, work-related activities and demands, and for children, other activities). Chapter 6 contains the report's overall conclusions.

REFERENCES

IOM (Institute of Medicine). 1991. *Disability in America: Toward a national agenda for prevention.* Edited by A. M. Pope and A. R. Tarlov. Washington, DC: The National Academies Press. https://doi.org/10.17226/1579.

IOM. 2010. *Cardiovascular disability: Updating the Social Security listings.* Washington, DC: The National Academies Press. https://doi.org/10.17226/12940.

Kaplan, D. 2000. The definition of disability: Perspective of the disability community. *Journal of Health Care Law & Policy* 3(2). https://digitalcommons.law.umaryland.edu/jhclp/vol3/iss2/5/.

Loeys, B. L., H. C. Dietz, A. C. Braverman, B. L. Callewaert, J. De Backer, R. B. Devereux, Y. Hilhorst-Hofstee, G. Jondeau, L. Faivre, D. M. Milewicz, R. E. Pyeritz, P. D. Sponseller, P. Wordsworth, and A. M. De Paepe. 2010. The revised Ghent nosology for the Marfan syndrome. *Journal of Medical Genetics* 47(7):476-485. https://doi.org/10.1136/jmg.2009.072785.

Malfait, F., C. Francomano, P. Byers, J. Belmont, B. Berglund, J. Black, L. Bloom, J. M. Bowen, A. F. Brady, N. P. Burrows, M. Castori, H. Cohen, M. Colombi, S. Demirdas, J. De Backer, A. De Paepe, S. Fournel-Gigleux, M. Frank, N. Ghali, C. Giunta, R. Grahame, A. Hakim, X. Jeunemaitre, D. Johnson, B. Juul-Kristensen, I. Kapferer-Seebacher, H. Kazkaz, T. Kosho, M. E. Lavallee, H. Levy, R. Mendoza-Londono, M. Pepin, F. M. Pope, E. Reinstein, L. Robert, M. Rohrbach, L. Sanders, G. J. Sobey, T. Van Damme, A. Vandersteen, C. van Mourik, N. Voermans, N. Wheeldon, J. Zschocke, and B. Tinkle. 2017. The 2017 international classification of the Ehlers-Danlos syndromes. *American Journal of Medical Genetics Part C: Seminars in Medical Genetics* 175(1):8-26. https://doi.org/10.1002/ajmg.c.31552.

NASEM (National Academies of Sciences, Engineering, and Medicine). 2017. *The promise of assistive technology to enhance activity and work participation*. Edited by A. M. Jette, C. M. Spicer, and J. L. Flaubert. Washington, DC: The National Academies Press. https://doi.org/10.17226/24740.

NASEM. 2019. *Functional assessment for adults with disabilities*. Edited by P. A. Volberding, C. M. Spicer, and J. L. Flaubert. Washington, DC: The National Academies Press. https://doi.org/10.17226/25376.

NASEM. 2021. *Childhood cancer and functional impacts across the care continuum*. Edited by P. A. Volberding, C. M. Spicer, T. Cartaxo, and L. Aiuppa. Washington, DC: The National Academies Press. https://doi.org/10.17226/25944.

SSA (U.S. Social Security Administration). 1999. *DI 24515.063 Exertional and nonexertional limitations*. http://policy.ssa.gov/poms.nsf/lnx/0424515063 (accessed January 24, 2022).

SSA. 2009. *SSR 09-1p: Title XVI: Determining childhood disability under the functional equivalence rule—The "whole child" approach*. https://www.ssa.gov/OP_Home/rulings/ssi/02/SSR2009-01-ssi-02.html#fn4 (accessed May 26, 2022).

SSA. 2021a. *Annual statistical report on the Social Security Disability Insurance program, 2020*. SSA Publication No. 13-11826. Washington, DC: SSA. https://www.ssa.gov/policy/docs/statcomps/di_asr/index.html (accessed May 23, 2022).

SSA. 2021b. *Annual statistical supplement, 2021—Supplemental Security Income: Summary (7.A)*. https://www.ssa.gov/policy/docs/statcomps/supplement/2021/7a.html (accessed January 26, 2022).

SSA. 2021c. *DI 24510.057 Sustainability and the residual functional capacity (RFC) assessment*. http://policy.ssa.gov/poms.nsf/lnx/0424510057 (accessed January 26, 2022).

SSA. 2022. *Substantial gainful activity*. https://www.ssa.gov/OACT/COLA/sga.html (accessed January 26, 2022).

SSA. n.d.-a. *Listing of impairments—Adult listings (Part A)*. https://www.ssa.gov/disability/professionals/bluebook/AdultListings.htm (accessed January 26, 2022).

SSA. n.d.-b. *Listing of impairments—Childhood listings (Part B)*. https://www.ssa.gov/disability/professionals/bluebook/ChildhoodListings.htm (accessed January 26, 2022).

WHO (World Health Organization). 2001. *International classification of functioning, disability and health*. Geneva, Switzerland: WHO. https://apps.who.int/iris/handle/10665/42407 (accessed July 22, 2022).

WHO. 2002. *Towards a common language for functioning, disability and health: ICF*. Geneva, Switzerland: WHO. https://www.who.int/publications/m/item/icf-beginner-s-guide-towards-a-common-language-for-functioning-disability-and-health (accessed July 22, 2022).

2

Overview of Hereditary Disorders of Connective Tissue

Heritable disorders of connective tissue (HDCTs) are a heterogeneous group of many inherited disorders and subtypes. Two of the most common HDCTs, Marfan syndrome (MFS) and the Ehlers-Danlos syndromes (EDS), are discussed in depth in Chapters 3 and 4, respectively, along with several related disorders. This chapter addresses the history, etiology, diagnosis, and management considerations common to all HDCTs.

HISTORY OF HEREDITARY DISORDERS OF CONNECTIVE TISSUE

Connective tissue—tissue that helps support, protect, and provide structure to other tissues and organs in the body—is the most abundant and diverse of tissues. Connective tissues vary with respect to their type of cells and cellularity (dense versus loose). Specialized connective tissues include bone, cartilage, ligaments, tendons, and adipose tissue (fat). The role of connective tissues in the vascular system, the gastrointestinal system, the intervertebral disc, and muscle is also recognized, and has furthered understanding of HDCT phenotypes and symptomatology.

The term "heritable disorder of connective tissue" was coined by Dr. Victor McKusick, who first wrote about the concept in his 1955 article "The Cardiovascular Aspects of Marfan's Syndrome: A Heritable Disorder of Connective Tissue" (McKusick, 1955). McKusick's thinking about HDCTs was influenced by the work of Follis, who studied a case of lethal osteogenesis imperfecta (OI) and demonstrated that the organic matrix of bone and the connective tissue of the skin and sclera were defective (Follis,

1952, 1953a,b). The first edition of McKusick's *Heritable Disorders of Connective Tissue*, published in 1956, included discussion of MFS, EDS, OI, pseudoxanthoma elasticum, and Morquio syndrome. By the time the fourth edition was published in 1972, chapters had been added on homocystinuria, alkaptonuria, Menkes disease, and cutis laxa, as well as the skeletal dysplasias or osteochondrodystrophies.

Since McKusick's initial writings in the 1950s, the concept of HDCTs has become firmly ingrained in the genetic lexicon. The 2002 volume *Connective Tissue and Its Heritable Disorders*, edited by Royce and Steinmann, includes 26 chapters, many of which subsume multiple distinct diagnoses (for example, Chapter 23 includes the skeletal dysplasias, of which there are now more than 450 well-delineated forms) (Mortier et al., 2019).

Two technological advances—the availability of genomic sequencing and ready access to information through the internet—have forever changed the way the medical community views HDCTs, as well as many other rare disorders. The ability of people affected by rare disorders to comb through online medical information and "ask Dr. Google" for information about their conditions has led to self-diagnosis in many cases. Affected people also are now able to share their experiences with a worldwide population of similarly affected individuals. Patient support groups, such as The Marfan Foundation and The Ehlers-Danlos Society, have encouraged and supported research, including basic, translational, and clinical research, that otherwise might not have been accomplished. Moreover, an increasing willingness, and even urgency, to understand the lived experience of people with these conditions has led to the development of a wide range of patient-reported outcome measures to help inform research on these conditions and the disability they cause.

EPIDEMIOLOGY

HDCTs are a complex group of disorders that can be difficult to diagnose. Since their genetic basis is heterogenous, the incidence of an individual HDCT can range from commonly occurring—for example, hypermobility spectrum disorders (HSD)—to rare recessively inherited disorders. Determining the true incidence of these conditions is challenging because it relies on recognition of the disorders, which is historically biased toward their more severe, and therefore recognizable, expressions, and on retrospective reviews and diagnosis codes.

Since many of these disorders are underappreciated, their precise prevalence is not established. For example, MFS is estimated to occur in 1 to 5 per 10,000 individuals (Judge and Dietz, 2005; NORD, 2021), while the prevalence of the phenotypically overlapping disorder Loeys-Dietz syndrome is unknown (Loeys and Dietz, 2018). The prevalence of HSD and different EDS types also varies significantly. Current research indicates that the EDS are thought to occur in about 1 in 5,000 people (Pyeritz, 2000; Steinmann et al., 2002). Among the EDS, hypermobile EDS (hEDS) is the most common type, while other types are much rarer. The estimated prevalence of vascular EDS, for example, is between 1/50,000 and 1/200,000 (Byers, 2019), while that of both musculocontractural EDS and dermatosparaxis EDS is less than 1/1,000,000 (Orphanet, 2022a,b).

GENETICS

For many years, the term "mutation" was used to describe changes in genes resulting in heritable conditions. As a result of the Human Genome Project and ready access to rapid genomic sequencing, new language has been adopted to describe the changes observed in human DNA; such changes are now referred to as "variants." The classification of sequence variations has been standardized according to guidelines published by the American College of Medical Genetics and Genomics and the Association for Molecular Pathology (Richards et al., 2015). It is recognized that some differences among the DNA sequences of humans have no discernable phenotypic consequences; such changes are termed "benign." Other changes are unequivocally disease-causing and are referred to as "pathogenic." Between these extremes are variants that are categorized as "likely benign" or "likely pathogenic." In addition, a wide array of variants are called "variants of unknown significance" because current knowledge is insufficient to classify them as benign or pathogenic. Study of the different types of variants in the human DNA sequence is ongoing, and variants are frequently reclassified as more information becomes available.

The concept of pleiotropism is central to the study of genetic disorders and is a universal feature of HDCTs. The term is used to describe how variation in a single gene may manifest in multiple organ systems. The specific organs affected by such a variation will be determined by the pattern of the gene's expression during embryological development, postnatal growth, and maintenance of tissue. For example, type I collagen is expressed in bone, skin, tendons, and ligaments; all of these tissues are impacted by the pathogenic variants of type I collagen that cause some forms of OI.

Variable expressivity, another standard concept in medical genetics, is also a hallmark of the HDCTs. This term denotes the different degrees of severity that may be seen in individuals carrying the same pathogenic DNA variant, even among members of the same family. Much work is still necessary to develop a full understanding of the gene–gene and gene–environment (e.g., tobacco use) interactions that contribute to the wide variation in expression seen in Mendelian genetic disorders.

CONNECTIVE TISSUE

Connective tissue is an integral component of every organ system and plays a crucial role in their function. Hence the physical and mental secondary impairments associated with HDCTs, which may develop and progress over time, manifest throughout the body and affect functioning in every body system. As disorders of connective tissue, HDCTs share many features because the molecules or genetic variants that produce disease are expressed in overlapping tissues. Thus, joint issues are seen in MFS, EDS, congenital contractural arachnodactyly (CCA), and the skeletal dysplasias since the respective genes that lead to these diseases are expressed in the tissues of the joints, as well as in other tissues. HDCTs arise from defects in the genes that encode extracellular matrix (ECM) molecules or molecules related to matrix biosynthesis and cell signaling. These molecules provide the physical structure for complex connective tissues, and are critical for appropriate physiological functions as they also dictate the functions of the cells within the tissues. There are two types of ECM—interstitial and pericellular. The interstitial matrix interconnects cells in connective tissues, while the pericellular matrix is a unique cell-adjacent matrix. The composition of the ECM varies among tissues based on each tissue's specialized functions. Bone ECM, for example, strongly expresses type I collagen, whereas in cartilage ECM, type II collagen predominates, and type I collagen is present at relatively low levels.

The components of connective tissue include cells, fibers, and ground substance (Nezwek and Varacallo, 2021). Figure 2-1 depicts the structure of connective tissue, which includes cells with receptors, such as integrins; fibers, such as collagen and elastin; and ground substances, such as proteoglycans. Ground substance is the amorphous gelatinous material in which the cells and fibers are embedded. It is composed primarily of water, along with hyaluronic acid, proteoglycans, and proteins (e.g., laminin and fibronectin) that function as glue for the cells in the ECM (Nezwek and Varacallo, 2021). This ground substance allows for the exchange of nutrients between cells and capillaries. Three basic types of fiber make up connective tissue: collagenous fibers, predominantly type I collagen that provides tensile strength to loose and dense connective tissues (Ricard-Blum, 2011); thin reticular fibers, composed of type III collagen that forms cross-links to generate a supportive mesh for tissues (Hayakawa et al., 1990); and branching elastic fibers, composed of elastin that allows tissues to stretch and recoil (Uitto, 1979).

Connective tissues help define the function of specialized tissues. Bone is composed of specialized cells that include osteoprogenitor cells, osteoblasts, osteocytes, and bone-lining cells. Ninety percent of bone ECM is composed primarily of type I collagen; the other 10 percent consists of

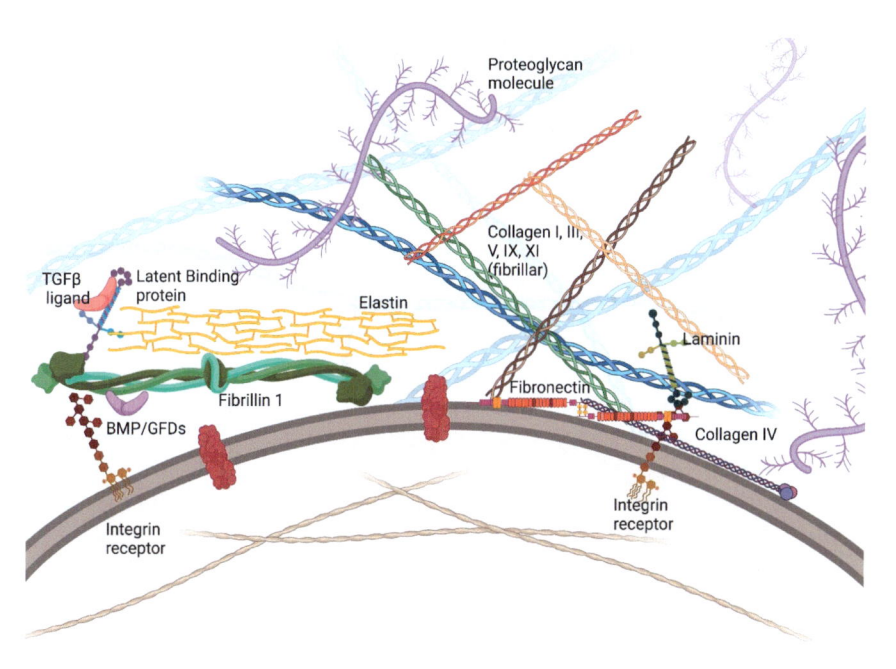

FIGURE 2-1 Connective tissue.
SOURCE: Generated by the committee.

noncollagenous proteins (Paiva and Granjeiro, 2017). In contrast with other connective tissues, bone ECM is mineralized, giving it strength and rigidity to sustain mechanical forces (Weatherholt et al., 2012).

Cartilage has multiple roles, including providing a template for linear growth and bone development, as well as covering for the surface of joints so bones can slide over each other. It comprises cartilage cells (chondrocytes) and a glycoprotein matrix supported by collagen fibers, predominantly type II collagen. Like bone, cartilage is a tough tissue that can withstand forces.

Tendons and ligaments are fibrous and dense connective tissues that connect muscle to bone (tendon) and bone to bone (ligament); they serve to stabilize the skeleton and allow movement by transmitting the mechanical force of muscle contractions to the bone (Ashara et al., 2017; Connizzo et al., 2013). Tendons and ligaments contain fibroblast-like cells, termed tenocytes, or ligament fibroblasts (Kannus, 2000). These cells are located between parallel chains of collagen fibrils. While these collagens are not specific to tendon and ligament, the protein tenomodulin is specifically expressed in these tissues (Shukunami et al., 2006).

Other musculoskeletal connective tissues, including muscle and fascia, have distinct ECMs that contribute to their function. Muscle fibers, made up of myocytes and progenitor cells, are embedded in a complex meshwork consisting of collagens, predominantly types I and III; glycoproteins; proteoglycans; and elastin. Muscle ECM plays an important role in development, as well as in muscle fiber force transmission, maintenance, and repair (Gillies and Lieber, 2011). Fascia is a generic term for a continuum of multiple types of connective tissue structures that traverse the entire body, from the surface to deeper (interior) anatomical layers. In recent years, it has been recognized that fascia is more than a packaging unit for the skin, muscle, and other organs. Like other connective tissue structures, it serves as a medium for transmitting forces, particularly those that come from muscle, and it is composed of cells, ground substance, and fibers that form a three-dimensional network. Fibroblasts and fibrocytes are the major cell types in fascia, which is composed predominantly of type I and III collagens, and proteoglycans and glycoproteins contribute to the formation of the ground substance. Newly identified cells in the fascia—telocytes and fasciacytes—are deemed responsible for the fascia's ability to glide (Dawidowicz et al., 2015; Stecco et al., 2018).

While the vascular system is not considered a connective tissue, the ECM that surrounds and is incorporated into the blood vessels plays an important role in multiple processes associated with their structure and function (del Monte-Nieto et al., 2020). The cardiovascular ECM is formed from more than 300 proteins that include collagens, elastins, fibulins, and laminins, among others. Importantly, the essential mechanical or viscoelastic properties of the vessels are provided by three main constituents: elastic fibers, fibrillar collagens, and large aggregating proteoglycans (Barallobre-Barreiro et al., 2020). The cardiovascular ECM is a highly dynamic structure, and alterations to these ECM molecules can affect the integrity of the cardiovascular system.

Connective tissue is also a structural and functional component of the central and peripheral nervous systems. The meninges provide a fibrovascular and ligamentous suspension system for the brain, the spinal cord, and vascular structures within the cranium and the spine, anchoring the cranial and spinal nerves as they merge with the peripheral nervous system. The meninges also have a role in the production and circulation of cerebrospinal fluid (CSF). The main functions of CSF are to provide a mechanical barrier against shock to the brain and spinal cord, remove metabolic waste products, and transport signaling neurotransmitters. The peripheral nerve fibers, made up of axons, are embedded in a complex framework of fibrocollagenous sheaths, also known as epi-, peri-, and endoneurium. These fibers form a network of corpuscle-like myelinated and unmyelinated axons and structured nerve endings that terminate in the connective tissue layers of the skin, the musculoskeletal system, and the ligaments and joints, where they are variably organized by collagen fibers and contiguous with collagen. The ultrastructure and function of those Ruffini bodies, Pacinian corpuscles, and Golgi or Merkel receptors have been widely studied, and shown to provide the nociceptive, mechanoreceptive, and proprioceptive network of the human body (Halata, 1977; Vandenabeele et al., 1997; Watanabe et al., 2004). Those units also harbor unmyelinated free-ending axon bundles having direct contact and an intricate relationship with individual collagen fibrils (Abdo et al., 2019).

The gastrointestinal tract consists of four layers—mucosa (innermost layer), submucosa, muscularis propria, and adventitia or serosa—the structure of which varies with their function in different areas throughout the system (University of Leeds, 2022). The submucosa and adventitia layers consist of loose connective tissue that contains blood vessels, lymphatic vessels, and nerves. The submucosa may also contain mucus-secreting cells. The mucosa itself comprises three layers: the epithelial lining; the lamina propria, a layer of loose connective tissue containing vasculature for the epithelium and often mucosal glands, lymphoid follicles, and plasma cells; and the muscularis mucosa, a double layer of smooth muscle (University of Leeds, 2022). Highly vascularized, the gastrointestinal tract is an interface of the nervous and immune systems and represents a confluence of processes impacted by many connective tissue disorders.

Cells of the immune system, such as lymphocytes, mast cells, and macrophages, are found within connective tissue. As the first line of defense in fighting illness and disease, the cells residing in the connective tissue in an activated or inactivated state account for a major part of the entire immune system (Krakower, 1972).

As noted above, genes encode the proteins that constitute the elements of connective tissue. While all connective tissues have the general types of ECM proteins (e.g., collagens, elastin, fibrillin) in common, their modifying genes, ECM organization, and differential gene expression contribute to variation in their function and in their presentation and phenotype in patients. In general, proteins that are more highly expressed in connective tissue have greater influence on tissue properties. Levels of gene expression can influence early development (embryogenesis), ongoing tissue maintenance, and the aging process as gene expression changes (Glass et al., 2013; Işıldak et al., 2020). Furthermore, gene variants can produce different effects in individuals and their connective tissues. For example, variants in a highly expressed protein in a connective tissue may produce mild to severe complications depending on the individual, and the same variant can produce different physical complications among family members. The interactions among genes, the proteins they encode, and environmental factors also can influence the behavior of connective tissues. For example, smoking negatively impacts the expression of type I and III collagen in skin and alters the balance of ECM turnover (Knuutinen et al., 2002), and may further contribute to disease progression in an at-risk individual with an HDCT.

Pathogenic variants in the genes encoding the structural constituents of connective tissue may result in HDCTs, with demonstrable abnormalities in the affected tissues. MFS, for example, results from pathogenic variants in the gene encoding fibrillin-1; this protein is expressed in microfibrils providing structural support in the lung, blood vessels, skin, ciliary zonules, tendon, cornea, and glomerulus. These microfibrils provide a framework for elastin deposition at the periphery of elastic fibers (Jensen and Handford, 2016). Thus, individuals with MFS manifest symptomatology and complications in fibrillin-1–expressing tissues. Examples include increased incidence of spontaneous pneumothoraxes, aortic root dilation with aneurysms, ectopia lentis, joint hypermobility, and renal cysts (Arnaud et al., 2021; Milewicz et al., 2021). Pathogenic variants in the fibrillin-1 gene can produce multiple other disorders as well, including those associated with short stature and limited joint mobility, such as Weill-Marchesani syndrome; geleophysic dysplasia; acromicric dysplasia (Sakai and Keene, 2019); and stiff skin syndrome—a rare disorder that presents in infancy or early childhood and is characterized by rock-hard skin, limited joint mobility, and mild hypertrichosis in the absence of other visceral involvement (Liu et al., 2008; Loeys et al., 2010).

Cartilage has a distinct cell type, the chondrocyte, that contributes to linear growth through a process of recruitment, proliferation, hypertrophy, and transition to bone formation. The chondrocyte also facilitates mobility by creating a low-friction environment and cushioning movement (Sophia Fox et al., 2009). The predominant collagen in cartilage is type II (Omelyanenko and Slutsky, 2014), which is also highly expressed in the vitreous of the eye (Deemter et al., 2009). Type II collagen is encoded by the *COL2A1* gene. HDCTs that include a spectrum of skeletal disorders due to pathogenic variants in *COL2A1* have significant cartilage involvement. Affected individuals often have significantly shorter stature, early-onset osteoarthritis, and retinal complications due to an abnormal vitreous (Savarirayan et al., 2019). These examples highlight that expression of an abnormal or decreased amount of protein in connective tissues that rely on a functional protein produces phenotypes that affect individuals in multiple organ systems.

DIAGNOSIS

As with many diseases, establishing an accurate diagnosis is an important first step in comprehensive care for individuals living with an HDCT. A specific diagnosis is key to understanding the expected natural history of the individual's condition, and allows for rational and informed decision making by the patient and clinician, anticipatory management, and optimized outcomes. In general, HDCTs are diagnosed through a combination of clinical findings, established clinical criteria, and family history, followed by confirmatory molecular genetic testing when the genes responsible for the suspected disorder have been identified.

For those HDCTs for which responsible genes and pathogenic variants have been identified, genetic testing is very specific and can establish a diagnosis. In some cases, genetic testing identifies "variants of uncertain significance" (VUS) that are not diagnostic in and of themselves. They have to be considered in a broader context, and no clinical decisions or genetic counseling should be based solely on the finding of a VUS. For some of the HDCTs for which a molecular cause is known, there is a small percentage of patients and families in whom pathogenic variants are not found. An example is Stickler syndrome, for which at least four different genes have been identified, but a small percentage of families with clinically diagnosed Stickler syndrome will not have identifiable variants in any of the known genes. Notably, the most common HDCTs—HSD/hEDS—currently have no known causative genes, so no genetic testing is available for these disorders.

A combination of clinical findings should lead the informed clinician to suspect a specific HDCT; for example, tall stature and arachnodactyly (long fingers and toes) should lead to a suspicion of MFS or Loeys-Dietz syndrome (LDS); generalized joint hypermobility in conjunction with significant skin hyperextensibility or fragility should lead to a suspicion of one of the varieties of EDS; and a personal or strong family history of early osteoarthritis is suggestive of Stickler syndrome, especially if the family history includes cleft palate, retinal detachment, and/or hearing loss. The first step in establishing a diagnosis is for the clinician to consider the possibility of an HDCT. Once that suspicion has been entertained, clinical algorithms and diagnostic criteria can help provide a specific diagnosis.

For most of the HDCTs, once a clinical diagnosis has been suspected or established, it can be confirmed through molecular genetic testing. At present, genetic testing is performed using a panel of genes that covers a wide range of potential causes for the phenotype in question. For example, if there is a personal or family history of thoracic aortic dissection, genetic testing using a panel of genes causing hereditary aortopathies would be the most rational course of action.

HDCT Diagnosis in Children and Adolescents

Many of the clinical findings associated with HDCTs can affect children and adolescents as well as adults, depending on the specific diagnosis and genetic basis. Manifestations of MFS, for example, can become apparent at any time between infancy and adulthood. Early-onset MFS is a very rare subtype of MFS that can present in the antenatal, neonatal, or infancy period (Abdel-Massih et al., 2002; Ardhanari et al., 2019). Likewise, some of the rare forms of EDS, such as the arthrochalasia type, present in early childhood (Byers et al., 1997). Hormonal influences that include the onset of puberty have been shown to influence hEDS/HSD; in a survey of women with hEDS/HSD, many reported the appearance or worsening of EDS/HSD symptoms with the onset of puberty (Blagowidow, 2021).

Delayed and Mistaken Diagnosis

Diagnosis of some HDCTs is difficult, potentially leading to delayed or mistaken diagnoses. EDS/HSD diagnosis, for example, is often delayed (mean of 14 years and as long as 28 years) (EURORDIS, 2009, p. 136). Multiple factors may contribute to such delays, including the multisystem, complex, and phenotypically variable nature of the disorders, which leads to a broadly "positive review of systems" such that medical providers are skeptical about patients' experience of the disorders (Clark, 2021; Halverson et al., 2021). Indeed, patients report experiencing denial among health care providers, as well as family members, as to the reality of their lived experience of certain manifestations of the disorders, such as pain, fatigue, and mild cognitive impairment, sometimes described as "brain fog," as well as limited treatment options (Clark, 2021; Langhinrichsen-Rohling et al., 2021; Palomo-Toucedo et al., 2020). Providers may mischaracterize the "subjective" experience of some gastrointestinal, neurological, and psychological symptoms as "functional" or "psychogenic" when they are in fact real and quite common neurobiological manifestations of the disorders (Barnum, 2014; Fikree et al., 2017). Research also has documented limited knowledge about HDCTs among health care providers, who often profess a lack of experience with the disorders and discomfort with diagnosing them (Schubart et al., 2021). In general, moreover, access to comprehensive, multidisciplinary care teams with expertise in HDCTs is lacking in terms of both geography and appropriate education (Halverson et al., 2021; Mittal et al., 2021). Finally, many health care professionals have inaccurate expectations that a diagnostic genetic test will be readily available for every HDCT, despite the fact that no such test is available for hEDS or any HSD (Bennett et al., 2021; Halverson et al., 2021).

Effects of Delayed or Mistaken Diagnosis

The long diagnostic odyssey experienced by many patients is often a source of distress and unnecessary hardship (Palomo-Toucedo et al., 2020). That experience may include inappropriate medical interventions and potential iatrogenic harm (EURORDIS, 2009, p. 137). Failure to diagnose an underlying HDCT may lead to inaccurate assessment of the risks and benefits associated with medical procedures, including such routine procedures as endoscopy or intubation, as well as reduced access to reasonable accommodations for the patient's condition at work or school.

Family stress and dysfunction may result from family members' failure to give credence to the symptoms reported by the patient (Halverson et al., 2021). Families may be subjected to stress associated with unexplained and repeated injuries and bruising, including inappropriate suspicion of child abuse (Castori, 2015). Patients report inappropriate assessments and inaccurate diagnoses, and many develop a mistrust of health care providers and negative expectations for future health care encounters, which may lead them to avoid further medical consultations (Halverson et al., 2021; Langhinrichsen-Rohling et al., 2021).

In the case of some of the HDCTs, such as MFS, LDS, and vascular EDS, failure to make the correct diagnosis may be life-threatening. Lack of monitoring for aortic root enlargement in MFS or LDS, for example, may lead to aortic dissection and death, while failure to recognize a characteristic phenotype (e.g., of MFS) in a patient presenting with chest pain may result in delayed diagnosis of aortic dissection, with potentially catastrophic results (Asouhidou and Asteri, 2009; Jarmulowicz and Phillips, 2001; Lovatt et al., 2022).

CLINICAL COURSE

HDCTs are lifelong disorders for which no curative treatments currently exist. Management involves supportive care, treatment of associated secondary impairments, and preventive measures to mitigate or prevent problems that may occur or worsen over time. The fact that HDCTs can manifest in a multitude of physical and mental secondary impairments in virtually any organ system can make the disorders difficult to recognize and manage. In addition, the clinical course of individuals with an HDCT is highly variable. Such variation relates not only to the disease-specific manifestations of each unique syndrome, as discussed above, but also to each individual and that person's comorbidities and/or underlying conditions. Nevertheless, the natural history of HDCTs as a general group demonstrates several commonalities, including the disorders' multisystem nature and potential secondary impairments.

Multiple connective tissues can work synchronously to form such structures as joints, where two bones make contact. Hinge joints, such as elbows, which allow for motion, are composed of bone, muscles, synovium, cartilage, and ligaments. These structures and connective tissues are often affected in HDCTs, making joint abnormalities common in most of the disorders. Joint laxity and dislocations are seen in MFS, OI, and EDS, as well as HSD. Joint contractures are seen in CCA, and early-onset degenerative osteoarthritis occurs with many types of EDS and skeletal dysplasia phenotypes (e.g., Stickler syndrome), illustrating how abnormally organized connective tissues can contribute to organ system dysfunction.

Instability of the joint between head and neck may lead to profound neurologic complications (Henderson et al., 2017). Other potential cranial and spinal neurologic complications are summarized by Debette and Germaine (2014) and Henderson and colleagues (2017). Dysautonomia—failure of the autonomic nervous system to balance properly between the "flight or fight" and "rest and digest" functions—is common in many of the HDCTs (Roma et al., 2018). Increasingly, dysfunction of the mast cells, which are first responders for the immune system, is recognized in several forms of EDS, as well as LDS (Brock et al., 2021). Gastrointestinal issues include motility and barrier dysfunction (i.e., altered intestinal permeability) (Alomari et al., 2020; Fikree et al., 2017; Wong et al., 2022). Mast cell activation and dysautonomia may play a role in gastrointestinal symptoms experienced by some individuals with EDS (Alomari et al., 2020; Wong et al., 2022). In some cases, gastrointestinal complications may lead to malabsorption and nutritional deficiencies (Beckers et al., 2017; Fikree et al., 2017; Wang et al., 2021). Any one or combination of these secondary impairments can contribute to the chronic pain and fatigue experienced by many individuals with HDCTs (Bowen et al., 2017; Hakim et al., 2017; Johansen et al., 2020; Speed et al., 2017; Syx et al., 2017; Tinkle et al., 2017). Mental manifestations (not only reactive) may also contribute to patients' experience of pain and fatigue. Anxiety, phobias, and depression in particular are very common, may affect the quality of life of individuals with these disorders, and therefore must be properly diagnosed and addressed (Bulbena et al., 2017).

The severity of an HDCT cannot be measured by a single genetic or laboratory test. Rather, the severity of the disorder in an individual is determined by the severity of the person's physical and mental secondary impairments, which may be measurable with existing clinical and function testing. Severity is also driven by the combined effects of multiple impairments, as well as the frequency, severity, and predictability of their fluctuations. The impact on the individual in terms of functional limitations and restrictions results from the combined effects of the multiple impairments in different body systems, which may be severe collectively even if they are individually graded as "less severe." This interplay among impairments and the multisystem nature of HDCTs can pose a major difficulty for the global assessment of disease severity.

The functional impairment in HDCTs is also linked to limitations and necessary restrictions due to vulnerability to specific environmental factors and other stressors. For many HDCTs, a patient's disease severity, manifestations, and clinical course may be adversely affected by specific environmental factors. In addition, physical and mental demands related to school or work may precipitate or exacerbate secondary impairments, perhaps further limiting activities and restricting participation. Beyond diagnosis of a specific HDCT, informed clinicians can help their patients substantially by being attuned to the many physical and mental secondary impairments with which these patients present. Recognizing the presence of these conditions and taking action to address them, even in the absence of confirmatory genetic testing, can mitigate their effects on the functional status and quality of life of individuals with HDCTs.

DISEASE STATE MANAGEMENT

Central to minimizing the impact of HDCTs on function is a coordinated multidisciplinary management strategy (Miklovic and Sieg, 2021; Mittal et al., 2021). Medical management needs to include a complete body-system review and assessment and periodic monitoring for areas of vulnerability. Functional management needs to address physical vulnerabilities and may require lifelong rehabilitation services. Psychosocial support of patients and families is also important. As noted previously, psychiatric manifestations, including anxiety and depression, are frequently seen in these conditions, as is the case in patients with other chronic conditions. Simple screening tools for depression and anxiety are available for use in the primary care setting. If these conditions are found to be present, a comprehensive mental health evaluation is important, and management may require ongoing assessment and treatment.

High-quality care for individuals with HDCTs relies on effective coordination among a team of providers across a broad range of disciplines (Miklovic and Sieg, 2021; Mittal et al., 2021). As discussed above, access to comprehensive, multidisciplinary care for the diagnosis and management of HDCTs can be limited by geography and other factors, including the availability of care teams with expertise in the disorders (Halverson et al., 2021; Mittal et al., 2021). In addition, access to multidisciplinary teams and relevant specialists is limited or nonexistent in rural areas; even many university centers lack multidisciplinary teams with expertise in HDCTs (Mittal et al., 2021). Education about HDCTs, including their multisystem physical and mental manifestations, diagnosis, and management, is important for all health care providers to increase recognition and earlier diagnosis of the disorders, as well as to improve coordination of their management (Miklovic and Sieg, 2021; Mittal et al., 2021; Schubart et al., 2021). With appropriate education, a variety of clinicians, including, for example, physicians, nurses, psychologists, neuropsychologists, rehabilitation specialists (e.g., physiatrists; physical, occupational, and speech therapists), nutritionists, and others, should be able to recognize HDCTs and direct affected individuals to the appropriate providers for management. Individuals with HDCTs and relevant support groups provide valuable education regarding the manifestations and lived experience of the disorders (Bloom et al., 2021). Education for patients and families is important to help them understand the multisystem nature of HDCTs and the options available for managing their disorder despite the lack of curative treatment. Information about lifestyle modifications; adherence to physical therapy, medication, and other medical interventions; and symptoms for which to seek immediate medical care can help reduce morbidity (Miklovic and Sieg, 2021). Increased recognition of the breadth and scope of HDCTs by health care professional education programs, professional organizations, and publishers of quality biomedical research is needed.

FINDINGS AND CONCLUSIONS

Findings

2-1. Heritable disorders of connective tissue (HDCTs) are a heterogeneous group of inherited disorders that affect connective tissues in organ systems throughout the body.

2-2. Connective tissues are an integral component of every organ system and play a crucial role in the function of those systems. Hence, the physical and mental secondary impairments associated with HDCTs, which may develop and potentially progress or wax and wane over time, manifest throughout the body and affect functioning in every body system.

2-3. HDCTs can be difficult to diagnose, and the true prevalence of many of these disorders is unknown.

2-4. Because HDCTs can cause a wide variety of physical and mental secondary impairments involving multiple organ systems, affected individuals often are referred to a succession of different specialists, resulting in delayed diagnosis of the underlying HDCT.

2-5. HDCTs are diagnosed through a combination of clinical findings and established clinical criteria, followed by confirmatory molecular genetic testing when specific genes have been identified for the suspected disorder.

2-6. HDCTs are lifelong disorders for which no curative treatments currently exist. Management involves supportive care, treatment of associated secondary impairments, and preventive measures to mitigate or prevent problems that may occur or worsen over time.

2-7. Individuals with HDCTs often experience difficulty with obtaining appropriate and integrated multidisciplinary care to address the wide range of physical and mental impairments associated with these disorders.

2-8. Access to comprehensive, multidisciplinary care for the diagnosis and management of HDCTs can be limited by geography and other factors, including the availability of care teams with expertise in the disorders.

2-9. The clinical course of HDCTs is highly variable and can be impacted not only by the disease-specific manifestations of each unique syndrome, but also by individuals' physical and mental secondary impairments, as well as environmental factors and physical and psychological demands.

2-10. The severity of HDCTs is linked to the severity of affected individuals' physical and mental secondary impairments, including the combined effects of multiple impairments, as well as the frequency, severity, and predictability of their fluctuations.

Conclusions

2-1. Consideration of a diagnosis of an HDCT is warranted for individuals who present with previously undiagnosed complex multisystem disorders.

2-2. Early diagnosis of HDCTs is important to reduce physical injury, reduce psychological harm to affected individuals and their family members, and prevent the risks associated with inappropriate medical care.

2-3. Appropriate multisystem assessments are important at the time of HDCT diagnosis and at intervals across a person's life.

2-4. Appropriate multidisciplinary understanding and management of HDCTs can reduce the frequency and severity of their manifestations and resulting functional limitations.

REFERENCES

Abdel-Massih, T., A. Goldenberg, P. Vouhé, F. Iserin, P. Acar, E. Villain, G. Agnoletti, D. Sidi, and D. Bonnet. 2002. Marfan syndrome in the newborn and infants less than 4 months: A series of 9 patients. *Archives des Maladies du Coeur et des Vaisseaux* 95(5):469-472.

Abdo, H., L. Calvo-Enrique, J. M. Lopez, J. Song, M. D. Zhang, D. Usoskin, A. El Manira, I. Adameyko, J. Hjerling-Leffler, and P. Ernfors. 2019. Specialized cutaneous schwann cells initiate pain sensation. *Science* 365(6454):695-699. https://doi.org/10.1126/science.aax6452.

Alomari, M., A. Hitawala, P. Chadalavada, F. Covut, L. A. Momani, S. Khazaaleh, F. Gosai, S. A. Ashi, A. Abushahin, and A. Schneider. 2020. Prevalence and predictors of gastrointestinal dysmotility in patients with hypermobile Ehlers-Danlos syndrome: A tertiary care center experience. *Cureus* 12(4):e7881. https://doi.org/10.7759/cureus.7881.

Ardhanari, M., D. Barbouth, and S. Swaminathan. 2019. Early-onset Marfan syndrome: A case series. *Journal of Pediatric Genetics* 8(2):86-90. https://doi.org/10.1055/s-0038-1675338.

Arnaud, P., O. Milleron, N. Hanna, J. Ropers, N. Ould Ouali, A. Affoune, M. Langeois, L. Eliahou, F. Arnoult, P. Renard, M. Michelon-Jouneaux, M. Cotillon, L. Gouya, C. Boileau, and G. Jondeau. 2021. Clinical relevance of genotype–phenotype correlations beyond vascular events in a cohort study of 1500 Marfan syndrome patients with FBN1 pathogenic variants. *Genetics in Medicine* 23(7):1296-1304. https://doi.org/10.1038/s41436-021-01132-x.

Asahara, H., M. Inui, and M. K. Lotz. 2017. Tendons and ligaments: Connecting developmental biology to musculoskeletal disease pathogenesis. *Journal of Bone and Mineral Research* 32(9):1773-1782. https://doi.org/10.1002/jbmr.3199.

Asouhidou, I., and T. Asteri. 2009. Acute aortic dissection: Be aware of misdiagnosis. *BMC Research Notes* 2:25. https://doi.org/10.1186/1756-0500-2-25.

Barallobre-Barreiro, J., B. Loeys, M. Mayr, M. Rienks, A. Verstraeten, and J. C. Kovacic. 2020. Extracellular matrix in vascular disease, part 2/4: JACC Focus Seminar. *Journal of the American College of Cardiology* 75(17):2189-2203. https://doi.org/10.1016/j.jacc.2020.03.018.

Barnum, R. 2014. Problems with diagnosing conversion disorder in response to variable and unusual symptoms. *Adolescent Health, Medicine and Therapeutics* 5:67-71. https://doi.org/10.2147/ahmt.S57486.

Beckers, A. B., D. Keszthelyi, A. Fikree, L. Vork, A. Masclee, A. D. Farmer, and Q. Aziz. 2017. Gastrointestinal disorders in joint hypermobility syndrome/Ehlers-Danlos syndrome hypermobility type: A review for the gastroenterologist. *Neurogastroenterology and Motility* 29(8):e13013. https://doi.org/10.1111/nmo.13013.

Bennett, S. E., N. Walsh, T. Moss, and S. Palmer. 2021. Understanding the psychosocial impact of joint hypermobility syndrome and Ehlers-Danlos syndrome hypermobility type: A qualitative interview study. *Disability and Rehabilitation* 43(6):795-804. https://doi.org/10.1080/09638288.2019.1641848.

Blagowidow, N. 2021. Obstetrics and gynecology in Ehlers-Danlos syndrome: A brief review and update. *American Journal of Medical Genetics Part C: Seminars in Medical Genetics* 187(4):593-598. https://doi.org/10.1002/ajmg.c.31945.

Bloom, L., J. Schubart, R. Bascom, A. Hakim, and C. A. Francomano. 2021. The power of patient-led global collaboration. *American Journal of Medical Genetics Part C: Seminars in Medical Genetics* 187(4):425-428. https://doi.org/10.1002/ajmg.c.31942.

Bowen, J. M., G. J. Sobey, N. P. Burrows, M. Colombi, M. E. Lavallee, F. Malfait, and C. A. Francomano. 2017. Ehlers-Danlos syndrome, classical type. *American Journal of Medical Genetics Part C: Seminars in Medical Genetics* 175(1):27-39. https://doi.org/10.1002/ajmg.c.31548.

Brock, I., W. Prendergast, and A. Maitland. 2021. Mast cell activation disease and immunoglobulin deficiency in patients with hypermobile Ehlers-Danlos syndrome/hypermobility spectrum disorder. *American Journal of Medical Genetics. Part C: Seminars in Medical Genetics* 187(4):473-481. https://doi.org/10.1002/ajmg.c.31940.

Bulbena, A., C. Baeza-Velasco, A. Bulbena-Cabré, G. Pailhez, H. Critchley, P. Chopra, N. Mallorquí-Bagué, C. Frank, and S. Porges. 2017. Psychiatric and psychological aspects in the Ehlers–Danlos syndromes. *American Journal of Medical Genetics Part C: Seminars in Medical Genetics* 175(1):237-245. https://doi.org/10.1002/ajmg.c.31544.

Byers, P. H. 2019. Vascular Ehlers-Danlos syndrome. In *GeneReviews® [Internet]*, edited by M. P. Adam, H. H. Ardinger, R. A. Pagon, S. E. Wallace, L. J. H. Bean, K. W. Gripp, G. M. Mirzaa, and A. Amemiya. Seattle, WA: University of Washington; 1993-2022. https://www.ncbi.nlm.nih.gov/books/NBK1494/.

Byers, P. H., M. Duvic, M. Atkinson, M. Robinow, L. T. Smith, S. M. Krane, M. T. Greally, M. Ludman, R. Matalon, S. Pauker, D. Quanbeck, and U. Schwarze. 1997. Ehlers-Danlos syndrome type VIIA and VIIB result from splice-junction mutations or genomic deletions that involve exon 6 in the COL1A1 and COL1A2 genes of type I collagen. *American Journal of Medical Genetics* 72(1):94-105. https://doi.org/10.1002/(sici)1096-8628(19971003)72:1<94::aid-ajmg20>3.0.co;2-o.

Castori, M. 2015. Ehlers-Danlos syndrome(s) mimicking child abuse: Is there an impact on clinical practice? *American Journal of Medical Genetics Part C: Seminars in Medical Genetics* 169(4):289-292. https://doi.org/10.1002/ajmg.c.31460.

Clark, S. 2021. Help me trust you after my misdiagnosis. *BMJ* 373:n1175. https://doi.org/10.1136/bmj.n1175.

Connizzo, B. K., S. M. Yannascoli, and L. J. Soslowsky. 2013. Structure-function relationships of postnatal tendon development: A parallel to healing. *Matrix Biology* 32(2):106-116. https://doi.org/10.1016/j.matbio.2013.01.007.

Dawidowicz, J., S. Szotek, N. Matysiak, Ł. Mielańczyk, and K. Maksymowicz. 2015. Electron microscopy of human fascia lata: Focus on telocytes. *Journal of Cellular and Molecular Medicine* 19(10):2500-2506. https://doi.org/10.1111/jcmm.12665.

Debette, S., and D. P. Germain. 2014. Chapter 37—Neurologic manifestations of inherited disorders of connective tissue. *Handbook of Clinical Neurology* 119:565-576. https://doi.org/10.1016/b978-0-7020-4086-3.00037-0.

del Monte-Nieto, G., J. W. Fischer, D. J. Gorski, R. P. Harvey, and J. C. Kovacic. 2020. Basic biology of extracellular matrix in the cardiovascular system, part 1/4: JACC Focus Seminar. *Journal of the American College of Cardiology* 75(17):2169-2188. https://doi.org/10.1016/j.jacc.2020.03.024.

EURORDIS. 2009. *The voice of 12,000 patients.* https://www.eurordis.org/publication/voice-12000-patients.

Fikree, A., G. Chelimsky, H. Collins, K. Kovacic, and Q. Aziz. 2017. Gastrointestinal involvement in the Ehlers-Danlos syndromes. *American Journal of Medical Genetics Part C: Seminars in Medical Genetics* 175(1):181-187. https://doi.org/10.1002/ajmg.c.31546.

Follis, R. H., Jr. 1952. Osteogenesis imperfecta congenita: A connective tissue diathesis. *The Journal of Pediatrics* 41(6):713-721. https://doi.org/10.1016/s0022-3476(52)80292-6.

Follis, R. H., Jr. 1953a. Histochemical studies on cartilage and bone. III. Osteogenesis imperfecta. *Bulletin of the Johns Hopkins Hospital* 93(6):386-399.

Follis, R. H., Jr. 1953b. Maldevelopment of the corium in the osteogenesis imperfecta syndrome. *Bulletin of the Johns Hopkins Hospital* 93(4):225-233.

Gillies, A. R., and R. L. Lieber. 2011. Structure and function of the skeletal muscle extracellular matrix. *Muscle & Nerve* 44(3):318-331. https://doi.org/10.1002/mus.22094.

Glass, D., A. Viñuela, M. N. Davies, A. Ramasamy, L. Parts, D. Knowles, A. A. Brown, Å. K. Hedman, K. S. Small, A. Buil, E. Grundberg, A. C. Nica, P. Di Meglio, F. O. Nestle, M. Ryten, the UK Brain Expression consortium, the MUther consortium, R. Durbin, M. I. McCarthy, P. Deloukas, E. T. Dermitzakis, M. E. Weale, V. Bataille, and T. D. Spector. 2013. Gene expression changes with age in skin, adipose tissue, blood and brain. *Genome Biology* 14(7):R75. https://doi.org/10.1186/gb-2013-14-7-r75.

Hakim, A., I. De Wandele, C. O'Callaghan, A. Pocinki, and P. Rowe. 2017. Chronic fatigue in Ehlers-Danlos syndrome-hypermobile type. *American Journal of Medical Genetics Part C: Seminars in Medical Genetics* 175(1):175-180. https://doi.org/10.1002/ajmg.c.31542.

Halata, Z. 1977. The ultrastructure of the sensory nerve endings in the articular capsule of the knee joint of the domestic cat (Ruffini corpuscles and Pacinian corpuscles). *Journal of Anatomy* 124(Pt 3):717-729. https://www.ncbi.nlm.nih.gov/pmc/articles/PMC1234668/.

Halverson, C. M. E., E. W. Clayton, A. Garcia Sierra, and C. Francomano. 2021. Patients with Ehlers–Danlos syndrome on the diagnostic odyssey: Rethinking complexity and difficulty as a hero's journey. *American Journal of Medical Genetics Part C: Seminars in Medical Genetics* 187(4):416-424. https://doi.org/10.1002/ajmg.c.31935.

Hayakawa, M., M. Kobayashi, and T. Hoshino. 1990. Microfibrils: A constitutive component of reticular fibers in the mouse lymph node. *Cell and Tissue Research* 262(1):199-201. https://doi.org/10.1007/bf00327763.

Henderson, F. C., Sr., C. Austin, E. Benzel, P. Bolognese, R. Ellenbogen, C. A. Francomano, C. Ireton, P. Klinge, M. Koby, D. Long, S. Patel, E. L. Singman, and N. C. Voermans. 2017. Neurological and spinal manifestations of the Ehlers-Danlos syndromes. *American Journal of Medical Genetics. Part C: Seminars in Medical Genetics* 175(1):195-211. https://doi.org/10.1002/ajmg.c.31549.

Işıldak, U., M. Somel, J. M. Thornton, and H. M. Dönertaş. 2020. Temporal changes in the gene expression heterogeneity during brain development and aging. *Scientific Reports* 10(1):4080. https://doi.org/10.1038/s41598-020-60998-0.

Jarmulowicz, M., and W. G. Phillips. 2001. Vascular Ehlers-Danlos syndrome undiagnosed during life. *Journal of the Royal Society of Medicine* 94(1):28-30. https://doi.org/10.1177/014107680109400108.

Jensen, S. A., and P. A. Handford. 2016. New insights into the structure, assembly and biological roles of 10–12 nm connective tissue microfibrils from fibrillin-1 studies. *Biochemical Journal* 473(7):827-838. https://doi.org/10.1042/BJ20151108.

Johansen, H., G. Velvin, and I. Lidal. 2020. Adults with Loeys–Dietz syndrome and vascular Ehlers–Danlos syndrome: A cross-sectional study of health burden perspectives. *American Journal of Medical Genetics Part A* 182(1):137-145. https://doi.org/10.1002/ajmg.a.61396.

Judge, D. P., and H. C. Dietz. 2005. Marfan's syndrome. *Lancet* 366(9501):1965-1976. https://doi.org/10.1016/s0140-6736(05)67789-6.

Kannus, P. 2000. Structure of the tendon connective tissue. *Scandinavian Journal of Medicine & Science in Sports* 10(6):312-320. https://doi.org/10.1034/j.1600-0838.2000.010006312.x.

Knuutinen, A., N. Kokkonen, J. Risteli, K. Vähäkangas, M. Kallioinen, T. Salo, T. Sorsa, and A. Oikarinen. 2002. Smoking affects collagen synthesis and extracellular matrix turnover in human skin. *British Journal of Dermatology* 146(4):588-594. https://doi.org/10.1046/j.1365-2133.2002.04694.x.

Krakower, C. 1972. The cells and tissues of the immune system: Structure, functions, interactions. *JAMA* 220(10):1366. https://doi.org/10.1001/jama.1972.03200100076031.

Langhinrichsen-Rohling, J., C. L. Lewis, S. McCabe, E. C. Lathan, G. A. Agnew, C. N. Selwyn, and M. E. Gigler. 2021. They've been BITTEN: Reports of institutional and provider betrayal and links with Ehlers-Danlos syndrome patients' current symptoms, unmet needs and healthcare expectations. *Therapeutic Advances in Rare Disease* 2:263300402110220. https://dx.doi.org/10.1177/26330040211022033.

Liu, T., T. H. McCalmont, I. J. Frieden, M. L. Williams, M. K. Connolly, and A. E. Gilliam. 2008. The stiff skin syndrome: Case series, differential diagnosis of the stiff skin phenotype, and review of the literature. *Archives of Dermatology* 144(10):1351-1359. https://doi.org/10.1001/archderm.144.10.1351.

Loeys, B. L., and H. C. Dietz. 2018. Loeys-Dietz syndrome. In *GeneReviews® [Internet]*, edited by M. P. Adam, H. H. Ardinger, R. A. Pagon, S. E. Wallace, L. J. H. Bean, K. W. Gripp, G. M. Mirzaa and A. Amemiya. Seattle, WA: University of Washington; 1993-2022. https://www.ncbi.nlm.nih.gov/books/NBK1133/.

Loeys, B. L., E. E. Gerber, D. Riegert-Johnson, S. Iqbal, P. Whiteman, V. McConnell, C. R. Chillakuri, D. Macaya, P. J. Coucke, A. De Paepe, D. P. Judge, F. Wigley, E. C. Davis, H. J. Mardon, P. Handford, D. R. Keene, L. Y. Sakai, and H. C. Dietz. 2010. Mutations in fibrillin-1 cause congenital scleroderma: Stiff skin syndrome. *Science Translational Medicine* 2(23):23ra20. https://doi.org/10.1126/scitranslmed.3000488.

Lovatt, S., C. W. Wong, K. Schwarz, J. A. Borovac, T. Lo, M. Gunning, T. Phan, A. Patwala, D. Barker, C. D. Mallen, and C. S. Kwok. 2022. Misdiagnosis of aortic dissection: A systematic review of the literature. *American Journal of Emergency Medicine* 53:16-22. https://doi.org/10.1016/j.ajem.2021.11.047.

McKusick, V. A. 1955. The cardiovascular aspects of Marfan's syndrome: A heritable disorder of connective tissue. *Circulation* 11(3):321-342. https://doi.org/10.1161/01.cir.11.3.321.

Miklovic, T., and V. Sieg. 2021. Ehlers Danlos syndrome. In *StatPearls [Internet]*. Treasure Island, FL: StatPearls Publishing. https://www.ncbi.nlm.nih.gov/books/NBK549814/.

Milewicz, D. M., A. C. Braverman, J. De Backer, S. A. Morris, C. Boileau, I. H. Maumenee, G. Jondeau, A. Evangelista, and R. E. Pyeritz. 2021. Marfan syndrome. *Nature Reviews: Disease Primers* 7(1):64. https://doi.org/10.1038/s41572-021-00298-7.

Mittal, N., D. S. Mina, L. McGillis, A. Weinrib, P. M. Slepian, M. Rachinsky, S. Buryk-Iggers, C. Laflamme, L. Lopez-Hernandez, L. Hussey, J. Katz, L. McLean, D. Rozenberg, L. Liu, Y. Tse, C. Parker, A. Adler, G. Charames, R. Bleakney, C. Veillette, C. J. Nielson, S. Tavares, S. Varriano, J. Guzman, H. Faghfoury, and H. Clarke. 2021. The GoodHope Ehlers Danlos Syndrome Clinic: Development and implementation of the first interdisciplinary program for multi-system issues in connective tissue disorders at the Toronto General Hospital. *Orphanet Journal of Rare Diseases* 16(1):357. https://doi.org/10.1186/s13023-021-01962-7.

Mortier, G. R., D. H. Cohn, V. Cormier-Daire, C. Hall, D. Krakow, S. Mundlos, G. Nishimura, S. Robertson, L. Sangiorgi, R. Savarirayan, D. Sillence, A. Superti-Furga, S. Unger, and M. L. Warman. 2019. Nosology and classification of genetic skeletal disorders: 2019 revision. *American Journal of Medical Genetics Part A* 179(12):2393-2419. https://doi.org/10.1002/ajmg.a.61366.

Nezwek, T. A., and M. Varacallo. 2021. Physiology, connective tissue. In *StatPearls [Internet]*. Treasure Island, FL: StatPearls Publishing. https://www.ncbi.nlm.nih.gov/books/NBK542226/.

NORD (National Organization for Rare Disorders). 2021. *Rare disease database: Marfan syndrome*. https://rarediseases.org/rare-diseases/marfan-syndrome/ (accessed February 9, 2022).

Omelyanenko, N. P., and L. I. Slutsky. 2014. *Connective tissue: Histophysiology, biochemistry, molecular biology*. 1st ed. Boca Raton, FL: CRC Press. https://doi.org/10.1201/b16297

Orphanet. 2022a. *Dermatosparaxis Ehlers-Danlos syndrome*. https://www.orpha.net/consor4.01/www/cgi-bin/Disease_Search.php?lng=EN&data_id=4045&Disease_Disease_Search_diseaseGroup=Dermatosparaxis-EDS&Disease_Disease_Search_diseaseType=Pat&Disease(s)/group%20of%20diseases=Dermatosparaxis-Ehlers-Danlos-syndrome&title=Dermatosparaxis%20Ehlers-Danlos%20syndrome&search=Disease_Search_Simple (accessed February 16, 2022).

Orphanet. 2022b. *Musculocontractural Ehlers-Danlos syndrome*. https://www.orpha.net/consor4.01/www/cgi-bin/Disease_Search.php?lng=EN&data_id=3480&Disease_Disease_Search_diseaseGroup=Musculocontractural-EDS&Disease_Disease_Search_diseaseType=Pat&Disease(s)/group%20of%20diseases=Musculocontractural-Ehlers-Danlos-syndrome&title=Musculocontractural%20Ehlers-Danlos%20syndrome&search=Disease_Search_Simple (accessed February 16, 2022).

Paiva, K. B. S., and J. M. Granjeiro. 2017. Chapter six—Matrix metalloproteinases in bone resorption, remodeling, and repair. *Progress in Molecular Biology and Translational Science* 148:203-303. https://doi.org/10.1016/bs.pmbts.2017.05.001.

Palomo-Toucedo, I. C., F. Leon-Larios, M. Reina-Bueno, M. D. C. Vázquez-Bautista, P. V. Munuera-Martínez, and G. Domínguez-Maldonado. 2020. Psychosocial influence of Ehlers-Danlos syndrome in daily life of patients: A qualitative study. *International Journal of Environmental Research and Public Health* 17(17). https://doi.org/10.3390/ijerph17176425.

Pyeritz, R. E. 2000. Ehlers-Danlos syndromes. In *Cecil textbook of medicine*. 21st ed. Vol. 1, edited by L. Goldman and J. C. Bennett. Philadelphia: W.B. Saunders. Pp. 1119-1120.

Ricard-Blum, S. 2011. The collagen family. *Cold Spring Harbor Perspectives in Biology* 3(1):a004978. https://doi.org/10.1101/cshperspect.a004978.

Richards, S., N. Aziz, S. Bale, D. Bick, S. Das, J. Gastier-Foster, W. W. Grody, M. Hegde, E. Lyon, E. Spector, K. Voelkerding, and H. L. Rehm. 2015. Standards and guidelines for the interpretation of sequence variants: A joint consensus recommendation of the American College of Medical Genetics and Genomics and the Association for Molecular Pathology. *Genetics in Medicine* 17(5):405-423. https://doi.org/10.1038/gim.2015.30.

Roma, M., C. L. Marden, I. De Wandele, C. A. Francomano, and P. C. Rowe. 2018. Postural tachycardia syndrome and other forms of orthostatic intolerance in Ehlers-Danlos syndrome. *Autonomic Neuroscience* 215:89-96. https://doi.org/10.1016/j.autneu.2018.02.006.

Sakai, L. Y., and D. R. Keene. 2019. Fibrillin protein pleiotropy: Acromelic dysplasias. *Matrix Biology* 80:6-13. https://doi.org/10.1016/j.matbio.2018.09.005.

Savarirayan, R., V. Bompadre, M. B. Bober, T.-J. Cho, M. J. Goldberg, J. Hoover-Fong, M. Irving, S. E. Kamps, W. G. Mackenzie, C. Raggio, S. S. Spencer, and K. K. White. 2019. Best practice guidelines regarding diagnosis and management of patients with type II collagen disorders. *Genetics in Medicine* 21(9):2070-2080. https://doi.org/10.1038/s41436-019-0446-9.

Schubart, J. R., R. Bascom, C. A. Francomano, L. Bloom, and A. J. Hakim. 2021. Initial description and evaluation of EDS ECHO: An international effort to improve care for people with the Ehlers-Danlos syndromes and hypermobility spectrum disorders. *American Journal of Medical Genetics Part C: Seminars in Medical Genetics* 187(4):609-615. https://doi.org/10.1002/ajmg.c.31960.

Shukunami, C., A. Takimoto, M. Oro, and Y. Hiraki. 2006. Scleraxis positively regulates the expression of tenomodulin, a differentiation marker of tenocytes. *Developmental Biology* 298(1):234-247. https://doi.org/10.1016/j.ydbio.2006.06.036.

Sophia Fox, A. J., A. Bedi, and S. A. Rodeo. 2009. The basic science of articular cartilage: Structure, composition, and function. *Sports Health* 1(6):461-468. https://doi.org/10.1177/1941738109350438.

Speed, T. J., V. A. Mathur, M. Hand, B. Christensen, P. D. Sponseller, K. A. Williams, and C. M. Campbell. 2017. Characterization of pain, disability, and psychological burden in Marfan syndrome. *American Journal of Medical Genetics Part A* 173(2):315-323. https://doi.org/10.1002/ajmg.a.38051.

Stecco, C., C. Fede, V. Macchi, A. Porzionato, L. Petrelli, C. Biz, R. Stern, and R. De Caro. 2018. The fasciacytes: A new cell devoted to fascial gliding regulation. *Clinical Anatomy* 31(5):667-676. https://doi.org/10.1002/ca.23072.

Steinmann, B., P. M. Royce, and A. Superti-Furga. 2002. The Ehlers-Danlos syndrome. In *Connective tissue and its heritable disorders: Molecular, genetic, and medical aspects*. 2nd ed., edited by B. Steinmann and P. M. Royce. New York: Wiley-Liss, Inc. Pp. 431-524. https://doi.org/10.1002/0471221929.ch9.

Syx, D., I. De Wandele, L. Rombaut, and F. Malfait. 2017. Hypermobility, the Ehlers-Danlos syndromes and chronic pain. *Clinical and Experimental Rheumatology* 35 Suppl 107(5):116-122.

Tinkle, B., M. Castori, B. Berglund, H. Cohen, R. Grahame, H. Kazkaz, and H. Levy. 2017. Hypermobile Ehlers-Danlos syndrome (a.k.a. Ehlers-Danlos syndrome type III and Ehlers-Danlos syndrome hypermobility type): Clinical description and natural history. *American Journal of Medical Genetics Part C: Seminars in Medical Genetics* 175(1):48-69. https://doi.org/10.1002/ajmg.c.31538.

Uitto, J. 1979. Biochemistry of the elastic fibers in normal connective tissues and its alterations in diseases. *Journal of Investigative Dermatology* 72(1):1-10. https://doi.org/10.1111/1523-1747.ep12530093.

University of Leeds. 2002. Oral: *Four layers of the G.I. tract*. https://www.histology.leeds.ac.uk/digestive/GI_layers.php (accessed July 19, 2022).

van Deemter, M., H. H. Pas, R. Kuijer, R. J. van der Worp, J. M. M. Hooymans, and L. I. Los. 2009. Enzymatic breakdown of type II collagen in the human vitreous. *Investigative Ophthalmology & Visual Science* 50(10):4552–4560. https://doi.org/10.1167/iovs.08-3125.

Vandenabeele, F., J. Creemers, I. Lambrichts, P. Lippens, and M. Jans. 1997. Encapsulated Ruffini-like endings in human lumbar facet joints. *Journal of Anatomy* 191(Pt 4):571-583. https://doi.org/10.1046/j.1469-7580.1997.19140571.x.

Wang, X. J., M. Babameto, D. Babovic-Vuksanovic, J. M. Bowen, and M. Camilleri. 2021. Audit of gastrointestinal manifestations in patients with Loeys-Dietz syndrome and vascular Ehlers-Danlos syndrome. *Digestive Diseases and Sciences* 66(4):1142-1152. https://doi.org/10.1007/s10620-020-06265-8.

Watanabe, T., Y. Hosaka, E. Yamamoto, H. Ueda, P. Tangkawattana, and K. Takehana. 2004. Morphological study of the Golgi tendon organ in equine superficial digital flexor tendon. *Okajimas Folia Anatomica Japonica* 81(2-3):33-37. https://doi.org/10.2535/ofaj.81.33.

Weatherholt, A. M., R. K. Fuchs, and S. J. Warden. 2012. Specialized connective tissue: Bone, the structural framework of the upper extremity. *Journal of Hand Therapy* 25(2):123-132. https://doi.org/10.1016/j.jht.2011.08.003.

Wong, S., S. Hasan, C. Parducci, and B. A. Riley. 2022. The gastrointestinal effects amongst Ehlers-Danlos syndrome, mast cell activation syndrome and postural orthostatic tachycardia syndrome. *AIMS Allergy and Immunology* 6(2):19-24. https://www.aimspress.com/article/doi/10.3934/Allergy.2022004.

3

Marfan Syndrome and Related Hereditary Aortopathies

Marfan syndrome (MFS) is an autosomal-dominant disorder that affects multiple organ systems, especially the ocular, cardiovascular, and skeletal systems. Absent appropriate diagnosis and management, severe disability and early death are common. MFS shares features with several related hereditary disorders of connective tissue (HDCTs) called hereditary aortopathies, including Loeys-Dietz syndrome (LDS), congenital contractural arachnodactyly (CCA; also known as Beals-Hecht syndrome), and Shprintzen-Goldberg syndrome (SGS), particularly in the cardiovascular and skeletal systems. This chapter describes the history, diagnosis, and characteristics of MFS and related hereditary aortopathies, and reviews their treatment, their management, and those disease manifestations that are potentially disabling. An overview of these disorders is provided in Annex Table 3-1 at the end of the chapter.

HISTORY OF MARFAN SYNDROME AND RELATED HEREDITARY AORTOPATHIES

In 1896, the French pediatrician Antoine Marfan described a young girl with unusually long digits (arachnodactyly) and joint contractures from birth. He did not note any problems with her heart or eyes. Soon after, his colleagues termed this condition "Marfan syndrome." Over the next five decades, some patients with arachnodactyly were also found to have dislocation of the lens of the eye (ectopia lentis); leakage of heart valves; and, most worrisome, enlargement (dilatation) of the aorta at the point where it exits the heart (aortic aneurysm). When the dilatation progressed to a severe degree, the wall of the aorta would tear (aortic dissection), which was often fatal. Consequently, it became clear that MFS resulted in a markedly reduced life expectancy, by one-third to one-half, with some patients dying in childhood. Of interest, by the 1960s it was clear that Marfan's original patient had a different but overlapping condition—CCA—which generally has none of the severe complications of MFS, particularly aortic dissection (Takeda et al., 2015). Since the late 1970s, steady progress has been made in the medical and surgical management of MFS.

The genetic cause of MFS was discovered in 1991 (Dietz et al., 1991; Lee et al., 1991). The syndrome is caused by pathogenic variants in the gene that encodes the connective tissue protein fibrillin-1 (*FBN1*). These variants are heterozygous—that is, alterations are seen in only one copy of the *FBN1* gene, while the other copy is unaffected. About three-quarters of patients have an affected parent (autosomal-dominant inheritance), while the remaining roughly 25 percent represent new pathogenic variants in a family. Each offspring of an affected individual has a 50 percent risk of inheriting the condition.

Over the past few decades, people with aortic aneurysms, often with a parental history of the same phenotype, have been found to demonstrate a wide spectrum of features sometimes overlapping with classic MFS. This observation has given rise to recognition of a separate set of syndromes called the aortopathies, the most severe of which is LDS. All share the risk of aortic dilatation and aortic dissection, although the risk varies within families and among individuals who carry a pathogenic variant in the same gene.

DIAGNOSIS OF MARFAN SYNDROME AND RELATED HEREDITARY AORTOPATHIES

Diagnosis of Marfan Syndrome

The current diagnostic criteria for MFS are based on clinical and molecular features, summarized most recently in the 2010 revised Ghent nosology, also known as the Ghent II criteria (Loeys et al., 2010). The Ghent II criteria address the presence of family history and aortic root dilatation, as well as pathogenic variants in *FBN1* (see Box 3-1), and include a scoring system that assigns points to defined clinical characteristics of MFS (see Box 3-2). Genetic testing involves analyzing *FBN1* for pathogenic and likely pathologic variants (mutations).

Diagnosis of Related Hereditary Aortopathies

As with MFS, the most severe hereditary aortopathies (e.g., LDS, CCA [see below]) can often be diagnosed on the basis of clinical examination and family history. Differences in clinical findings may be subtle, however, and final diagnosis and management depend on the results of genetic testing. Currently, pathogenic variants in more than two dozen genes other than *FBN1* have been discovered to be causative of the aortopathies. To date, pathogenic variants in five different genes have been found to cause different types of LDS: *TGFBR1* (LDS1) (Loeys et al., 2005), *TGFBR2* (LDS2) (Loeys et al., 2005), *SMAD3* (LDS3) (Regalado et al., 2011), *TGFB2* (LDS4) (Lindsay et al., 2012), and *TGFB3* (LDS5) (Bertoli-Avella et al., 2015; Matyas et al., 2014; Rienhoff et al., 2013). CCA is caused by pathogenic variants in the *FBN2* gene (Gupta et al., 2002), and Shprintzen-Goldberg syndrome results from pathogenic variants in the *SKI* gene (Doyle et al., 2012).

CHARACTERISTICS OF MARFAN SYNDROME AND RELATED HEREDITARY AORTOPATHIES

Marfan Syndrome

Clinical Picture

The majority of MFS patients have notable involvement of the cardiovascular, musculoskeletal, and ocular systems, as well as abnormalities in the respiratory and central nervous systems (Loeys et al., 2010). Although MFS typically manifests in multiple body systems, the severity of the manifestations may vary among body systems within a given individual (Bruno et al., 1984). In other words, within a given patient, there may be a lack of correlation between, for example, the severity of aortic dilatation and the degree of joint hypermobility. In addition, the range and timing of clinical symptoms experienced by individual patients can be broad. For example, some patients present in the neonatal period with rapidly progressive or severe multisystem disease, whereas others with more limited manifestations may go undiagnosed until they experience a sentinel event, such as aortic dissection, in adulthood (Dietz, 2022). Musculoskeletal and ocular abnormalities in patients with MFS are often identified in childhood, while respiratory abnormalities typically manifest in adulthood. The age at time of diagnosis ranges from the prenatal period to the eighth decade of life (Groth et al., 2015). Most patients demonstrate joint laxity throughout life, although paradoxically, some have reduced mobility in certain joints, such as the digits or elbows (Dietz, 2022). Investigation for MFS is

> **BOX 3-1**
> **Revised Ghent Criteria for Diagnosis of Marfan Syndrome and Related Conditions**
>
> In the absence of family history:
>
> 1. Aortic root dilatation (Z score ≥ 2) AND ectopia lentis = Marfan syndrome*
>   - "The presence of aortic root dilatation (Z-score ≥ 2 when standardized to age and body size) or dissection and ectopia lentis allows the unequivocal diagnosis of Marfan syndrome, irrespective of the presence or absence of systemic features except where these are indicative of Shprintzen-Goldberg syndrome, Loeys-Dietz syndrome, or vascular Ehlers-Danlos syndrome" (Loeys et al., 2010, p. 478).
> 2. Aortic root dilatation (Z score ≥ 2) AND *FBN1* = Marfan syndrome
>   - "The presence of aortic root dilatation (Z ≥ 2) or dissection and the identification of a bona fide *FBN1* mutation is sufficient to establish the diagnosis, even when ectopia lentis is absent" (Loeys et al., 2010, p. 478).
> 3. Aortic root dilatation (Z score ≥ 2) AND systemic score [see Box 3-2] ≥ 7 points = Marfan syndrome*
>   - "Where aortic root dilatation (Z ≥ 2) or dissection is present, but ectopia lentis is absent and the *FBN1* status is either unknown or negative, a Marfan syndrome diagnosis is confirmed by the presence of sufficient systemic findings (≥ 7 points, according to a scoring system). However, features suggestive of Shprintzen-Goldberg syndrome, Loeys-Dietz syndrome, or vascular Ehlers-Danlos syndrome must be excluded and appropriate alternative

warranted in young people with unexplained aortic dissection, as data from the International Registry of Acute Aortic Dissection have shown that MFS accounts for half of patients under age 40 with this condition (Januzzi et al., 2004). When diagnosed early, and with appropriate management, most people with classic MFS have a relatively normal life expectancy. However, many of the other findings in the condition (e.g., ectopia lentis, glaucoma, joint laxity, pes planus/planovalgus, scoliosis, acetabular protrusion, dural ectasia, and pulmonary complications) contribute to the risk of long-term disabling clinical issues, only some of which, such as ectopia lentis, can be reliably managed by medical and surgical intervention (Esfandiari et al., 2019).

> genetic testing (*TGFBR1/2,* collagen biochemistry, *COL3A1,* and other relevant genetic testing when indicated and available upon the discovery of other genes) should be performed" (Loeys et al., 2010, p. 478).
> 4. Ectopia lentis AND an *FBN1* mutation with known aortic root dilatation = Marfan syndrome
>   • "In the presence of ectopia lentis, but absence of aortic root dilatation/dissection, the identification of an *FBN1* mutation previously associated with aortic disease is required before making the diagnosis of Marfan syndrome" (Loeys et al., 2010, p. 478).
>
> In the presence of family history:
>
> 5. Ectopia lentis AND family history of Marfan syndrome (as defined above) = Marfan syndrome
> 6. A systemic score (≥ 7 points) AND family history of Marfan syndrome (as defined above) = Marfan syndrome*
> 7. Aortic root dilatation (Z score ≥ 2 above 20 yrs. old, ≥ 3 below 20 yrs. old) + family history of Marfan syndrome (as defined above) = Marfan syndrome*
>
> ---
>
> * Caveat: without discriminating features of Shprintzen-Goldberg syndrome, Loeys-Dietz syndrome or vascular Ehlers-Danlos syndrome AND after *TGFBR1/2,* collagen biochemistry, *COL3A1* testing if indicated. Other conditions/genes will emerge with time.
> SOURCE: Loeys et al., 2010. Adapted by permission from BMJ Publishing Group Limited. "The revised Ghent nosology for the Marfan syndrome," B. L. Loeys, H. C. Dietz, A. C. Braverman, B. L. Callewaert, J. De Backer, R. B. Devereux, Y. Hilhorst-Hofstee, G. Jondeau, L. Faivre, D. M. Milewicz, R. E. Pyeritz, P. D. Sponseller, P. Wordsworth, and A. M. De Paepe, 47(1), p. 477, 2010.

Epidemiology

MFS affects males and females with equal frequency, although overall severity may be somewhat greater in males (Roman et al., 2017). The true prevalence of MFS is unclear, but current estimates are 1 to 5 per 10,000 population (Judge and Dietz, 2005; NORD, 2021), with no gender, race, or ethnic origin preference (Chiu et al., 2014).

Given the wide range of organ systems potentially affected by MFS and the marked variability in expression of pathologic variants in *FBN1*, there is no "average age" of appearance of manifestations. In the most severe form of MFS (often termed "neonatal MFS"), severe ocular, skeletal, and cardiovascular features are present at birth, and life expectancy is markedly reduced, even with early and aggressive treatment. In less severe forms, some features (e.g., aortic dilatation, disproportionately tall stature) may

> **BOX 3-2**
> **Ghent II Criteria for Scoring of Systemic Features**
>
> Systemic features excluding aortic disease, ectopia lentis and family history for the diagnosis of Marfan syndrome
>
> - Wrist and thumb signs (3 points)
> - Wrist or thumb sign (1 point)
> - Anterior chest deformity (2 points)
> - Hind foot deformity (2 points)
> - Pneumothorax (2 points)
> - Dural ectasia (2 points)
> - Protrusio acetabuli (2 points)
> - Reduced upper segment [to] lower segment and increased arm span to height ratio (1 point)
> - Reduced elbow extension (1 point)
> - Facial features: dolichocephaly, enophthalmos, downslanting palpebral fissures, malar hypoplasia, and retrognathia (1 point if 3 out 5 features are present)
> - Skin striae other than due to pregnancy or obesity (1 point)
> - Myopia > 3 diopters (1 point)
> - Mitral valve prolapse (1 point)
>
> The total score of the systemic features is used in the diagnostic criteria.
>
> SOURCE: Excerpted from Milewicz et al., 2021, p. 8. Reprinted by permission from Springer Nature: Springer Nature, *Nature Reviews: Disease Primers*, "Marfan syndrome," M. D. Milewicz, A. C. Braverman, J. De Backer, S. A. Morris, C. Boileau, I. H. Maumenee, G. Jondeau, A. Evangelista, and R. E. Pyeritz, 2021.

be present in infancy and worsen with age, while others are not evident until childhood (e.g., ectopia lentis, scoliosis) or even adulthood (e.g., dural ectasia, weaking of the covering of the spinal root).

Manifestations

This section describes some of the physical and mental manifestations associated with MFS and how they may interfere with daily life. Chapter 5 contains additional information related to the physical and mental secondary impairments associated with and functional implications of MFS and related hereditary aortopathies (see Annex Tables 5-3–5-16 at the end of that chapter).

Cardiovascular features of MFS include aortic root aneurysm, aortic root dissection, mitral valve prolapse, premature calcification of the mitral annulus, and pulmonary artery dilation (Loeys et al., 2010; Stuart and Williams, 2007). Echocardiography findings demonstrate aortic root dilation in most pediatric MFS patients by the age of 19 and adult MFS patients (Aburawi and O'Sullivan, 2007). Aortic root dilation typically increases with age and is often accompanied by aortic regurgitation (Jeremy et al., 1994; Jondeau et al., 1999). Aortic pathology may lead to aneurysmal formation; dilation; and ultimately dissection, the primary cause of patient morbidity and mortality (Adams and Trent, 1998). Mitral valve prolapse with elongated leaflets also occurs frequently in patients with MFS, although it is considered a nonspecific finding given the frequent observation of mitral valve prolapse in the general population (Rybczynski et al., 2010). Associated mitral valve regurgitation may be present and progressive, sometimes leading to heart failure in children with the most severe presentation. Less commonly, patients may have cardiomyopathy unrelated to valvular disease (Alpendurada et al., 2010). The increased risk of aortic aneurysm and dissection limits many physical activities, in particular those that elevate heart rate or blood pressure and/or involve impact (Bitterman and Sponseller, 2017). Aortic or mitral regurgitation, if severe and untreated, may lead to chronic heart failure. Management of MFS requires lifestyle modifications, and it is recommended that physical activity be reduced to about 50 percent of capacity (Milewicz et al., 2021). Aortic root dilatation is more common in males than in females, whereas mitral valve prolapse is more common in females than in males (Roman et al., 2017).

Clinical musculoskeletal features in MFS typically include tall stature, disproportionately long limbs and digits, abnormal curvature of the spine (scoliosis), indentation or protrusion of the breast bone (pectus excavatum or carinatum, respectively), medial displacement of the head of the femur within the hip joint (protrusio acetabuli), unusual flexibility and/or restriction of joints, flat feet (pes planus/planovalgus), reduced elbow extension, and finger contractures (Bitterman and Sponseller, 2017). Musculoskeletal manifestations may contribute to pain and are likely to increase over time. Scoliosis and arachnodactyly are more prevalent in females than in males (Roman et al., 2017). Scoliosis can limit the ability to bend at the waist or chest. Joint laxity contributes to progressive degenerative arthritis, especially with repetitive bending or carrying under strain.

Ocular involvement is seen in the majority of MFS patients. Ectopia lentis is seen in 50–80 percent of patients; this condition is progressive, can impair vision, and often requires surgical intervention (Agarwal and Narang, 2014; Dietz, 2022; Sandvik et al., 2019). Other ophthalmologic abnormalities include amblyopia, strabismus (Izquierdo et al., 1994), myopia, increased globe length, and corneal flattening (Loeys et al., 2010). An elongated globe contributes to severe myopia and a risk of retinal detachment, which may lead to visual impairment or permanent blindness. Early cataract formation may also be observed (Dietz, 2022). In addition, the risk of developing glaucoma, a known complication of MFS, is significantly increased after surgical repair of retinal detachment (Tranos et al., 2004). High-impact activities can lead to lens displacement or dislocation (Bitterman and Sponseller, 2017).

Neurologic manifestations commonly include dural ectasia, an enlargement of the dural sac around the spinal cord, and spinal arachnoid cysts or diverticula (Meester et al., 2017). Severe dural ectasia and meningoceles can cause lower back and radicular pain and leg weakness, especially with prolonged standing and walking.

Other findings include facial manifestations (high arched palate, teeth crowding, flattening of the midface, small and receding lower jaw). Lung or pulmonary complications can result from chest wall abnormalities (pectus excavatum) that contribute to restrictive lung disease. Widening of the lung spaces can result in spontaneous pneumothorax that in turn can lead to cardiopulmonary instability (Huang et al., 2014). MFS patients may develop emphysematous changes in the airway as they age, with histologic evidence of pathology apparent in early or middle adulthood (Dyhdalo and Farver, 2011). Respiratory involvement may also cause sleep-disordered breathing in adults with MFS, ultimately contributing to mental impairment and disability (Sowho et al., 2020). Skin abnormalities include changes in the skin due to thinning of the underlying connective tissues, otherwise known as "stretch marks" (striae atrophicae).

Chronic pain is experienced by 47–92 percent of patients with MFS (Velvin et al., 2016a) and may significantly impair daily functioning. Participants in a study by Speed and colleagues (2017) reported poor physical and mental health functioning and moderate pain-related disability. And while 89 percent of respondents reported experiencing pain, 41 percent reported never receiving a pain diagnosis. Chronic fatigue is another common manifestation of MFS, frequently comorbid with chronic pain and orthostatic intolerance; MFS patients with versus those without chronic pain report higher levels of chronic fatigue (Bathen et al., 2014). Chronic fatigue may in turn result in impaired cognitive functioning. Chronic fatigue has been found to interfere with daily functioning and to be associated with less participation in the workforce, younger age at retirement, and increased likelihood of receiving disability benefits (Bathen et al., 2014; Velvin et al., 2015).

MFS affects many organ systems, in particular the cardiovascular, nervous, respiratory, musculoskeletal, and ocular systems, and can result in impairments in daily functioning. The chronic pain and chronic fatigue experienced by many MFS patients can affect work participation and education-related activities; Rao and colleagues (2016), for example, found that chronic fatigue was associated with reduced work capacity. Research has shown that children and adolescents with MFS may be unable to participate in many physical activities as a result of the physical manifestations of their disease, and these limitations can in turn affect their psychosocial functioning (Nielsen et al., 2019). Additional research on the relative benefits versus risks of participation in common childhood activities (e.g., contact sports, gymnastics, dance) would inform management of the disease in this area. Severe back and neck pain, in addition to frequent headaches, may result from a number of manifestations of MFS, also affecting physical and mental functioning (Nielsen et al., 2019). Common as well among those with MFS are cardiac problems; spine issues, including back pain; and generalized fatigue (Rao et al., 2016). MFS may also result in difficulties with executive function, particularly mental fatigue (Ratiu et al., 2018) and cognitive difficulties, that diminish quality of life and affect a patient's ability to work (Nielsen et al., 2019). Several studies of a Norwegian cohort of men and women with MFS have shown that both physical and mental impairments associated with the disease result in poorer quality of life that increases with age (Rand-Hendriksen et al., 2010; Vanem et al., 2020; Velvin et al., 2016b). MFS has been associated with less employment, younger age at retirement, more disability benefits (Velvin et al., 2015), and reduced work hours (Rao et al., 2016). Studies in other populations with MFS have also found increased pain, anxiety and depression, and reduced mobility compared with patients with other chronic conditions (Andonian et al., 2021).

Loeys-Dietz Syndrome

Clinical Picture

The clinical findings of LDS are similar to those of MFS, and these syndromes show a considerable degree of phenotypical overlap, particularly in cardiovascular, skeletal, and cutaneous findings. Overlapping features include cardiac complications, scoliosis, pes planus, anterior chest deformity, spontaneous pneumothorax, and dural ectasia (Meester et al., 2017).

There are, however, important differences between the two syndromes. Individuals with LDS can experience aortic dissection earlier in life and with smaller aortic diameters relative to those with MFS. Other cardiovascular manifestations seen in LDS but not in MFS include tortuous arteries in multiple anatomic locations (Loeys and Dietz, 2018). Certain craniofacial features of LDS (e.g., widely spaced eyes [hypertelorism] and cleft palate [bifid uvula]), as well as the absence of ectopia lentis, also distinguish it from MFS (Meester et al., 2017). Additionally, skeletal overgrowth is less pronounced and arachnodactyly less common with LDS than with MFS (Erkula et al., 2010).

Epidemiology

LDS occurs without regard to gender, race, or ethnic origin (Loeys and Dietz, 2018). Its true prevalence is unknown. As with MFS, the onset of secondary impairments associated with LDS can range from childhood (typically severe cases) to adulthood.

Manifestations

In addition to hypertelorism and bifid uvula, craniofacial features of LDS include strabismus and craniosynostosis. Craniosynostosis may involve any of the suture lines, but most often affects the sagittal suture, leading to dolicocephaly (long narrow-shaped head) (Loeys and Dietz, 2018). Other facial features include retrognathia (receding jaw), malar flattening (midface), tall and broad forehead, downsloping palpebral fissures, and frontal bossing with a high anterior hairline.

The vascular features of LDS include rapidly progressive aortic and peripheral arterial aneurysmal disease that can lead to dissection (Loeys and Dietz, 2018; Loughborough et al., 2018). Patients with LDS show diffuse arterial involvement, and a large proportion of patients develop aneurysms of the iliac, mesenteric, and intracranial arteries (Loughborough et al., 2018). Additionally, bicuspid aortic valve, atrial septal defect, and patent ductus arteriosus are observed more frequently in LDS than in the general population (MacCarrick et al., 2014).

Neurologic manifestations of LDS may include dural ectasia and Chiari malformation, as well as migraines, intracranial hypertension and hypotension, and spinal disorders (atlanto-occipital instability, atlanto-axial instability, basilar invagination, and instability/malformation of the cervical spine).

Skeletal features of LDS include an indented or protruding sternum, scoliosis, joint laxity, arachnodactyly, club foot (talipes equinovarus), and cervical spine malformation and/or instability (Loeys and Dietz, 2018). Cutaneous features of LDS include velvety and translucent skin, easy bruising, and dystrophic scars (Loeys and Dietz, 2018).

Other important manifestations of LDS include a high incidence of allergic or inflammatory diseases such as asthma, eczema, and food or environmental allergies (Frischmeyer-Guerrerio et al., 2013). Patients with LDS also show an increased predisposition to gastrointestinal inflammation, including eosinophilic esophagitis and gastritis or inflammatory bowel disease (Wang et al., 2021). In addition, the disease carries an increased risk of pregnancy complications (MacCarrick et al., 2014; Meester et al., 2017).

A study from Norway reports on a combined cohort of persons with vascular Ehlers-Danlos syndrome (vEDS) and LDS who responded to a questionnaire on physical function and psychosocial aspects of hereditary thoracic aortic disease (Johansen et al., 2020). The authors found that 21/34 respondents with LDS were receiving disability pensions, rehabilitation benefits, partial disability pensions, or were retired; 29/34 respondents reported chronic musculoskeletal pain. No associations were found between age or gender and chronic musculoskeletal pain in the combined cohort with LDS and vEDS. A score for the respondents' multi–organ system burden, including chronic musculoskeletal pain, neck instability, joint problems, scoliosis, vision problems, hearing problems, pneumothorax, hernia, rupture of internal organs, skin problems, allergies, and abdominal pain, was calculated based on a range from 0 (least burden) to 12 (greatest). The median score for LDS1 and 2 was 5, for LDS3 was 3.5, and for LDS4 was 6.

Congenital Contractural Arachnodactyly

Clinical Picture

The features of CCA often overlap with those of the other disorders discussed in this chapter. CCA is characterized by external ear anomalies, arachnodactyly, camptodactyly, contractures, muscle weakness, a high arched palate, and occasional cardiovascular complications (Callewaert et al., 2009).

Epidemiology

Inheritance is autosomal-dominant, and males and females are equally affected. The true prevalence of CCA is unknown (Callewaert, 2019), but its distinctive physical features often result in earlier diagnosis relative to other HDCTs. One study found the mean age of diagnosis to be 10.6 years (Callewaert et al., 2009).

Manifestations

The most prominent skeletal features of CCA are malformations of the hands and spine (Callewaert et al., 2009). Contractures of joints (typically elbows, fingers, and knees), elongated fingers and toes, external ear malformation, and protruding sternum are often detected at birth (Tunçbilek and Alanay, 2006). Contractures for individuals with CCA generally improve over time, while scoliosis and kyphosis are usually progressive (Callewaert et al., 2009), necessitating aggressive management.

Cardiovascular malformations have been identified with CCA, but with less frequency than with MFS and LDS (Callewaert et al., 2009). Aortic root dilation has been reported in as many as 10–15 percent of cases of CCA with fibrillin-2 (*FBN2*) pathogenic variants (Callewaert, 2019).

Shprintzen-Goldberg Syndrome

Clinical Picture

SGS shows considerable phenotypic overlap with MFS and LDS, but also manifests in developmental delays, mild to moderate intellectual disability, and severe skeletal muscle hypotonia (Greally, 2020). It is characterized by a marfanoid habitus; craniosynostosis; and skeletal, neurologic, and cardiovascular abnormalities (Doyle et al., 2012; Greally, 2020).

Epidemiology

Inheritance of SGS is autosomal-dominant, and males and females are equally affected, with no ethnic predisposition (NORD, 2017). Its prevalence is unknown (Greally, 2020).

Manifestations

This disorder is often recognized early in life (Adès et al., 1995). Clinical findings include marfanoid habitus, craniosynostosis, hydrocephalous, arachnodactyly, camptodactyly (bent fingers), undersized lower jaw, protruding eyes, abnormal external ears, indented or protruding sternum, scoliosis, mitral valve prolapse, occasional aortic root dilatation and aneurysms, occasional aneurysms beyond the aorta, multiple abdominal wall hernias, infantile hypotonia, intellectual disability, bone loss, decreased subcutaneous tissues, and obstructive sleep apnea (Greally, 2020; Loeys et al., 2005; Robinson et al., 2005).

TREATMENT AND MANAGEMENT

MFS and related hereditary aortopathies manifest in multiple body systems, and individuals with these disorders may experience a variety of secondary impairments that, individually or in combination, can cause functional limitations of varying severity. Appropriate management of the HDCTs and treatment of associated secondary impairments are important for managing functional limitations and reducing HDCT-related disability. This section addresses the management of MFS, LDS, CCA, and SGS. Chapter 5 addresses the relationship among secondary impairments associated with these disorders, their potential effects on function, and considerations relevant to Social Security Administration disability.

Management of MFS and related hereditary aortopathies involves specialists in numerous physical and mental health disciplines. For example, cardiologists and cardiovascular surgeons diagnose, monitor, and treat mitral valve prolapse and aortic root dilatation. Orthopedists monitor and manage the development of scoliosis, protrosio acetabuli, pes planus, and associated issues of joint hypermobility. If necessary, thoracic surgeons manage and treat deformity of the anterior chest wall, particularly if it causes chest pain or affects breathing. Ophthalmologists diagnose and manage ectopia lentis, myopia, and strabismus in childhood, and monitor adults for the development of cataracts, glaucoma, and retinal tears. Physical and occupational therapists can provide interventions to mediate impairments and functional limitations. Overall management should be coordinated by a medical geneticist or physician with knowledge of and experience with these disorders.

Marfan Syndrome

No curative treatment currently exists for MFS. Management of the disorder involves early recognition and aggressive monitoring and treatment of manifestations in multiple organ systems, treatment of associated secondary impairments present at the time of diagnosis, and measures to reduce or prevent problems that may occur with age. Management is lifelong (as summarized in Milewicz et al., 2021), including routine eye examinations and imaging of the aorta. Pharmacologic therapies and prophylactic surgeries can prevent aortic dissections. Skeletal complications should be treated as they arise (Milewicz et al., 2021). Conservative treatment of musculoskeletal manifestations is preferred whenever possible because of higher complication rates following surgical intervention among persons with MFS relative to the general population (Bitterman and Sponseller, 2017). An important component of lifelong management is genetic counseling, as there is about a 50 percent chance of transmitting the pathologic *FBN1* variant to offspring with each pregnancy.

The types of treatment necessary for a given patient vary widely based on the severity of the disease complications and the age at which they present. Severe, progressive scoliosis, for example, requires early and aggressive bracing, as well as careful clinical and radiologic monitoring during childhood and adolescence and when necessary, surgical stabilization of the vertebral column to prevent progression (Bitterman and Sponseller, 2017).

The most life-threatening complication of MFS is dilatation of the ascending aorta, which predisposes to aortic dissection. Monitoring of the diameter of the ascending aorta, typically with echocardiography, should be initiated as soon as the diagnosis of MFS is established; the frequency of monitoring depends on the severity and pace of progression of enlargement.

Prophylactic treatment with beta-adrenergic blockade, angiotensin receptor blockade, or both should be considered as soon as the diagnosis of MFS is made. Once the aortic diameter has reached a certain size (typically 45–50 mm in an adult), prophylactic aortic root replacement is recommended (Hiratzka et al., 2010; Hoskoppal et al., 2018).

Management of patients with MFS changes over time, as many features associated with the disease worsen or become apparent only with aging. Some manifestations (e.g., sleep apnea, central obesity, dural ectasia) do not appear or cause problems until adulthood. Some features become apparent only because life expectancy for persons with MFS has been increasing as a result of effective management of cardiovascular complications (Pyeritz, 2019).

Loeys-Dietz Syndrome

The management of LDS and other hereditary aortopathies is similar to that of MFS. The more aggressive nature of aortic root dilatation and dissection in LDS warrants close monitoring, and surgery is recommended at an earlier stage of aortic dilation because of the increased likelihood of catastrophic events. Unlike management of MFS, management of LDS includes diagnostic or baseline vascular imaging with magnetic resonance angiography or computed tomography angiography of the head, neck, chest, abdomen, and pelvis to assess for aneurysms throughout the aorta and arterial tree and to look for arterial tortuosity (MacCarrick et al., 2014). Some individuals with an abdominal aortic aneurysm may require surgery before root replacement, underscoring the need for whole-body surveillance (Beaulieu, et al., 2017). Since LDS patients have a strong predisposition toward allergic and inflammatory diseases, appropriate management of those conditions should be included in care plans for these patients. Cutaneous findings in LDS are more severe than those seen in MFS, and wound healing can be delayed, with atrophic scars resulting.

Congenital Contractural Arachnodactyly

During childhood, spinal deformity resulting from CCA should be followed closely by physical examination and radiography. If it is severe or progressive, an orthopedist with special expertise in abnormal spinal curvature should be consulted. Bracing should be considered, as should surgery if bracing is ineffective. Because of the increased incidence of aortic root dilatation with CCA, periodic echocardiography is recommended.

Shprintzen-Goldberg Syndrome

Management of SGS is currently limited to symptom treatment. Patients should be monitored with echocardiograms and bone scans. Treatments include surgical repairs as necessary for the cardiovascular and skeletal systems. Medications may be considered if the patient shows abnormal aortic growth. Patients should be assessed and receive early intervention for developmental delays, and may need occupational, physical, and speech therapy. Because of the severe muscle hypotonia associated with SGS, bracing of the feet and spine may be necessary to help with ambulation. A feeding tube may be required for adequate nutrition. Continuous positive airway pressure is recommended for obstructive sleep apnea. Individuals with SGS may also need to avoid contact sports and other activities that stress their cardiovascular system or may result in injury or pain in their joints (Greally, 2020).

EMERGING TREATMENTS

Better medications to protect the aorta remain an important and ongoing goal of research in MFS and related hereditary aortopathies; at present, beta blockers and angiotensin-converting enzyme blockage remain the mainstay of treatment. Surgical approaches to repair aortic aneurysms are highly effective, but aortic dissection remains a difficult problem to treat. Efforts are under way to develop noninvasive methods for assessing the strength of the enlarged aorta to identify those patients most at risk of dissection (Baliga et al., 2014). ClinicalTrials.gov (NLM, 2022) is a database of more than 400,000 clinical trials being conducted in the 50 U.S. states and 220 other countries and territories. As of May 2022, more than 20 clinical trials related to MFS, 5 trials related to LDS, and 1 trial related to CCA were either recruiting, actively ongoing, or completed.

FINDINGS AND CONCLUSIONS

Findings

3-1. Marfan syndrome (MFS), Loeys-Dietz syndrome (LDS), congenital contractural arachnodactyly (CCA; also known as Beals-Hecht syndrome), and Shprintzen-Goldberg syndrome (SGS) affect multiple body systems, often with cardiovascular, skeletal, and ocular manifestations.
3-2. Diagnosis of MFS, LDS, CCA, and SGS is based on established clinical criteria and can be confirmed through genetic testing.

3-3. Many manifestations of hereditary aortopathies worsen over time, with some not appearing until adulthood.

3-4. No curative treatments currently exist for MFS, LDS, CCA, SGS, or other hereditary aortopathies. Management of these disorders involves early diagnosis and aggressive monitoring and treatment of manifestations in multiple organ systems, including treatment of associated physical and mental secondary impairments present at the time of identification and measures to reduce or prevent problems that may occur with age.

3-5. Management of MFS and related hereditary aortopathies is lifelong and involves specialists across multiple physical and mental health disciplines.

3-6. As the life spans of patients with these syndromes increase with improvements in management of previously fatal complications (e.g., aortic rupture, spontaneous pneumothorax), concurrent increases are seen in the occurrence and severity of age-related secondary impairments.

3-7. Hereditary aortopathies can affect individuals' everyday physical and mental functioning, often impacting multiple body systems. MFS frequently manifests in cardiovascular, nervous, respiratory, musculoskeletal, and ocular system impairments. LDS and CCA manifest particularly in cardiovascular, cerebrovascular, respiratory, musculoskeletal, craniofacial, ocular, and neurological impairments. SGS manifests in developmental delays and intellectual disability, as well as impairments associated with the other hereditary aortopathies.

3-8. Pregnancy can be a high-risk condition in some individuals with hereditary aortopathies.

Conclusions

3-1. MFS and related hereditary aortopathies have multiple physical and mental manifestations that, individually or in combination, can cause functional limitations of varying severity. Some manifestations may become apparent only with age, and the severity of manifestations may, and often does, progress with age. Treatment can be successful in reducing impairments in selected cases.

3-2. Management of MFS and related hereditary aortopathies requires a multidisciplinary approach and involves early diagnosis of the multisystem findings associated with these syndromes, treatment of associated physical and mental secondary impairments, and measures to reduce or prevent problems that may present with aging.

REFERENCES

Aburawi, E. H., and J. O'Sullivan. 2007. Relation of aortic root dilatation and age in Marfan's syndrome. *European Heart Journal* 28(3):376-379. https://doi.org/10.1093/eurheartj/ehl457.

Adams, J. N., and R. J. Trent. 1998. Aortic complications of Marfan's syndrome. *Lancet* 352(9142):1722-1723. https://doi.org/10.1016/s0140-6736(05)79822-6.

Adès, L. C., L. L. Morris, R. G. Power, M. Wilson, E. A. Haan, J. F. Bateman, D. M. Milewicz, and D. O. Sillence. 1995. Distinct skeletal abnormalities in four girls with Shprintzen-Goldberg syndrome. *American Journal of Medical Genetics* 57(4):565-572. https://doi.org/10.1002/ajmg.1320570410.

Alpendurada, F., J. Wong, A. Kiotsekoglou, W. Banya, A. Child, S. K. Prasad, D. J. Pennell, and R. H. Mohiaddin. 2010. Evidence for Marfan cardiomyopathy. *European Journal of Heart Failure* 12(10):1085-1091. https://doi.org/10.1093/eurjhf/hfq127.

Agarwal, A., and P. Narang. 2014. Ectopia lentis a major ocular manifestion of Marfan syndrome. *Ocular Surgey News* (September 10). https://www.healio.com/news/ophthalmology/20140910/ectopia-lentis-a-major-ocular-manifestation-of-marfan-syndrome (accessed May 5, 2022).

Andonian, C., S. Freilinger, S. Achenbach, P. Ewert, U. Gundlach, H. Kaemmerer, N. Nagdyman, R. C. Neidenbach, L. Pieper, J. Schelling, M. Weyand, and J. Beckmann. 2021. Quality of life in patients with Marfan syndrome: A cross-sectional study of 102 adult patients. *Cardiovascular Diagnosis and Therapy* 11(2):602-610. https://cdt.amegroups.com/article/view/63061.

Baliga, R. R., C. A. Nienaber, E. Bossone, J. K. Oh, E. M. Isselbacher, U. Sechtem, R. Fattori, S. V. Raman, and K. A. Eagle. 2014. The role of imaging in aortic dissection and related syndromes. *Journal of Cardiovascular Imaging* 7(4):406-424. https://doi.org/10.1016/j.jcmg.2013.10.015.

Bathen, T., G. Velvin, S. Rand-Hendriksen, and H. S. Robinson. 2014. Fatigue in adults with Marfan syndrome, occurrence and associations to pain and other factors. *American Journal of Medical Genetics Part A* 164(8):1931-1939. https://doi.org/10.1002/ajmg.a.36574.

Bertoli-Avella, A. M., E. Gillis, H. Morisaki, J. M. A. Verhagen, B. M. de Graaf, G. van de Beek, E. Gallo, B. P. T. Kruithof, H. Venselaar, L. A. Myers, S. Laga, A. J. Doyle, G. Oswald, G. W. A. van Cappellen, I. Yamanaka, R. M. van der Helm, B. Beverloo, A. de Klein, L. Pardo, M. Lammens, C. Evers, K. Devriendt, M. Dumoulein, J. Timmermans, H. T. Bruggenwirth, F. Verheijen, I. Rodrigus, G. Baynam, M. Kempers, J. Saenen, E. M. Van Craenenbroeck, K. Minatoya, R. Matsukawa, T. Tsukube, N. Kubo, R. Hofstra, M. J. Goumans, J. A. Bekkers, J. W. Roos-Hesselink, I. M. B. H. van de Laar, H. C. Dietz, L. Van Laer, T. Morisaki, M. W. Wessels, and B. L. Loeys. 2015. Mutations in a TGF-β ligand, *TGFB3*, cause syndromic aortic aneurysms and dissections. *Journal of the American College of Cardiology* 65(13):1324-1336. https://doi.org/10.1016/j.jacc.2015.01.040.

Beaulieu R. J., J. Lue, B. A. Ehlert, J. C. Grimm, C. W. Hicks, and J. H. Black III. 2017. Surgical management of peripheral vascular manifestations of Loeys-Dietz syndrome. *Annals of Vascular Surgery* 38:10-16. https://doi.org/10.1016/j.avsg.2016.06.007.

Bitterman, A. D., and P. D. Sponseller. 2017. Marfan syndrome: A clinical update. *Journal of the American Academy of Orthopaedic Surgeons* 25(9):603-609. https://doi.org/10.5435/jaaos-d-16-00143.

Bruno, L., S. Tredici, M. Mangiavacchi, V. Colombo, G. F. Mazzotta, and C. R. Sirtori. 1984. Cardiac, skeletal, and ocular abnormalities in patients with Marfan's syndrome and in their relatives. Comparison with the cardiac abnormalities in patients with kyphoscoliosis. *British Heart Journal* 51(2):220-230. https://doi.org/10.1136/hrt.51.2.220.

Callewaert, B. 2019. Congenital contractural arachnodactyly. In *GeneReviews® [Internet]*, edited by M. P. Adam, H. H. Ardinger, R. A. Pagon, S. E. Wallace, L. J. H. Bean, K. W. Gripp, G. M. Mirzaa, and A. Amemiya. Seattle, WA: University of Washington; 1993-2022. https://www.ncbi.nlm.nih.gov/books/NBK1386/?report=classic.

Callewaert, B. L., B. L. Loeys, A. Ficcadenti, S. Vermeer, M. Landgren, H. Y. Kroes, Y. Yaron, M. Pope, N. Foulds, O. Boute, F. Galán, H. Kingston, N. Van der Aa, I. Salcedo, M. E. Swinkels, C. Wallgren-Pettersson, O. Gabrielli, J. De Backer, P. J. Coucke, and A. M. De Paepe. 2009. Comprehensive clinical and molecular assessment of 32 probands with congenital contractural arachnodactyly: Report of 14 novel mutations and review of the literature. *Human Mutation* 30(3):334-341. https://doi.org/10.1002/humu.20854.

Chiu, H. H., M. H. Wu, H. C. Chen, F. Y. Kao, and S. K. Huang. 2014. Epidemiological profile of Marfan syndrome in a general population: A national database study. *Mayo Clinic Proceedings* 89(1):34-42. https://doi.org/10.1016/j.mayocp.2013.08.022.

Dietz, H. C. 2022. *FBN1*-related Marfan syndrome. In *GeneReviews® [Internet]*, edited by M. P. Adam, H. H. Ardinger, R. A. Pagon, S. E. Wallace, L. J. H. Bean, K. W. Gripp, G. M. Mirzaa and A. Amemiya. Seattle, WA: University of Washington; 1993-2022. https://www.ncbi.nlm.nih.gov/books/NBK1335.

Dietz, H. C., C. R. Cutting, R. E. Pyeritz, C. L. Maslen, L. Y. Sakai, G. M. Corson, E. G. Puffenberger, A. Hamosh, E. J. Nanthakumar, S. M. Curristin, G. Stetten, D. A. Meyers, and C. A. Francomano. 1991. Marfan syndrome caused by a recurrent *de novo* missense mutation in the fibrillin gene. *Nature* 352(6333):337-339. https://doi.org/10.1038/352337a0.

Doyle, A. J., J. J. Doyle, S. L. Bessling, S. Maragh, M. E. Lindsay, D. Schepers, E. Gillis, G. Mortier, T. Homfray, K. Sauls, R. A. Norris, N. D. Huso, D. Leahy, D. W. Mohr, M. J. Caulfield, A. F. Scott, A. Destrée, R. C. Hennekam, P. H. Arn, C. J. Curry, L. Van Laer, A. S. McCallion, B. L. Loeys, and H. C. Dietz. 2012. Mutations in the TGF-β repressor *SKI* cause Shprintzen-Goldberg syndrome with aortic aneurysm. *Nature Genetics* 44(11):1249-1254. https://doi.org/10.1038/ng.2421.

Dyhdalo, K., and C. Farver. 2011. Pulmonary histologic changes in Marfan syndrome: A case series and literature review. *American Journal of Clinical Pathology* 136(6):857-863. https://doi.org/10.1309/ajcp79sndhgkqfin.

Erkula, G., P. D. Sponseller, L. C. Paulsen, G. L. Oswald, B. L. Loeys, and H. C. Dietz. 2010. Musculoskeletal findings of Loeys-Dietz syndrome. *Journal of Bone and Joint Surgery (American Volume)* 92(9):1876-1883. https://doi.org/10.2106/jbjs.I.01140.

Esfandiari, H., S. Ansari, H. Mohammad-Rabei, and M. B. Mets. 2019. Management strategies of ocular abnormalities in patients with Marfan syndrome: Current perspective. *Journal of Ophthalmic & Vision Research* 14(1):71-77. https://www.ncbi.nlm.nih.gov/pmc/articles/PMC6388525/.

Frischmeyer-Guerrerio, P. A., A. L. Guerrerio, G. Oswald, K. Chichester, L. Myers, M. K. Halushka, M. Oliva-Hemker, R. A. Wood, and H. C. Dietz. 2013. TGFβ receptor mutations impose a strong predisposition for human allergic disease. *Science Translational Medicine* 5(195):195ra194. https://doi.org/10.1126/scitranslmed.3006448.

Greally, M. T. 2020. Shprintzen-Goldberg syndrome. In *GeneReviews® [Internet]*, edited by M. P. Adam, H. H. Ardinger, R. A. Pagon, S. E. Wallace, L. J. Bean, K. W. Gripp, G. M. Mirzaa, and A. Amemiya. Seattle, WA: University of Washington; 1993-2022. https://www.ncbi.nlm.nih.gov/books/NBK1277/.

Groth, K. A., H. Hove, K. Kyhl, L. Folkestad, M. Gaustadnes, N. Vejlstrup, K. Stochholm, J. R. Østergaard, N. H. Andersen, and C. H. Gravholt. 2015. Prevalence, incidence, and age at diagnosis in Marfan syndrome. *Orphanet Journal of Rare Diseases* 10(1):153. https://doi.org/10.1186/s13023-015-0369-8.

Gupta, P. A., E. A. Putnam, S. G. Carmical, I. Kaitila, B. Steinmann, A. Child, C. Danesino, K. Metcalfe, S. A. Berry, E. Chen, C. V. Delorme, M. K. Thong, L. C. Adès, and D. M. Milewicz. 2002. Ten novel FBN2 mutations in congenital contractural arachnodactyly: Delineation of the molecular pathogenesis and clinical phenotype. *Human Mutation* 19(1):39-48. https://doi.org/10.1002/humu.10017.

Hiratzka L. F., G. L. Bakris, J. A. Beckman, R. M. Bersin, V. F. Carr, D. E. Casey Jr, K. A. Eagle, L. K. Hermann, E. M. Isselbacher, E. A. Kazerooni, N. T. Kouchoukos, B. W. Lytle, D. M. Milewicz, D. L. Reich, S. Sen, J. A. Shinn, L. G. Svensson, and D. M. Williams, 2010. ACCF/AHA/AATS/ACR/ASA/SCA/SCAI/SIR/STS/SVM guidelines for the diagnosis and management of patients with thoracic aortic disease: A report of the American College of Cardiology Foundation/American Heart Association Task Force on Practice Guidelines, American Association for Thoracic Surgery, American College of Radiology, American Stroke Association, Society of Cardiovascular Anesthesiologists, Society for Cardiovascular Angiography and Interventions, Society of Interventional Radiology, Society of Thoracic Surgeons, and Society for Vascular Medicine. *Circulation* 121(13):e266-e369. https://doi.org/10.1161/CIR.0b013e3181d4739e.

Hoskoppal, A., S. Menon, F. Trachtenberg, K. M. Burns, J. De Backer, B. D. Gelb, M. Gleason, J. James, W. W. Lai, A. Liou, L. Mahony, A. K. Olson, R. E. Pyeritz, A. M. Sharkey, M. Stylianou, S. B. Wechsler, L. Young, J. C. Levine, E. S. S. Tierney, R. V. Lacro, and T. J. Bradley, on behalf of Pediatric Heart Network Investigators. 2018. Predictors of rapid aortic root dilation and referral for aortic surgery in Marfan syndrome. *Pediatric Cardiology* 39(7):1453-1461. https://doi.org/10.1007/s00246-018-1916-6.

Huang, Y., H. Huang, Q. Li, R. F. Browning, S. Parrish, J. F. Turner, Jr., K. Zarogoulidis, I. Kougioumtzi, G. Dryllis, I. Kioumis, G. Pitsiou, N. Machairiotis, N. Katsikogiannis, N. Courcoutsakis, A. Madesis, K. Diplaris, T. Karaiskos, and P. Zarogoulidis. 2014. Approach of the treatment for pneumothorax. *Journal of Thoracic Disease* 6(Suppl 4):S416-S420. https://doi.org/10.3978/j.issn.2072-1439.2014.08.24.

Izquierdo, N. J., E. I. Traboulsi, C. Enger, and I. H. Maumenee. 1994. Strabismus in the Marfan syndrome. *American Journal of Ophthalmology* 117(5):632-635. https://doi.org/10.1016/S0002-9394(14)70069-8.

Januzzi, J. L., E. M. Isselbacher, R. Fattori, J. V. Cooper, D. E. Smith, J. Fang, K. A. Eagle, R. H. Mehta, C. A. Nienaber, and L. A. Pape. 2004. Characterizing the young patient with aortic dissection: Results from the International Registry of Aortic Dissection (IRAD). *Journal of the American College of Cardiology* 43(4):665-669. https://doi.org/10.1016/j.jacc.2003.08.054.

Jeremy, R. W., H. Huang, J. Hwa, H. McCarron, C. F. Hughes, and J. G. Richards. 1994. Relation between age, arterial distensibility, and aortic dilatation in the Marfan syndrome. *American Journal of Cardiology* 74(4):369-373. https://doi.org/10.1016/0002-9149(94)90405-7.

Johansen, H., G. Velvin, and I. Lidal. 2020. Adults with Loeys–Dietz syndrome and vascular Ehlers–Danlos syndrome: A cross-sectional study of health burden perspectives. *American Journal of Medical Genetics Part A* 182(1):137-145. https://doi.org/10.1002/ajmg.a.61396.

Jondeau, G., P. Boutouyrie, P. Lacolley, B. Laloux, O. Dubourg, J.-P. Bourdarias, and S. Laurent. 1999. Central pulse pressure is a major determinant of ascending aorta dilation in Marfan syndrome. *Circulation* 99(20):2677-2681. https://doi.org/10.1161/01.CIR.99.20.2677.

Judge, D. P., and H. C. Dietz. 2005. Marfan's syndrome. *Lancet* 366(9501):1965-1976. https://doi.org/10.1016/s0140-6736(05)67789-6.

Lee, B., M. Godfrey, E. Vitale, H. Hori, M.-G. Mattei, M. Sarfarazi, P. Tsipouras, F. Ramirez, and D. W. Hollister. 1991. Linkage of Marfan syndrome and a phenotypically related disorder to two different fibrillin genes. *Nature* 352(6333):330-334. https://doi.org/10.1038/352330a0.

Lindsay, M. E., D. Schepers, N. A. Bolar, J. J. Doyle, E. Gallo, J. Fert-Bober, M. J. Kempers, E. K. Fishman, Y. Chen, L. Myers, D. Bjeda, G. Oswald, A. F. Elias, H. P. Levy, B. M. Anderlid, M. H. Yang, E. M. Bongers, J. Timmermans, A. C. Braverman, N. Canham, G. R. Mortier, H. G. Brunner, P. H. Byers, J. Van Eyk, L. Van Laer, H. C. Dietz, and B. L. Loeys. 2012. Loss-of-function mutations in *TGFB2* cause a syndromic presentation of thoracic aortic aneurysm. *Nature Genetics* 44(8):922-927. https://doi.org/10.1038/ng.2349.

Loeys, B. L., J. Chen, E. R. Neptune, D. P. Judge, M. Podowski, T. Holm, J. Meyers, C. C. Leitch, N. Katsanis, N. Sharifi, F. L. Xu, L. A. Myers, P. J. Spevak, D. E. Cameron, J. De Backer, J. Hellemans, Y. Chen, E. C. Davis, C. L. Webb, W. Kress, P. Coucke, D. B. Rifkin, A. M. De Paepe, and H. C. Dietz. 2005. A syndrome of altered cardiovascular, craniofacial, neurocognitive and skeletal development caused by mutations in *TGFBR1* or *TGFBR2*. *Nature Genetics* 37(3):275-281. https://doi.org/10.1038/ng1511.

Loeys, B. L., H. C. Dietz, A. C. Braverman, B. L. Callewaert, J. De Backer, R. B. Devereux, Y. Hilhorst-Hofstee, G. Jondeau, L. Faivre, D. M. Milewicz, R. E. Pyeritz, P. D. Sponseller, P. Wordsworth, and A. M. De Paepe. 2010. The revised Ghent nosology for the Marfan syndrome. *Journal of Medical Genetics* 47(7):476-485. https://doi.org/10.1136/jmg.2009.072785.

Loughborough, W. W., K. S. Minhas, J. C. L. Rodrigues, S. M. Lyen, H. E. Burt, N. E. Manghat, M. J. Brooks, G. Stuart, and M. C. K. Hamilton. 2018. Cardiovascular manifestations and complications of Loeys-Dietz syndrome: CT and MR imaging findings. *Radiographics* 38(1):275-286. https://doi.org/10.1148/rg.2018170120.

MacCarrick, G., J. H. Black, 3rd, S. Bowdin, I. El-Hamamsy, P. A. Frischmeyer-Guerrerio, A. L. Guerrerio, P. D. Sponseller, B. Loeys, and H. C. Dietz, 3rd. 2014. Loeys-Dietz syndrome: A primer for diagnosis and management. *Genetics in Medicine* 16(8):576-587. https://doi.org/10.1038/gim.2014.11.

Matyas, G., P. Naef, M. Tollens, and K. Oexle. 2014. De novo mutation of the latency-associated peptide domain of *TGFB3* in a patient with overgrowth and Loeys-Dietz syndrome features. *American Journal of Medical Genetics Part A* 164a(8):2141-2143. https://doi.org/10.1002/ajmg.a.36593.

Meester, J. A. N., A. Verstraeten, D. Schepers, M. Alaerts, L. Van Laer, and B. L. Loeys. 2017. Differences in manifestations of Marfan syndrome, Ehlers-Danlos syndrome, and Loeys-Dietz syndrome. *Annals of Cardiothoracic Surgery* 6(6):582-594. https://doi.org/10.21037/acs.2017.11.03.

Milewicz, D. M., A. C. Braverman, J. De Backer, S. A. Morris, C. Boileau, I. H. Maumenee, G. Jondeau, A. Evangelista, and R. E. Pyeritz. 2021. Marfan syndrome. *Nature Reviews: Disease Primers* 7(1):64. https://doi.org/10.1038/s41572-021-00298-7.

Nielsen, C., I. Ratiu, M. Esfandiarei, A. Chen, and E. S. Selamet Tierney. 2019. A review of psychosocial factors of Marfan syndrome: Adolescents, adults, families, and providers. *Journal of Pediatric Genetics* 08(03):109-122. https://doi.org/10.1055/s-0039-1693663.

NLM (U.S. National Library of Medicine). 2022. *Clinicaltrails.gov*. https://clinicaltrials.gov/ (accessed February 11, 2022).

NORD (National Organization for Rare Disorders). 2017. *Rare disease database: Shprintzen Goldberg syndrome*. https://rarediseases.org/rare-diseases/marfan-syndrome/ (accessed May 11, 2022).

NORD. 2021. *Rare disease database: Marfan syndrome*. https://rarediseases.org/rare-diseases/marfan-syndrome/ (accessed February 9, 2022).

Pyeritz, R. E. 2019. Marfan syndrome: Improved clinical history results in expanded natural history. *Genetics in Medicine* 21(8):1683-1690. https://doi.org/10.1038/s41436-018-0399-4.

Rand-Hendriksen, S., H. Johansen, S. O. Semb, O. Geiran, J. K. Stanghelle, and A. Finset. 2010. Health-related quality of life in Marfan syndrome: A cross-sectional study of short form 36 in 84 adults with a verified diagnosis. *Genetics in Medicine* 12(8):517-524. https://doi.org/10.1097/GIM.0b013e3181ea4c1c.

Rao, S. S., K. D. Venuti, H. C. Dietz, 3rd, and P. D. Sponseller. 2016. Quantifying health status and function in Marfan syndrome. *Journal of Surgical Orthopaedic Advances* 25(1):34-40.

Ratiu, I., T. B. Virden, H. Baylow, M. Flint, and M. Esfandiarei. 2018. Executive function and quality of life in individuals with Marfan syndrome. *Quality of Life Research* 27(8):2057-2065. https://doi.org/10.1007/s11136-018-1859-7.

Regalado, E. S., D. C. Guo, C. Villamizar, N. Avidan, D. Gilchrist, B. McGillivray, L. Clarke, F. Bernier, R. L. Santos-Cortez, S. M. Leal, A. M. Bertoli-Avella, J. Shendure, M. J. Rieder, D. A. Nickerson, and D. M. Milewicz. 2011. Exome sequencing identifies *SMAD3* mutations as a cause of familial thoracic aortic aneurysm and dissection with intracranial and other arterial aneurysms. *Circulation Research* 109(6):680-686. https://doi.org/10.1161/circresaha.111.248161.

Rienhoff, H. Y., Jr., C. Y. Yeo, R. Morissette, I. Khrebtukova, J. Melnick, S. Luo, N. Leng, Y. J. Kim, G. Schroth, J. Westwick, H. Vogel, N. McDonnell, J. G. Hall, and M. Whitman. 2013. A mutation in *TGFB3* associated with a syndrome of low muscle mass, growth retardation, distal arthrogryposis and clinical features overlapping with Marfan and Loeys-Dietz syndrome. *American Journal of Medical Genetics Part A* 161a(8):2040-2046. https://doi.org/10.1002/ajmg.a.36086.

Robinson, P. N., L. M. Neumann, S. Demuth, H. Enders, U. Jung, R. König, B. Mitulla, D. Müller, P. Muschke, L. Pfeiffer, B. Prager, M. Somer, and S. Tinschert. 2005. Shprintzen-Goldberg syndrome: Fourteen new patients and a clinical analysis. *American Journal of Medical Genetics Part A* 135(3):251-262. https://doi.org/10.1002/ajmg.a.30431.

Roman, M. J., R. B. Devereux, L. R. Preiss, F. M. Asch, K. A. Eagle, K. W. Holmes, S. A. LeMaire, C. L. Maslen, D. M. Milewicz, S. A. Morris, S. K. Prakash, R. E. Pyeritz, W. J. Ravekes, R. V. Shohet, H. K. Song, and J. W. Weinsaft. 2017. Associations of age and sex with Marfan phenotype: The National Heart, Lung, and Blood Institute GenTAC (Genetically Triggered Thoracic Aortic Aneurysms and Cardiovascular Conditions) Registry. *Circulation: Cardiovascular Genetics* 10(3). https://doi.org/10.1161/circgenetics.116.001647.

Rybczynski, M., T. S. Mir, S. Sheikhzadeh, A. M. Bernhardt, C. Schad, H. Treede, S. Veldhoen, E. F. Groene, K. Kühne, D. Koschyk, P. N. Robinson, J. Berger, H. Reichenspurner, T. Meinertz, and Y. von Kodolitsch. 2010. Frequency and age-related course of mitral valve dysfunction in the Marfan syndrome. *American Journal of Cardiology* 106(7):1048-1053. https://doi.org/10.1016/j.amjcard.2010.05.038.

Sandvik, G. F., T. T. Vanem, S. Rand-Hendriksen, S. Cholidis, M. Sæthre, and L. Drolsum. 2019. Ten-year reinvestigation of ocular manifestations in Marfan syndrome. *Clinical & Experimental Ophthalmology* 47(2):212-218. https://doi.org/10.1111/ceo.13408.

Sowho, M. O., S. Patil, H. Schneider, G. MacCarrick, J. P. Kirkness, L. F. Wolfe, L. Sterni, P. A. Cistulli, and E. R. Neptune. 2020. Sleep disordered breathing in Marfan syndrome: Value of standard screening questionnaires. *Molecular Genetics & Genomic Medicine* 8(1):e1039. https://doi.org/10.1002/mgg3.1039.

Speed, T. J., V. A. Mathur, M. Hand, B. Christensen, P. D. Sponseller, K. A. Williams, and C. M. Campbell. 2017. Characterization of pain, disability, and psychological burden in Marfan syndrome. *American Journal of Medical Genetics Part A* 173(2):315-323. https://doi.org/10.1002/ajmg.a.38051.

Stuart, A. G., and A. Williams. 2007. Marfan's syndrome and the heart. *Archives of Disease in Childhood* 92(4):351-356. https://doi.org/10.1136/adc.2006.097469.

Takeda, N., H. Morita, D. Fujita, R. Inuzuka, Y. Taniguchi, Y. Imai, Y. Hirata, and I. Komuro. 2015. Congenital contractural arachnodactyly complicated with aortic dilatation and dissection: Case report and review of literature. *American Journal of Medical Genetics Part A* 167a(10):2382-2387. https://doi.org/10.1002/ajmg.a.37162.

Tan, E. W., R. U. Offoha, G. L. Oswald, R. L. Skolasky, A. K. Dewan, G. Zhen, J. R. Shapiro, H. C. Dietz, X. Cao, and P. D. Sponseller. 2013. Increased fracture risk and low bone mineral density in patients with Loeys-Dietz syndrome. *American Journal of Medical Genetics Part A* 161a(8):1910-1914. https://doi.org/10.1002/ajmg.a.36029.

Tranos, P., R. Asaria, W. Aylward, P. Sullivan, and W. Franks. 2004. Long term outcome of secondary glaucoma following vitreoretinal surgery. *British Journal of Ophthalmology* 88(3):341. https://doi.org/10.1136/bjo.2003.028076.

Tunçbilek, E., and Y. Alanay. 2006. Congenital contractural arachnodactyly (Beals syndrome). *Orphanet Journal of Rare Diseases* 1(1):20. https://doi.org/10.1186/1750-1172-1-20.

Van Hemelrijk, C., M. Renard, and B. Loeys. 2010. The Loeys-Dietz syndrome: An update for the clinician. *Current Opinion in Cardiology* 25(6):546-551. https://doi.org/10.1097/HCO.0b013e32833f0220.

Vanem, T. T., S. Rand-Hendriksen, C. Brunborg, O. R. Geiran, and C. Røe. 2020. Health-related quality of life in Marfan syndrome: A 10-year follow-up. *Health and Quality of Life Outcomes* 18(1):376. https://doi.org/10.1186/s12955-020-01633-4.

Velvin, G., T. Bathen, S. Rand-Hendriksen, and A. Ø. Geirdal. 2015. Work participation in adults with Marfan syndrome: Demographic characteristics, MFS related health symptoms, chronic pain, and fatigue. *American Journal of Medical Genetics Part A* 167(12):3082-3090. https://doi.org/10.1002/ajmg.a.37370.

Velvin, G., T. Bathen, S. Rand-Hendriksen, and A. Geirdal. 2016a. Systematic review of chronic pain in persons with Marfan syndrome. *Clinical Genetics* 89(6):647-658. https://doi.org/10.1111/cge.12699.

Velvin, G., T. Bathen, S. Rand-Hendriksen, and A. Ø. Geirdal. 2016b. Satisfaction with life in adults with Marfan syndrome (MFS): Associations with health-related consequences of MFS, pain, fatigue, and demographic factors. *Quality of Life Research* 25(7):1779-1790. https://doi.org/10.1007/s11136-015-1214-1.

Wang, X. J., M. Babameto, D. Babovic-Vuksanovic, J. M. Bowen, and M. Camilleri. 2021. Audit of gastrointestinal manifestations in patients with Loeys-Dietz syndrome and vascular Ehlers-Danlos syndrome. *Digestive Diseases and Sciences* 66(4):1142-1152. https://doi.org/10.1007/s10620-020-06265-8.

Annex Table 3-1
Overview of Marfan Syndrome and Related Hereditary Aortopathies

Selected HDCTs	Description	Documentation (e.g., laboratory tests, diagnostic criteria)
Marfan syndrome	Marfan syndrome is a heritable genetic disorder associated with multiorgan syndrome dysfunctions and inherited in an autosomal dominant manner. Abnormalities seen in this disorder include ectopia lentis, myopia, corneal flatness, retinal detachment, early-onset glaucoma and cataracts, trabeculodysgenesis, strabismus, aortic valve regurgitation, mitral valve regurgitation and prolapse, congestive heart failure, tricuspid valve prolapse, premature calcification of the mitral annulus, aortic root dilatation and dissection, ascending aortic root aneurysm, pulmonary artery dilatation, emphysema, pneumothorax, pulmonary blebs, pectus abnormalities, recurrent hernias, scoliosis, spondylolithesis, lumbar dural ectasia, protrusion acetabulae, long-bone overgrowth, joint hypermobility and contractures, hammer toes, pes planus and pes cavus, and decreased muscle mass.	**Diagnostic criteria** 2010 Revised Ghent Nosology **Laboratory** genetic (mutation) testing *Fibrillin 1 (FBN1)*
Loeys-Dietz syndrome	Loeys-Dietz syndrome is an autosomal dominant inherited arthropathy syndrome with widespread systemic involvement. Abnormalities seen in this disorder include micrognathia, hypertelorism, exotropia, blue sclerae, proptosis, malar hypoplasia, bifid uvula, cleft palate, atrial septal defect (uncommon), bicuspid aortic valve (uncommon), bicuspid pulmonary valve (rare), mitral valve prolapse (uncommon), arterial tortuosity (generalized), patent ductus arteriosus, ascending aortic aneurysm and dissection, pulmonary artery aneurysm, descending aortic aneurysm, cerebral aneurysm, pectus deformity, joint laxity, craniosynostosis (uncommon), scoliosis, arachnodactyly, camptodactyly, postaxial polydactyly (rare), talipes equinovarus, velvety textured and translucent skin, mental retardation (uncommon), developmental delay (uncommon), Chiari malformation (uncommon), hydrocephalus (uncommon), headaches, asthma, food allergy, eczema, allergic rhinitis, increased incidence of eosinophilic gastrointestinal disease and other gastrointestinal complaints, pneumothorax and restrictive lung disease, and increased fracture risk.	**Diagnostic criteria** Heterozygous mutation in one of the genes listed below and either of the following: (1) aortic root enlargement (defined as an aortic root z-score ≥2.0) or type A dissection, or (2) compatible systemic features, including characteristic craniofacial, skeletal, cutaneous, and/or vascular manifestations found in combination, and particularly arterial tortuosity. **Laboratory** genetic (mutation) testing *TGFBR1; TGFBR2; SMAD2; SMAD3; TGFB2; TGFB3*

Congenital contractural arachnodactyly (also known as Beals-Hecht syndrome)	Congenital contractural arachnodactyly is an autosomal dominant disorder characterized primarily by contractures and musculoskeletal and cardiac complications. Abnormalities seen in this disorder include marfanoid habitus (dolichostenomelia); dolichocephaly; micrognathia; crumpled appearing ears; ectopia lentis; myopia; high-arched palate; mitral valve prolapse; mitral regurgitation; atrial and ventricular septal defect; bicuspid aortic valve; patent ductus arteriosus; aortic root dilatation; interrupted aortic arch; pectus carinatum; duodenal or esophageal atresia (including intestinal malrotation); osteopenia; congenital kyphoscoliosis; hip, elbow, and knee contractures; subluxation of patella; arachnodactyly; camptodactyly; adducted thumbs; flexion contractures of proximal interphalangeal joints; metatarsus varus; talipes equinovarus; and motor developmental delay.	**Diagnostic criteria** Arachnodactyly (wrist and thumb sign) Marfanoid habitus (dolichostenomelia)—decreased upper to lower segment ratio (<0.85 in white adults; <0.78 in black adults) **Laboratory** genetic (mutation) testing *Fibrillin 2 (FBN2)*
Shprintzen Goldberg syndrome	Shprintzen Goldberg syndrome is an ultrarare autosomal dominant disorder characterized by craniofacial, skeletal, and cardiovascular abnormalities. Clinical findings include craniosynostosis (premature fusion of cranial bones in infancy), craniofacial features (maxillary hypoplasia, micrognathia, ptosis), mitral valve prolapse, aortic dilation, rare arterial tortuosity, obstructive apnea, pectus excavatum or carinatum, marfanoid habitus, joint laxity and/or contractures, umbilical and abdominal hernias, scoliosis, osteopenia, talipes equinovarus, pes planus, hyperelastic skin, lack of subcutaneous tissue, intellectual disability, Chiari malformation, hydrocephalus, and severe muscle hypotonia.	**Diagnostic criteria** No formal diagnostic criteria Considerable phenotypic overlap with Marfan syndrome and Loeys-Dietz syndrome with additional findings of intellectual disabilities and severe muscle hypotonia **Laboratory** genetic (mutation) testing *SKI Protooncogene (SKI)*

NOTE: HDCT = heritable disorder of connective tissue and disability.

SOURCES: Bertoli-Avella et al., 2015; Callewaert, 2019; Doyle et al., 2012; Frischmeyer-Guerrerio et al., 2013; Greally, 2020; Gupta et al., 2002; Lindsay et al., 2012; Loeys and Dietz, 2018; Loeys et al., 2005, 2010; Matyas et al., 2014; Regalado et al., 2011; Rienhoff et al., 2013; Tan et al., 2013; Van Hemelrijk et al., 2010.

4

Ehlers-Danlos Syndromes and Hypermobility Spectrum Disorders

The Ehlers-Danlos syndromes (EDS) are a group of heritable disorders of connective tissue (HDCTs) that share joint hypermobility and skin involvement. Other organ systems are involved to greater or lesser degrees, depending on the type of EDS. Hypermobility spectrum disorders (HSD) are included in this discussion because of their similarities with EDS, especially hypermobile EDS (hEDS), although they do not meet the diagnostic criteria for EDS. This chapter describes the history, diagnosis, and characteristics of EDS/HSD, and reviews their treatment, management, and selected associated physical and mental secondary impairments, many of which can limit activities and restrict participation of affected individuals in work and school. An overview EDS and HSD is provided in Annex Table 4-1 at the end of the chapter. Throughout this chapter, hEDS and HSD are considered together as "hEDS/HSD" because of their clinical similarities. Diagnostic criteria prior to 2017 would not have distinguished between hEDS and HSD, so much of the research on these disorders cited in this report is based on a mix of the two. The term "EDS/HSD" includes HSD with other types of EDS when it encompasses hEDS.

HISTORY OF EHLERS-DANLOS SYNDROMES AND HYPERMOBILITY SPECTRUM DISORDERS

Parapia and Jackson (2008) present a historical review of EDS/HSD. The first report of a patient with joint hypermobility and skin laxity was published in 1892 by Tschernogobow, who presented two patients to the Moscow and Venereology and Dermatology Society (Tschernogobow,

1892). Other cases of joint hypermobility and skin laxity were subsequently reported by Gould and Pyle (1897) and Wile (1883).

In 1901, Ehlers described a patient with joint laxity; unusually stretchy skin; and a history of easy bruising, frequent knee subluxations, and delayed walking (Beighton, 1970). In 1908, Danlos collaborated with Pautier to further explore the physical manifestations of what came to be known as Ehlers-Danlos syndrome (Beighton, 1970).

In the United States, Tobias (1934) reported the first case of EDS/HSD; Ronchese (1936) reported on 24 cases in the literature and 3 whom he had seen personally. McKusick's first edition of *Heritable Disorders of Connective Tissue* (1956) chronicled fewer than 100 reports in the literature; this number had risen to 300 by 1966, when the third edition was published. The first suggestion that the condition was inherited as an autosomal-dominant trait was published by Johnson and Falls (1949), who studied a large family with 32 affected members. As described by Parapia and Jackson (2008), Jansen (1955) reviewed all the extant published pedigrees at the time and suggested that a genetic defect of collagen most likely explained the EDS/HSD phenotype; support for this conclusion was later published by Sestak (1962).

By the late 1960s, different forms of EDS/HSD had begun to be recognized (Beighton, 1970; McKusick, 1972). Pinnell and colleagues (1972) described lysyl hydroxylase deficiency in an autosomal-recessive form of EDS presenting with rupture of the ocular globe and scoliosis. This observation represented the first identified molecular causation of a type of EDS. By 1988, nine different types of EDS/HSD had been proposed in an international nosology of HDCTs—the Beighton criteria (Beighton et al., 1988). A simplified classification was later proposed in what was called the Villefranche nosology (Beighton et al., 1998). Almost 20 years would transpire before an updated nosology would be published in 2017, identifying 13 distinct types of EDS, including hEDS (Malfait et al., 2017) (Table 4-1).

By 2017, the molecular cause of 12 of the then 13 types of EDS/HSD had been identified (Table 4-1). In 2018, another gene associated with classical-like EDS (type 2) was identified: bi-allelic alterations in the *AEBP1* gene lead to defective collagen assembly and abnormal connective tissue structure (Blackburn et al., 2018). Identification and understanding of the genetic basis of the 13 EDS types, several of which have two or more subtypes, continue to evolve. While joint hypermobility is common to all types of EDS, as well as HSD, other presenting factors may vary among types and individuals. Only one type of EDS (the most common type, hEDS) and HSD remain without a known genetic cause. In an effort to accelerate the search for the hEDS gene(s) and increase the likelihood of finding

TABLE 4-1
Clinical Classification of the Ehlers-Danlos Syndromes, Inheritance Pattern, and Genetic Basis

	Clinical EDS subtype	Abbreviation	IP	Genetic basis	Protein
1	Classical EDS	cEDS	AD	Major: COL5A1, COL5A1	Type V collagen
				Rare: COL1A1 c.934C>T, p.(Arg312Cys)	Type I collagen
2	Classical-like EDS	clEDS	AR	TNXB	Tenascin XB
3	Cardiac-valvular	cvEDS	AR	COL1A2 (biallelic mutations that lead to COL1A2 NMD and absence of pro α2(I) collagen chains)	Type I collagen
4	Vascular EDS	vEDS	AD	Major: COL3A1	Type III collagen
				Rare: COL1A1 c.934C>T, p.(Arg312Cys) c.1720C>T, p.(Arg574Cys) c.3227C>T, p.(Arg1093Cys)	Type I collagen
5	Hypermobile EDS	hEDS	AD	Unknown	Unknown
6	Arthrochalasia EDS	aEDS	AD	COL1A1, COL1A2	Type I collagen
7	Dermatosparaxis EDS	dEDS	AR	ADAMTS2	ADAMTS-2
8	Kyphoscoliotic EDS	kEDS	AR	PLOD1	LH1
				FKBP14	FKBP22
9	Brittle Cornea syndrome	BCS	AR	ZNF469	ZNF469

continued

TABLE 4-1 Continued

	Clinical EDS subtype	Abbreviation	IP	Genetic basis	Protein
10	Spondylodysplastic EDS	spEDS	AR	*B4GALT7*	β4GalT7
				B3GALT6	β3GalT6
				SLC39A13	ZIP13
11	Musculocontractural EDS	mcEDS	AR	*CHST14*	D4ST1
				DSE	DSE
12	Myopathic EDS	mEDS	AD or AR	*COL12A1*	Type XII collagen
13	Periodontal EDS	pEDS	AD	*C1R*	C1r
				C1S	C1s

SOURCE: Malfait et al., 2017, p. 10. © 2017 Wiley Periodicals, Inc.
NOTE: AD, autosomal dominant; AR, autosomal recessive, IP, inheritance pattern; NMD, nonsense-mediated mRNA decay.

them, the International Consortium on the Ehlers-Danlos Syndromes & Hypermobility Spectrum Disorders convened in 2016 to refine the diagnostic criteria for hEDS. These new criteria were significantly more rigorous than the previously defined criteria for what was called the hypermobility type under the Villefranche criteria. Consortium members, led by Castori, recognized that some people who met the Villefranche criteria for the hypermobility type would not meet the new, more restrictive criteria under the 2017 nosology; thus, the concept of "hypermobility spectrum disorders" emerged (Castori et al., 2017). Castori and colleagues (2017) proposed that joint hypermobility exists on a spectrum in the human population. Individuals who meet the established clinical criteria for hEDS receive that diagnosis, while those who do not meet those criteria but manifest symptomatic hypermobility are considered to have HSD. The diagnostic distinction between HSD and hEDS may not be clinically meaningful, however, as both groups may experience the same types of physical and mental impairments and potential functional limitations (Aubry-Rozier et al., 2021).

While the early reports of EDS/HSD focused on the unusual joint and skin findings observed in these patients, clinicians began to recognize the multisystem nature of these disorders, such that they affect virtually every organ system in the body. Secondary impairments include chronic pain (Castori, 2016), gastrointestinal dysmotility (Fikree et al., 2017), chronic fatigue (Hakim et al., 2017a), mental manifestations (Bulbena et al., 2017), dysautonomia (Roma et al., 2018), and cranial and spinal neurologic complications (Henderson et al., 2017). Recent reports suggest that immune dysfunction and mast cell activation are more common in hEDS/HSD than in the general population (Brock et al., 2021). Elevated tryptase levels are present in an estimated 6 percent of the general population. Hereditary alpha tryptasemia (HAT) is associated with an elevated serum tryptase, and persons with HAT may manifest joint hypermobility similar to that seen in other HDCT phenotypes (National Institute of Allergy and Infectious Diseases, 2018). The spectrum of mast cell dysregulation in these disorders is increasingly recognized. Prevalence estimates for these disorders are currently lacking, but this is an area of active investigation (Seneviratne et al., 2017).

Research has shown that individuals who meet the diagnostic criteria for hEDS and HSD have similar extra-articular manifestations and disease severity (Aubry-Rozier et al., 2021), contradicting the initial diagnostic description of HSD as being purely musculoskeletal. Therefore, patients diagnosed with HSD must not be assumed to have a milder condition or problems related only to the musculoskeletal system, as initially presumed when the diagnostic criteria were first established in 2017. These observations have prompted a call for further studies to reassess the 2017 diagnostic criteria and develop evidence-based diagnostic criteria for hEDS and HSD (Tinkle, 2020). Some such studies are currently under way.

Recent investigations have demonstrated that individuals meeting the diagnostic criteria for hEDS and those diagnosed with HSD have comparable rates of secondary impairments, such as chronic pain, dysautonomia, and gastrointestinal dysmotility. Research also shows that while there are two distinct groups among individuals with hEDS and HSD with respect to the severity of the secondary impairments they experience, the severity groups do not correspond to diagnosis (Copetti et al., 2019).

DIAGNOSIS OF EHLERS-DANLOS SYNDROMES AND HYPERMOBILITY SPECTRUM DISORDERS

Each type of EDS, as well as HSD, has its own set of specific diagnostic criteria (see Annex Table 4-1). Most important in making the diagnosis is the clinician's awareness that EDS/HSD should be considered. Once a patient has been recognized as having joint hypermobility, the differential diagnosis should consider the various forms of EDS/HSD. Because the genes underlying the hEDS phenotype are not yet identified, diagnosis of hEDS rests entirely on the clinical criteria. Castori and colleagues (2017) present one widely used diagnostic algorithm for hEDS (see also International Consortium, 2017). These diagnostic criteria incorporate data from the Beighton scoring system used to assess hypermobility (Juul-Kristensen et al., 2017). Table 4-2 lists a number of additional hypermobility scales that can be used to assess hypermobility and diagnose generalized joint hypermobility associated with EDS/HSD.

The clinical diagnostic criteria for 12 other types of EDS are provided on the Ehlers-Danlos Society website,[1] but because of the overlap of symptoms among many types of EDS and HSD, definitive diagnosis includes confirmation through genetic testing of those types for which the responsible genes have been identified. The classical type (cEDS) and vascular type (vEDS) of EDS have their own sets of diagnostic criteria (Byers et al., 2017); diagnostic criteria for the 10 rarer types were published in 2017 (Malfait et al., 2017).

Research consistently describes the challenges and delays involved in establishing a correct diagnosis and receiving proper management for hEDS/HSD (Halverson et al., 2021; Knight, 2015). People with hEDS/HSD commonly report receiving incorrect or incomplete diagnoses, and studies

TABLE 4-2
Selected Hypermobility Assessment Scales

Scale	Reference
Carter and Wilkinson Scale	Carter and Wilkinson, 1964
Beighton and Horan Scale	Beighton and Horan, 1970
Beighton Scoring System	Beighton et al., 1973
Rotés Querol	Bulbena et al., 1992; Rotés Querol, 1983
Contompasis	McNerney and Johnston, 1979
Hospital del Mar	Bulbena et al., 1992
Lower Limb Assessment Score	Meyer et al., 2017
Upper Limb Hypermobility Assessment Tool	Nicholson and Chan, 2018
5-Item Questionnaire (self-report)	Hakim and Grahame, 2003
7-Item Questionnaire (self-report)	Bulbena et al., 2014

---

[1] See https://www.ehlers-danlos.com/eds-types (accessed May 25, 2022).

document an average 11–12 years' delay in establishing a correct diagnosis (Halverson et al., 2021; Knight, 2015; Terry et al., 2015). Even once diagnosed, individuals often report receiving inappropriate interventions from clinicians who are not knowledgeable about EDS/HSD. Because symptoms of hEDS/HSD are not always visible, affected individuals may experience high levels of distress and isolation as a result of actually or fearing not being believed about their signs and symptoms (Halverson et al., 2021; Knight, 2015; Langhinrichsen-Rohling et al., 2021; Palomo-Toucedo et al., 2020). Psychosocial support is important for patients with these disorders to help them face the challenges associated with the variety of symptoms they experience, as well as the potential effects of those symptoms on daily activities (Miklovic and Sieg, 2022; Palomo-Toucedo et al., 2020).

EDS/HSD are a complex set of disorders in large part because of their manifestations in multiple body systems. Some of the symptoms experienced by affected individuals are not clearly attributable to a single impairment in a specific body system. A well-functioning body depends on the proper functioning of all of its parts together, not just as individual components, operating as a complete system in which all of the parts interact with one another. Accordingly, a malfunction in one part inevitably affects other parts as well. The relationships among body systems are complex and not fully understood by science, a fact that becomes particularly apparent in disorders that, like EDS/HSD, affect tissues throughout the body. Problems in the immune system, for example, such as mast cell activation disease (MCAD), can manifest as symptoms in other body systems, such as gastrointestinal disorders, respiratory difficulties, nonmigraine headaches, and cognitive dysfunction or impairment, sometimes referred to as "brain fog" (Maitland, 2020). Dysfunction of the autonomic nervous system (dysautonomia) also affects the entire body (Maxwell, 2020; Vernino et al., 2021). In EDS/HSD, a variety of factors, including MCAD and dysautonomia, likely contribute to such symptoms as abdominal (gastrointestinal) distress and cognitive impairment (Maxwell, 2020). In addition to cognitive impairment, dysautonomia can manifest as symptoms of anxiety, attention deficit, and insomnia (Maxwell, 2020).

This clinical picture highlights the complex relationship not only among the physical parts of the body and their functioning but also between physical functioning and mental symptoms and functioning (e.g., cognitive function, mood disorders, anxiety). Moreover, individuals with chronic pain have a higher risk of developing symptoms of anxiety or depression, while those with anxiety or depression are more likely to experience chronic or intensified pain (Anxiety & Depression Association of America, 2022; Harvard Health Publishing, 2017).

The historical dichotomy between physical and mental disorders and the medical specialties that address them, combined with the complex nature of HDCTs and a general lack of knowledge about these disorders among health care providers, undoubtedly contributes to the delayed diagnosis and misdiagnosis often experienced by individuals with EDS/HSD. The problem is bidirectional, with patients caught in the middle. Clinicians trained to address "physical" disorders may inappropriately refer a patient presenting with "unexplained" symptoms to a mental health care provider. Similarly, mental health care providers may not consider the possibility that symptoms commonly associated with a condition such as depression or anxiety may be caused, or exacerbated, by physical disorders.

The question of whether the symptoms commonly associated with a variety of mental disorders (e.g., anxiety disorders, eating disorders, attention-deficit/hyperactivity disorder) are manifestations of a physical disorder (e.g., dysautonomia), a comorbid mental disorder, or a mix of the two is a topic of debate. Two types of literature investigate the relationship between EDS/HSD and various mental disorders: some studies look at the prevalence of specific mental disorders among a population of individuals diagnosed with EDS/HSD, while others look at the prevalence of EDS/HSD or joint hypermobility more generally among a population of individuals diagnosed with a specific mental disorder. For example, the literature contains reports of an increased prevalence of eating disorders among individuals with EDS/HSD (Baeza-Velasco et al., 2022). The researchers posit that oral and gastrointestinal symptoms experienced by some people with EDS/HSD can lead to an aversion to eating, which in turn can develop into an eating disorder. On the other hand, it has been reported that most patients diagnosed with anorexia nervosa also meet the criteria for EDS/HSD (Baeza-Velasco et al., 2022).

The concern is that many individuals with EDS/HSD are inappropriately diagnosed with a psychiatric condition as the sole explanation for their symptoms, while the HDCT goes undiagnosed, and the associated physical impairments go untreated. While science works to establish a better diagnostic process or to define set of concurrent diagnoses, along with more effective standards of care, it is important to acknowledge that clinical assessment of these patients often falls short in investigating and identifying of the underlying causes of their symptoms. It is therefore critical for health care providers to be educated about such disorders as EDS/HSD and the constellation of symptoms with which they present (Miklovic and Sieg, 2022; Mittal et al., 2021). In addition, just as mental health care providers need to be aware of the physical disorders that may accompany symptoms attributable to psychiatric diagnoses, clinicians in primary care and the medical specialties need to be alert to the mental and emotional health of their patients.

Failure to recognize the complex relationships among body systems can lead to inappropriate or incomplete treatment. Treatment of symptoms without identification and treatment of contributing factors is likely to be successful only partially if at all. For example, appropriate treatment of gastrointestinal symptoms could involve treatment for immune system dysfunction *and* dysautonomia. Appropriate treatment for pain requires identification and treatment of underlying pathology, as well as interventions to control the pain. Appropriate treatment for symptoms of anxiety could involve treatment of dysautonomia in addition to interventions to address the anxiety. It is clear that individuals with multisystem disorders such as HDCTs require care from multidisciplinary teams to investigate all of the potential causes of their symptoms (both physical and mental) (Miklovic and Sieg, 2022; Mittal et al., 2021).

CHARACTERISTICS OF EHLERS-DANLOS SYNDROMES AND HYPERMOBILITY SPECTRUM DISORDERS

Clinical Picture

The natural history of EDS/HSD is variable. The range and severity of clinical course are best understood in the context of each specific type of EDS and HSD. Nevertheless, as a group, patients with EDS/HSD share general features of joint hypermobility, skin hyperextensibility, and tissue fragility that may affect organ systems, blood vessels, skin, joints, and ligaments (Bloom et al., 2017). It is important to note that specific manifestations may depend on the type of EDS/HSD, with hallmark features, such as vascular rupture (seen in vEDS), being specific to a particular type. Additional features of pain; fatigue; cognitive dysfunction; dysautonomia; and gastrointestinal, respiratory, and immune dysfunction are often underappreciated in EDS/HSD, particularly given their waxing and waning nature in affected individuals. Results of a large survey of patients' lived experience with hEDS/HSD show the multimorbidity nature of these conditions, with individuals reporting 15–25 symptoms involving different organ systems and having substantial impact on daily functioning (Murray et al., 2013). Schubart and colleagues (2019a) identified three symptom clusters: a pain-dominant cluster, a high symptom burden cluster, and a mental fatigue cluster. The percentage of participants in the pain-dominant subgroup was similar in all EDS/HSD diagnostic subtypes, while the percentage in the high symptom burden subgroup was higher in the cEDS and hEDS/HSD subtypes, and the percentage in the mental fatigue subgroup was higher in the vEDS and "rare/unclassified" EDS subtypes (Schubart et al., 2019a).

EDS/HSD patients often appear healthy but report a constellation of symptoms that may be difficult for clinicians to recognize as being related. Therefore, as described previously, delayed or misdiagnosis is common, and may significantly and negatively impact the clinical course. At the time of diagnosis, patients are likely to have a history of multiple articular dislocations or subluxations, poor wound healing, easy bruising, and atypical scarring. Such features are often present in childhood but may be considered "normal" for the family or attributed to external factors; in severe cases, child abuse may be suspected. Severe types may also present in relatively young patients with such dramatic manifestations as spontaneous organ rupture or vascular dissection, as is seen in patients with vEDS (Shalhub et al., 2019). Often children show hypersensitivity; difficulties in eating, which may lead to eating disorders; and more fears and anxiety than are found in the general population (Baeza-Velasco et al., 2022; Ezpeleta et al., 2018).

Profound changes in body composition that occur with puberty include, for example, increased musculoskeletal growth and changes in brain development (including cognitive maturation and psychosocial maturation) and in the cardiovascular system. These changes are mediated by hormones that can affect all organ systems. In many individuals with EDS/HSD, particularly those types manifesting hypermobility, puberty is associated with the onset or worsening of secondary impairments, especially in females, and may be a period of disease amplification (Tinkle et al., 2017). These impairments include increased gastrointestinal dysmotility (Dhingra et al., 2021a), respiratory complications (Bascom et al., 2021b), postural tachycardia syndrome (POTS) (Coupal et al., 2019), MCAD (Zierau et al., 2012), increased musculoskeletal pain (Dhingra et al., 2021b; Feldman et al., 2020; Mu et al., 2019), chronic fatigue (Pacey et al., 2015), and neuropsychiatric diagnoses (Kindgren et al., 2021; Tran et al., 2020), among others. Importantly, one study found that in vEDS, mortality was increased 3-fold in males under age 20 as a result of unanticipated vascular events (Pepin et al., 2014).

A recent study assessed the health-related quality of life (HRQoL) and mental health of children and adolescents aged 4–18 with a variety of HDCTs—MFS, LDS, hEDS, and other EDS types—through child- and parent-reported questionnaires (Warnink-Kavelaars, et al., 2022). Parents also reported on the impact of their child's condition on the family and themselves. Overall, children and adolescents with HDCTs reported "increased pain, decreased physical functioning and general health, a negative mental health state, [and] limitations in school-related and leisure activities and participation with friends and family"; those with hEDS also reported low self-esteem compared with representative general-population samples (Warnink-Kavelaars, et al., 2022, p. 6). With respect to parental and family impact, parents of children with hEDS reported increased distress and limitations on their personal time and family activities relative to the comparison sample. Children and adolescents with hEDS and their parents had the lowest scores on all but a few of the HRQoL subscales. Mu and colleagues (2019) also found that children and adolescents with hEDS/HSD had lower

HRQoL scores compared with healthy controls, and that pain and fatigue were the primary predictors of HRQoL. These findings emphasize the need for psychosocial support among children diagnosed with EDS/HSD and their families.

Epidemiology

Epidemiology addresses the distribution and determinants of health-related states or events in specified populations and the impact of approaches for treating or controlling health problems (Last, 2001, p. 61). This discipline provides a framework for answering many of the questions posed in the committee's statement of task: the prevalence of HDCTs; the status of diagnosis, treatment, and prognosis for those disorders; their age at onset and gender distribution; laboratory and diagnostic tests for the disorders; their usual clinical course for adults and children; the likelihood, frequency, and duration of changes in the clinical or medical severity of symptoms, such as flare-ups or remissions; the possibility and likelihood of reducing the work-related severity of symptoms; the treatments or circumstances that may lead to vocationally relevant improvement; and secondary impairments that result from either the disorders or their treatments.

Incidence

By definition, all HDCTs are present at birth, as the underlying causative genetic variant exists within an individual's genome. Some HDCTs are recognized at birth because of their distinct and severe manifestations, whereas the manifestations of many HDCTs evolve over time, with shifting distributions in the population. As discussed previously, delays in diagnosis are well recognized.

Prevalence

As reported in Chapter 2, all types of EDS combined are thought to occur in about 1 in 5,000 people (Pyeritz, 2000; Steinmann et al., 2002). Among all types of EDS, hEDS likely accounts for 80–90 percent of cases (Tinkle et al., 2017). Rarer EDS types include vEDS, with an estimated prevalence of 1/50,000 (Byers, 2019). All other EDS types are extremely rare (Steinmann et al., 2002); musculocontractural EDS and dermatosparaxis EDS, for example, are estimated to have a prevalence of less than 1/1,000,000 (Orphanet, 2022a,b).

Preferred sources of epidemiologic information include large case series and population-based datasets. Current inferences of prevalence are subject to ascertainment and referral bias, and must be viewed with caution.

There is now a genetic test with which to identify many, although not all, of the EDS subtypes (Malfait et al., 2017). An epidemiologic approach to estimating the population prevalence of each EDS subtype with identified pathogenic variants would be to test for this variant in a general-population sample.

As noted in Chapter 2, there currently is no identified gene (pathogenic variant) for hEDS/HSD. Estimates of the prevalence of these disorders therefore derive from screening using standardized tests, such as the Beighton scoring system, and other clinical criteria (Castori et al., 2017). Mulvey and colleagues (2013) estimate a general-population prevalence of joint hypermobility of 18 percent, determined using a validated self-administered screening tool (Hakim and Grahame, 2003), with chronic widespread pain being present in a subset of these cases, perhaps indicating that the true prevalence of hEDS/HSD is much higher than 1/5,000.

A recent estimate of the prevalence of EDS/HSD derives from a national electronic cohort study and nested case control study conducted in Wales, United Kingdom. To derive this estimate, the researchers identified persons who were assigned a coded diagnosis of EDS/HSD or joint hypermobility syndrome (an older diagnostic term that includes both HSD and hEDS) between 1990 and 2017, finding a point prevalence of 10 cases in a practice of 5,000 patients (Demmler et al., 2019). Outpatient records were classified according to the READ 2 criteria and inpatient records according to the *International Classification of Diseases*, 10th edition (ICD-10).

Age and Gender Effects

hEDS/HSD are recognized in equal proportions in boys and girls. Increased joint hypermobility is seen in pubertal females (Quatman et al., 2008). Clinicians have observed the emergence of a female predominance in symptomatic EDS in the peripubertal period. The above-cited national cohort study of individuals with EDS/HSD in Wales, United Kingdom, showed a gender difference of 8.5 years in the mean age at diagnosis: the highest proportion of males was first identified at ages 5–9, while the highest proportion of females was diagnosed at ages 15–19 (Demmler et al., 2019). Overall, among 6,021 identified individuals, 30 percent were male and 70 percent female. This finding is supported by large case control studies of U.S. private insurers showing increased prescription drug claims for females beginning peripubertally (Bascom et al., 2021b; Dhingra et al., 2021a). Of note, a community-based survey conducted by Mulvey and colleagues (2013) found a progressive decline in the prevalence of joint hypermobility throughout adulthood (Mulvey et al., 2013).

Manifestations

The 2017 report of the International Consortium on Ehlers-Danlos Syndromes & Hypermobility Spectrum Disorders provides a detailed review of clinical findings for EDS/HSD, organized by organ system and derived from clinical experience, case series, and some large population samples (Bloom et al., 2017; Hakim et al., 2021). Annex Tables 5-3–5-12 list many of the physical and mental impairments associated with EDS/HSD. Studies cited below provide epidemiologic evidence for specific organ system manifestations associated with these disorders. This research shows greater prevalence of symptoms and diagnoses involving diverse organ systems among persons with EDS/HSD than was previously thought. These findings provide growing evidence that EDS/HSD should be viewed as a disorder not only with musculoskeletal manifestations but also with diverse, multi–organ system manifestations, including orthostatic intolerance (De Wandele et al., 2014a,b; 2014b; Hakim et al., 2017b; Roma et al., 2018; Rowe et al., 1999; Rowe, 2022), gastrointestinal symptoms, neurologic manifestations, respiratory manifestations (Bascom et al., 2021a,b; Chohan et al., 2021), and psychiatric manifestations (Bulbena et al., 2017). Notably, the pathophysiologic relationship between EDS/HSD and many of these manifestations and comorbid conditions is unclear, and the evidence linking them is primarily associative; many are also common in chronic conditions that are not characterized by connective tissue dysfunction. Further research is needed to understand the pathogenetic sequence for these manifestations and the implications for primary/secondary/tertiary prevention and disease state management.

Multisystem manifestations are often significant, but may vary both among individuals and throughout an affected individual's lifetime. Not only do the physical and mental secondary impairments experienced by individuals with EDS/HSD differ from person to person, but the presence and severity of the impairments also may fluctuate (wax and wane) over time. A growing body of literature suggests that comorbid conditions, such as orthostatic intolerance and immune dysregulation, collectively contribute to disease severity and thus to an individual's experience and associated disability (Copetti et al., 2019; Kalisch et al., 2020; Krahe et al., 2018). Individuals with versus those without hEDS/HSD also develop migraines earlier, have more days with migraines per month, and experience more accompanying symptoms (Puledda et al., 2015).

Patients will likely experience musculoskeletal and other disease manifestations throughout life. Joint hypermobility contributes to articular instability, with subluxation or dislocation leading to pain and premature degenerative arthritis over time. Hand and wrist pain can compromise fine motor skills, making it difficult to perform such activities as keyboarding and other fine motor tasks that may be required for work or school. Pes planus (flat feet, usually associated with ankle pronation) is common in all forms of EDS/HSD and may further contribute to joint instability and pain; moderate to severe pes planus has been associated with knee and intermittent lower back pain (Kosashvili et al., 2008). Clinically significant and progressive scoliosis may develop, particularly in the kyphoscoliotic, classical, and arthrochalasia types of EDS as well as hEDS/HSD (Yonko et al., 2021). In addition, EDS/HSD patients are at increased risk of craniocervical and other spinal instability and such central nervous system pathologies as Chiari 1 malformation, intracranial hypertension, tethered cord syndrome, and syringomyelia (Henderson et al., 2017; Klinge et al., 2021, 2022). Myopia is common but nonspecific, and there is an increased risk for retinal detachment, glaucoma, strabismus, cataract, amblyopia, cornea scarring or rupture, and blindness (Louie et al., 2020). EDS/HSD is also associated with immune dysfunction, including MCAD, as well as primary immune deficiencies, which in turn can contribute to immune-mediated pathology in one or multiple organ systems (Brock et al., 2021; Sordet et al., 2005). Acute catastrophic events experienced during the course of disease are most likely to be seen in patients with vEDS, cEDS, or kyphoscoliotic EDS (kEDS) (Bowen et al., 2017; Brady et al., 2017; Byers et al., 2017). Such events include stroke, arterial dissection, spontaneous cerebrospinal fluid leak, ruptured aneurysm, spontaneous rupture of bladder, diverticulum, incarcerated hernia, intestinal intussusception, gastric perforation, and peripartum uterine rupture (Castori et al., 2015; Gilliam et al., 2020).

Gastrointestinal problems can be pronounced and contribute to high levels of health impairment and functional limitations in patients with hEDS/HSD. Individuals who experience frequent episodes of gastroinstestinal distress require access to a restroom whenever necessary at work or school. These problems are amplified by the presence of POTS or MCAD (Chelimsky and Chelimsky, 2018; Hsieh, 2018; Inayet et al., 2018; Lam et al., 2021; Mehr et al., 2018; Tai et al., 2020; Wilder-Smith et al., 2019). Genitourinary conditions are also common and can affect activities and participation (Nee et al., 2019). For example, urinary incontinence can make it difficult to stand for extended periods of time without leakage. A study of gynecologic symptoms in hEDS/HSD indicated high frequencies of menorrhagia, dysmenorrhea, and dyspareunia (Hugon-Rodin et al., 2016). Urogynecological problems are amplified by comorbid POTS and MCAD, and hEDS/HSD symptoms may increase before and during menses (Patel and Khullar, 2021; Peggs et al., 2012). Adolescents with EDS/HSD may also experience severe gynecological symptoms (Hernandez and Dietrich, 2020).

Since the first clinical report in 1988, several psychopathological conditions, especially anxiety and depression, have been reported consistently in individuals with EDS/HSD (Baeza-Velasco et al., 2011; Bathen et al.,

2013; Berglund et al., 2015; Bulbena et al., 2017; Bulbena et al., 1988; Bulbena et al., 2015). Chronic pain is also common among individuals with EDS/HSD (Voermans et al., 2010a), with studies finding a prevalence of between 43 percent (Kalisch et al., 2020) and 99 percent (Murray et al., 2013). Individuals with EDS/HSD commonly experience severe fatigue as well (Voermans et al., 2010b). Depression is common among individuals with other chronic conditions, including pain, and dysautonomias can cause symptoms commonly associated with anxiety.

As noted, EDS/HSD may manifest in several organ systems, and these manifestations can result in impaired quality of life (Berglund et al., 2015) and employment difficulties. A survey of 455 persons with hEDS/HSD showed that 55 percent were currently employed, and 24 percent were working only part-time as a result of their disorder (Murray et al., 2013), while 12 percent (54 of 466 respondents) indicated they were not working because of hEDS/HSD-associated limitations. Among those who were working, half had to change roles or take on less responsibility because of their diagnosis. Of the 119 student respondents, 18 percent were unable to attend school full-time, and 32 percent reported not being enrolled in school at all because of their EDS/HSD diagnosis.

The most common manifestations of EDS/HSD that impact quality of life are chronic pain (joint and limb), chronic fatigue, and hypermobility (Murray et al., 2013). Other organ systems that may be affected by EDS/HSD include the gastrointestinal, nervous, ocular, respiratory, and urogenital systems. All of these manifestations, along with anxiety, depression, and fibromyalgia, can affect an individual's participation in work, school, and other activities (Murray et al., 2013). In particular, hEDS/HSD appear to be associated with greater pain and work impairment (De Baets et al., 2021), whereas cEDS has a greater effect on activities of daily living; both types of EDS/HSD were found to result in greater perceived disability than is evident in the general population (Bogni et al., 2015). hEDS/HSD are also associated with mobility disability, which was found to be more prevalent among individuals who are older, have more fatigue, and have a higher body mass index (Kalisch et al., 2020). Mobility issues can be an impediment to working for individuals with hEDS/HSD who need a wheelchair or have difficulty accessing public transportation, and some pain medications used for EDS/HSD have sedative side effects that preclude driving. Obstructive sleep apnea occurs among those with EDS/HSD more frequently than in the general population and is associated with greater fatigue, particularly during the day, and poorer quality of life (Gaisl et al., 2017); daytime sleepiness can affect an individual's ability to work regular hours. POTS, a frequent manifestation of EDS/HSD, is associated with a variety of persistent symptoms, such as cognitive impairments (e.g., in attention and recall), fatigue, low energy, headaches, and sleep disturbances, and can have substantial effects on various aspects of quality of life (Mathias et al., 2021; Vernino et al., 2021), including employment and household tasks. Individuals with EDS/HSD report that their pain and fatigue can make working difficult, requiring reduced hours or different jobs, and in some cases leading them to leave a job or be terminated (Palomo-Toucedo et al., 2020).

TREATMENT AND MANAGEMENT

There is no cure for EDS/HSD, and management strategies rely on preventing and mitigating symptoms and treating associated physical and mental secondary impairments; these interventions are important for managing functional limitations and reducing HDCT-related disability. This section addresses the management of EDS/HSD; Chapter 5 addresses the relationship among secondary impairments associated with these disorders, their potential effects on function, and considerations relevant to Social Security Administration disability determinations.

Given the paucity of clinical trials or large-scale studies of specific therapeutic options for EDS/HSD, experts caring for patients with these disorders have developed management algorithms. The International Consortium on the Ehlers-Danlos Syndromes & Hypermobility Spectrum Disorders is the leading authority on EDS/HSD diagnosis, classification, and management, and as noted earlier, in 2017 published clinical practice guidance (Bloom et al., 2017; Malfait et al., 2017). More recent clinical guidance was published in the December 2021 issue of the *American Journal of Medical Genetics* (Hakim et al., 2021).

The treatment burden for EDS/HSD includes high numbers of clinician encounters to manage multisystem manifestations. Demmler and colleagues (2019) found that adults with EDS/HSD had significantly more diagnoses in 16 of 20 Read Code disease categories compared with controls, as well as more prescriptions for 15/17 Read Codes. A large proportion of persons with EDS/HSD require medications chronically, with a subset meeting criteria for polypharmacy—a substantial medication burden. Numbers of surgical procedures can be very high as well, as are the need for and use of allied health professional services. Durable medical equipment, including braces and mobility assistive devices, also may be required.

Education is particularly important for optimal EDS/HSD management, not only for patients and families but also for members of their health care team so they can appropriately identify and manage disease manifestations and coordinate multidisciplinary care (Miklovic and Sieg, 2021; Mittal et al., 2021). Patients and providers should understand how to recognize EDS/HSD-related disease manifestations and what monitoring practices may be beneficial in assessing the development of complications seen generally in EDS/HSD or specific to a certain EDS type. In addition, multidisciplinary care teams should include a clinical geneticist to provide guidance on the implications of EDS/HSD for family members and the risk of recurrence within the family. Patients should be counseled on strategies for preventing or mitigating symptoms, as well as the risks associated with certain activities that may result in physical trauma, such as physically demanding activities or pregnancy and childbirth. Moreover, their hypersensitivity may cause individuals with EDS/HSD to have poor tolerance for pharmacologic treatments, a possibility clinicians need to consider when prescribing such drugs as corticoids, antidepressants, and some antibiotics. Given the lack of clinical experience with EDS/HSD in most clinical settings, it is important for those with expertise in EDS/HSD to educate other members of the patient's care team regarding the disorders and develop monitoring and treatment plans collaboratively. Anyone newly diagnosed with vEDS or some other rare EDS type that is considered to pose a high risk of significant cardiovascular involvement should be referred to a clinical center with experience and expertise in EDS management (Byers et al., 2017).

Once a diagnosis of EDS/HSD has been made, patients should be counseled regarding potential disease-associated manifestations that necessitate immediate care. Acute, sometimes atraumatic dislocations are common. In certain types of EDS, urgent conditions may be signaled by the sudden onset of severe pain, including chest pain, or bleeding that can occur with vascular or organ (spleen, liver, colon, gravid uterus) rupture. Acute ruptures are most commonly seen in vEDS or kEDS, and more rarely in other types of EDS (D'Hondt et al., 2018; Lum et al., 2011). Any acute reduction in vision or increase in ocular discomfort requires emergency ophthalmic evaluation. Rapidly progressing neurologic signs may indicate central nervous system involvement requiring urgent management (Henderson et al., 2017, 2019). Finally, the sudden onset of shortness of breath may indicate spontaneous pneumothorax, for which immediate evaluation and treatment are required.

Monitoring for the presence of certain disease manifestations can be helpful in preventing the above emergencies by identifying early signs of pathology in asymptomatic patients. Specifically, all adult and pediatric EDS patients should undergo baseline cardiovascular evaluation. Cardiovascular assessment should include echocardiography to determine the presence and degree of cardiovascular involvement, such as valvular disease or aortic dilation (Atzinger et al., 2011). Patients with normal baseline studies and an EDS type considered low-risk for cardiovascular involvement may require fewer repeat evaluations, although no standardized interval for repeat testing has been established. Patients with abnormal findings or those with an EDS type considered high-risk for cardiovascular involvement (such as vEDS or kEDS) should be managed by a cardiovascular specialist to provide frequent monitoring and initiate specific interventions (e.g., pharmacologic, surgical) as needed. In addition, patients with many of the rarer forms of EDS have cardiovascular involvement with functional consequences necessitating lifelong specialist management (Brady et al., 2017).

Given the risk of retinal detachment, lens luxation, and cornea breakdown, all EDS patients should undergo baseline ophthalmologic evaluation that is repeated at regular intervals to assess for evidence of corneal, lenticular, scleral, or retinal involvement. Although patients with kEDS are at the greatest risk for disease-related manifestations involving the eye, including retinal detachment, scleral fragility, globe rupture, and glaucoma, patients with other EDS types may be affected by these conditions and benefit from regular evaluation as well.

Several management considerations apply broadly to EDS/HSD, and strategies for mitigating certain symptoms can be used in patients with any EDS/HSD type. Evidence suggests that similar management strategies can be used for patients with hEDS and HSD (Aubry-Rozier et al., 2021). Joint hypermobility is a common feature in both, and preventive measures to minimize recurrent dislocations and/or the early onset of osteoarthritis are advised for individuals with either disorder. Preservation of joint function may be supported if the patient limits certain high-risk activities, such as contact sports or gymnastics, while engaging in joint-sparing, appropriate muscle-strengthening activities, such as water exercises or Pilates (Bowen et al., 2017). Joint management should include consultation with physical and occupational therapists, as well as evaluation by an orthotist. Although robust data are lacking, one study found that the majority of EDS/HSD patients enrolled in a physical therapy program reported benefit (Rombaut et al., 2011). For patients experiencing musculoskeletal pain related to joint hypermobility, pharmacologic treatment can be helpful but should be monitored by a clinician experienced in EDS/HSD management. Over-the-counter and prescription pain medications, as well as supplements, are more likely to cause adverse reactions in this population than in the general population (Agarwal et al., 2007; Bonadonna et al., 2016; Drugs.com, 2021; Song et al., 2020; Tahir et al., 2020; Vernino et al., 2021).

Spinal disease is a common feature of many forms of EDS/HSD. Scoliosis may be diagnosed in both children and adults, and clinically significant scoliosis may necessitate bracing or surgical intervention, especially in patients with kEDS but also in those with the cEDS, hEDS/HSD, and arthrochalasia EDS types. Experts in spine care should be involved in the care of EDS/HSD patients experiencing neck pain; headaches; migraines; or signs and symptoms suggestive of Chiari I malformation, intracranial hypertension, craniocervical or atlantoaxial instability, tethered cord, syringomyelia, dystonias, or Tarlov cysts (Henderson et al., 2017). Evaluation should include advanced imaging, such as magnetic resonance imaging.

Additional manifestations of EDS/HSD vary but may warrant specialty referral and assessment. Patients with gastrointestinal complaints should undergo a complete evaluation, including evaluation for extraluminal conditions. Upper endoscopy and colonoscopy should be approached with caution in individuals with EDS/HSD because of their underlying tissue fragility and increased risk of mucosal bleeding and complications from sedation (Kilaru et al., 2019). Immunologic involvement, particularly in patients with recurrent infections or those with symptoms of mast cell activation, requires consultation with a provider with expertise in allergy and immunology. Dysautonomia may be present, particularly in patients with hEDS/HSD. It may cause orthostatic intolerance, as well as tachycardia and/or palpitations, and contribute to a number of secondary neurological manifestations, such as fatigue, dizziness, syncope, and memory and concentration problems (Tinkle et al., 2017). Patients experiencing these complications, as well as those affected by recurrent headache, a common feature in patients with hEDS/HSD, should receive a neurologic evaluation. Patients with respiratory symptoms should receive a baseline assessment—spirometry with flow-volume loops and assessment of bronchodilator responsiveness.

Psychological assessment is important to screen for the presence of anxiety, phobic features, and depression since they frequently go unnoticed, and can interfere with daily life functions and even adherence to treatments. Individuals with EDS/HSD often have been classified as "somatizers" by clinicians unfamiliar with the disorders (Bulbena-Cabré et al., 2021). However, research on the biological and clinical basis of EDS/HSD is improving understanding of their physiology and psychopathology. The literature confirms that psychological processes, such as fear, emotional distress, or negative emotions, in EDS/HSD have a significant impact on patients' outcomes (Bulbena-Cabré et al., 2021) and can interfere with daily activities and participation in work or school (see Chapter 5). ESD/HSD have common systemic associations with anxiety disorders, as well as significant correlations with neurodevelopmental, eating, mood, and sleep disorders (Bulbena-Cabré et al., 2021). All of these psychological issues need to be addressed in the assessment and management of individuals with EDS/HSD. It is important to reiterate that the relationships (associative or causal) among the different manifestations of EDS/HSD, as well as the relationships of those manifestations to the underlying disorder, are not fully understood. The presence and treatment of comorbid psychological disorders should not preclude the assessment and treatment of physical conditions that may underlie or contribute to symptoms associated with the psychological disorders.

Management of EDS/HSD patients should also include special consideration of specific transient states, such as the perioperative or peripartum periods. Patients undergoing surgical interventions are more likely than the general population to experience adverse events associated with both soft-tissue fragility and anesthesia reactions/intolerance. Determining the presence and severity of patient-specific and EDS/HSD type–specific manifestations, such as bleeding, poor wound healing, cardiovascular involvement, or increased risk of joint subluxation or dislocation and cervical spine injury, is crucial during preoperative consultation. Tissue fragility associated with HDCTs motivated a recent assessment of surgical risk associated with EDS/HSD (and Marfan syndrome) as compared with controls in a national database (Jayarajan et al., 2020). The overall complication rate for all inpatient vascular surgery procedures was statistically greater for EDS/HSD patients (52.2 percent) than for controls (44.6 percent) ($p < 0.0001$). Patients with EDS/HSD showed an increased risk of postoperative hemorrhage (39 percent versus 22 percent for controls), but not of respiratory failure (8.7 percent versus 10.7 percent for controls).

Anecdotal reports beginning in 1990 (Arendt-Nielsen et al., 1990) and corroborated in 2005 (Hakim et al., 2005) indicate insufficient effect of local analgesics among persons with hEDS/HSD. Accordingly, preprocedure screening with a simple questionnaire (Hakim and Grahame, 2003) has been recommended to detect hypermobility and alert proceduralists intending to use local anesthetics for pain control in these patients. In 2017, the Patient-Centered Outcomes Research Institute–funded EDS Comorbidity Coalition conducted a research prioritization exercise; among 80 research ideas proposed, one of the 3 highest priorities was the issue of local anesthetic resistance (Bloom et al., 2021; Hakim et al., 2005). To assess the prevalence of this problem, Schubart and colleagues (2019b) conducted an online survey, finding that 88 percent of people with versus 33 percent of those without EDS/HSD reported inadequate response to local anesthesias. Postoperative pain management also is often inadequate in EDS/HSD patients, and the pain they experience may seem out of proportion. Clinicians need to understand nociception is altered in these patients, and they may require more pain medication and different combinations of medications. A recent study of hEDS/HSD patients undergoing craniocervical fixation surgery found that opioid-free anesthesia in addition to postoperative administration of lidocaine, ketamine, and dexmedetomidine significantly reduced postoperative pain and the need of methadone rescues compared with opioid-based anesthesia and postsurgical management (Ramírez-Paesano et al., 2021).

The examples given above, supported by the committee members' experience, indicate that persons with EDS/HSD have particular risks associated with procedures. A number of preoperative and preprocedural screening tools can be used to identify, quantify, communicate, and manage these risks (Moonesinghe et al., 2013). There remains, however, a need to better understand and quantify procedural and surgical risks in EDS/HSD, as well as the other HDCTs. Needed as well are simple screening tools that can be used by anesthesiologists and proceduralists, particularly given the likelihood that a substantial proportion of persons with EDS/HSD are undiagnosed, but the lack of diagnosis does not remove the risk.

Use of desmopressin, a synthetic form of vasopressin, may be helpful in achieving hemostasis during and after invasive procedures (Castori, 2012). Patients with easy bruising and those demonstrating skin fragility, a notable feature in cEDS and vEDS, may benefit from daily ascorbic acid (Bowen et al., 2017). Surgical incisions (or wounds following trauma) should be closed without tension, deep stitches should be applied generously and closely, and cutaneous stitches should be left in place twice as long as in non-EDS patients; additional fixation of adjacent skin with adhesive tape can help prevent stretching of the scar (Castori, 2012, 2013b). Mast cells play a role in wound healing (Komi et al., 2020) and tolerance of adhesives; notably, their activation can be common and poorly controlled after such stressors as surgery. In addition, it may be advisable to counsel patients that, regardless of the best surgical interventions, they may have an elevated risk of postoperative complications (Guier et al., 2020; Kulas Søborg et al., 2017; Louie et al., 2020; Yonko et al., 2021) and decreased likelihood of surgical success (Rombaut et al., 2011; Yonko et al., 2021). In addition to those risks, moreover, surgical intervention and anesthesia may provoke POTS and MCAD. To limit surgical morbidity, all conservative (i.e., nonsurgical) measures should be exhausted before surgery for individuals with EDS/HSD is contemplated (see Table 4-3).

Patients contemplating pregnancy should be counseled about the risk of obstetrical complications (Byers, 2019; Byers et al., 2017; Eagleton, 2016; Karthikeyan and Venkat-Raman, 2018; Pepin et al., 2000; Pezaro et al., 2018). Preterm labor or premature rupture of membranes may occur in pregnant patients with EDS/HSD (Byers, 2019; Pezaro et al., 2018). Delivery may be precipitous and complicated by postpartum hemorrhage, extensive laceration, or extension of episiotomy incisions, or contribute to genitourinary complications, such as pelvic organ prolapse (Karthikeyan and Venkat-Raman, 2018; Pezaro et al., 2018). Similar to individuals with Loeys-Dietz syndrome, women with vEDS are at increased risk for uterine rupture and peripartum hemorrhage (Byers, 2019; Eagleton, 2016; Meester et al., 2017).

As discussed in Chapter 5, chronic pain and fatigue each have different, multifactorial causes. Management of each of these symptoms requires identification of and interventions to address the root cause. For example, management of fatigue caused by dysautonomia, MCAD, or sleep apnea requires treatment of that cause. Once the cause has been managed, relaxation techniques and mindfulness-based exercises can be helpful.

TABLE 4-3
Surgical and Anesthetic Recommendations for Joint Hypermobility Syndrome/Ehlers-Danlos Syndrome Hypermobility Type (JHS/EDS-HT)

Evidence		Ref.	Recommendation
Surgical procedure			
(1)	Orthopedic surgery is paradoxically associated with pain worsening in JHS/EDS-HT; anecdotal observations suggest a low success rate for abdominal surgery in functional disorders.	Voermans et al., 2010a	Consider more conservative treatments as an alternative to non-life-threatening operations.
(2)	Although soft tissue fragility is not severe in JHS/EDS-HT, delayed wound healing with consequent suture widening, suture dehiscence and postsurgical hernias are possible complications.	Burcharth and Rosenberg, 2012; Castori, 2013a	(a) Perform skin closure in two layers (cutaneous and subcutaneous) without excessive tension. (b) Use generous sutures, deep stitches and steri-strips as reinforcement devices. (c) Leave sutures twice as long as normally recommended.
(3)	Minor bleeding disorders are common in JHS/EDS-HT.	Jackson et al., 2013	Consider preoperative prophylaxis with desmopressin (1-deamino-8-D-arginine vasopressin), especially in patients with a positive history for mucosal bleeding (nose, gingivae, bowel, bladder, etc.) and/or easy bruising.
(4)	Episiotomy is associated with an increased risk for pelvic prolapses in JHS/EDS-HT women.	Castori et al., 2012b	Consider cesarean section as first-choice delivery procedure.
Anesthetic procedure			
(5)	Dysautonomia is a major feature in JHS/EDS-HT and may need special anesthetic considerations.	Mathias et al., 2011	(a) Consider to carry out appropriate investigations (e.g. tilt test) before any intervention in order to properly plan the anesthetic procedure, especially in patients with cardiovascular symptoms. (b) In case of confirmed dysautonomia, consider prophylactic early fluid loading and phenylephrine infusion.
(6)	JHS/EDS-HT patients often display resistance to intradermal lidocaine infiltrations and topical EMLA cream.	Arendt-Nielsen et al., 1990; Hakim et al., 2005	Consider alternative anesthetic procedures or double the anesthetic dose.

TABLE 4-3
Continued

Evidence	Ref.	Recommendation
(7) Epi/peridural anesthesia may be hampered by severe spondylosis and/or scoliosis, and could be complicated by intraspinal hypotension due to increased meningeal weakness in JHS/EDS-HT.	None[1]	Favor total anesthesia in case of major surgery.
(8) Temporomandibular joint dysfunction and occipitoatlantoaxial instability may be more common in JHS/EDS-HT.	De Coster et al., 2005; Milhorat et al., 2007	Perform intubation with care and consider the use of pediatric devices also in adults.
Postsurgery recovery		
(9) Muscle deconditioning due to inactivity rapidly worsens chronic pain and fatigue in JHS/EDS-HT.	Castori et al., 2012a	Consider early physical therapy support in case of surgery with postoperative bed rest for >7 days.

[1] Reports specifically describing such likely complications are lacking. However, mild scoliosis and premature spondylosis are commonly encountered in the JHS/EDS-HT clinic, while some preliminary studies indicate that generalized joint hypermobility is associated with orthostatic headache.

SOURCE: Castori, 2013b. Copyright © 2013 Karger Publishers, Basel, Switzerland.

Psychosocial support and education are cornerstones of EDS/HSD management. The Ehlers-Danlos Society provides an abundance of information for both providers and patients, including community resources and support groups (www.ehlers-danlos.com).

PROGNOSIS

The prognosis and clinical course of EDS/HSD depend on individual patient factors (e.g., personal factors in the International Classification of Functioning, Disability and Health [ICF] model of disability described in Chapter 1), which vary greatly among affected individuals and are often related to the severity of disease-related physical and mental impairments, as well as the EDS/HSD type. As discussed previously, HDCTs are lifelong disorders. Recent longitudinal data from a well-characterized cohort of individuals with different types of EDS, assessed with repeated administration of standardized instruments (Schubart et al., 2022), support the clinical impression of heterogeneity in clinical course. For many, EDS/HSD symptoms and disease burdens are chronic. Some persons with EDS/HSD experience a marked worsening over time, while a few see a decrease in the intensity and severity of manifestations. Overall, large cross-sectional case control studies of national prescription claims databases as a proxy for disease indicate an increase in multiple prescribed medications over the life course in persons with EDS/HSD compared with controls (Bascom et al., 2021b; Dhingra et al., 2021b).

It is important to note that patients with vEDS have a decreased life expectancy, with a median survival age of 46 for males and 54 for females (Pepin et al., 2014). The gender difference, which closes by age 40, appears attributable to a greater proportion of deaths among males, especially in the second decade of life: one study found that 18 percent of deaths among males compared with 7 percent of females occurred by age 20 (Pepin et al., 2014). Appropriate surveillance and management of at-risk individuals can be expected to improve life expectancy (NORD, 2017). Although patients with the most common forms of EDS/HSD do not have decreased life expectancy, the disorders may profoundly impact their quality of life. Longitudinal studies of individuals with different types of EDS/HSD would increase understanding of the clinical course of the disorders; their effects on functioning; and potentially the impact of interventions, including reasonable accommodations, on participation in work and school.

EMERGING TREATMENTS

Emerging treatments or interventions for EDS/HSD are limited; clinical trials evaluating the efficacy of various treatments, aimed not only at the underlying disease but also at the specific disease-associated manifestations, are generally lacking. Several ongoing clinical trials have been registered in ClinicalTrials.gov (NLM, 2022). As of early February 2022, the database included a total of 46 active clinical trials for EDS, almost all of them in the United States and Europe (mainly France). Some trials target specific subtypes of EDS. Several trials have been completed; their results have not yet been published, but it is reasonable to expect this to occur in the next couple of years. Participants are actively being recruited for still other trials. All of these trials have been designed to address basic mechanisms of disease, secondary impairments, and/or the efficacy of various interventions with respect to function. A wide variety of interventions are being tested, including drugs, rehabilitation strategies, behavioral interventions, and assistive devices, among others.

FINDINGS AND CONCLUSIONS

Findings

4-1. The Ehlers-Danlos syndromes (EDS) are a group of multisystem, heritable disorders of connective tissue (HDCTs) that share common elements of joint hypermobility and skin and soft tissue involvement. Hypermobility spectrum disorders (HSD) are also multisystem connective tissue disorders that are clinically similar to hypermobile EDS (hEDS) with respect to their manifestations and management.

4-2. Many factors, including underdiagnosis, lead to an underestimate of the prevalence of EDS/HSD.

4-3. EDS/HSD can manifest in physical and mental secondary impairments in any organ system and often in multiple organ systems in a given individual.

4-4. The type and severity of physical and mental manifestations associated with EDS/HSD often vary both among individuals and throughout an affected individual's lifetime. Epidemiologic evidence supports multi–organ system manifestations, high treatment burden, and high disease burden.

4-5. The pathophysiologic relationships between EDS/HSD and many of their manifestations and comorbid conditions are unclear, and the evidence linking them is primarily associative.

4-6. Diagnosis of EDS/HSD is based on established clinical criteria, and most, though not all, types can be confirmed through genetic testing.

4-7. Diagnosis of hEDS and HSD is based solely on clinical criteria, since neither has a known genetic test. Understanding of and diagnostic criteria for hEDS and HSD continue to evolve.

4-8. There are currently no curative treatments for EDS or HSD. Management of the disorders involves early diagnosis and recognition; monitoring; and treatment of the manifestations in multiple organ systems, including treatment of associated physical and mental secondary impairments present at the time of identification and preventive measures to lessen or prevent problems that may develop over time.

4-9. The prognosis and clinical course of EDS/HSD depend on individual patient factors, which vary greatly among affected individuals and are often related to the severity of disease-associated physical and mental impairments, as well as the EDS/HSD type.

4-10. Individuals with vascular EDS (vEDS) have a decreased life expectancy, with a median survival age of 46 for males and 54 for females.

4-11. Diagnosis and management of EDS and HSD involve specialists across multiple physical and mental health disciplines.

4-12. Delayed diagnosis may result in a lack of or inappropriate management that may exacerbate physical and mental manifestations of EDS/HSD. Unanticipated risks and harms may attend routine procedures and therapies that carry EDS/HSD-specific risks, such as tissue fragility and physiologic reactivity resulting from autonomic and immune dysregulation.

4-13. EDS/HSD can affect individuals' everyday physical and mental functioning, particularly as a result of limitations associated with pain, fatigue, and anxiety.

4-14. Secondary impairments in any of the body systems can be severe and affect the functioning of individuals with EDS/HSD.

4-15. Physical and mental secondary impairments associated with EDS/HSD often manifest or worsen during puberty, especially in females. Males with vEDS are at higher risk for complications during puberty.

4-16. Pregnancy can be a high-risk condition in some individuals with EDS; women with vEDS have an increased risk of uterine rupture or peripartum hemorrhage.

4-17. Following trauma or surgery, individuals with versus those without EDS/HSD often have a worse trajectory in terms of both length of recovery and frequency of complications.

Conclusions

4-1. EDS and HSD have multiple clinical manifestations that, individually or in combination, can cause functional limitations of varying severity. Some manifestations may become apparent only with age, and the types and severity of manifestations may vary throughout an affected individual's lifetime.

4-2. Development of a screening tool to identify EDS/HSD could provide timely diagnosis of the disorders and help mitigate the negative effects of delayed diagnosis and EDS/HSD-specific risks that may attend routine procedures and therapies.

4-3. Management of EDS/HSD requires a multidisciplinary approach and involves early diagnosis of the multisystem findings, treatment of associated physical and mental secondary impairments, and measures to reduce or prevent problems that may present over time.

4-4. More research is needed on the pathophysiological mechanisms of EDS/HSD and their comorbid conditions and the implications for appropriate management and outcomes of the many secondary impairments associated with EDS/HSD.

4-5. Longitudinal studies of individuals with different types of EDS/HSD would increase understanding of the clinical course of the disorders; their effects on physical and mental functioning; and potentially the impact of interventions, including reasonable accommodations, on participation in work and school.

4-6. Health care providers need to be aware of the EDS/HSD-specific risks that may attend routine procedures and therapies.

REFERENCES

Abu, A., M. Frydman, D. Marek, E. Pras, U. Nir, H. Reznik-Wolf, and E. Pras. 2008. Deleterious mutations in the zinc-finger 469 gene cause brittle cornea syndrome. *American Journal of Human Genetics* 82(5):1217-1222. https://doi.org/10.1016/j.ajhg.2008.04.001.

Agarwal, A. K., R. Garg, A. Ritch, and P. Sarkar. 2007. Postural orthostatic tachycardia syndrome. *Postgraduate Medical Journal* 83(981):478-480. https://doi.org/10.1136/pgmj.2006.055046.

Anxiety & Depression Association of America. 2022. *Chronic pain*. https://adaa.org/understanding-anxiety/related-illnesses/other-related-conditions/chronic-pain (accessed March 7, 2022).

Arendt-Nielsen, L., S. Kaalund, P. Bjerring, and B. Høgsaa. 1990. Insufficient effect of local analgesics in Ehlers Danlos type III patients (connective tissue disorder). *Acta Anaesthesiologica Scandinavica* 34(5):358-361. https://doi.org/10.1111/j.1399-6576.1990.tb03103.x.

Atzinger, C. L., R. A. Meyer, P. R. Khoury, Z. Gao, and B. T. Tinkle. 2011. Cross-sectional and longitudinal assessment of aortic root dilation and valvular anomalies in hypermobile and classic Ehlers-Danlos syndrome. *Journal of Pediatrics* 158(5):826-830.e821. https://doi.org/10.1016/j.jpeds.2010.11.023.

Aubry-Rozier, B., A. Schwitzguebel, F. Valerio, J. Tanniger, C. Paquier, C. Berna, T. Hügle, and C. Benaim. 2021. Are patients with hypermobile Ehlers–Danlos syndrome or hypermobility spectrum disorder so different? *Rheumatology International* 41(10):1785-1794. https://doi.org/10.1007/s00296-021-04968-3.

Baeza-Velasco, C., P. Espinoza, A. Bulbena, A. Bulbena-Cabré, M. Seneque, and S. Guillaume. 2022. Hypermobility spectrum disorders/Ehlers–Danlos syndrome and disordered eating behavior. In *Hidden and Lesser-known Disordered Eating Behaviors in Medical and Psychiatric Conditions*, edited by E. Manzato, M. Cuzzolaro and L. M. Donini. Switzerland: Springer Nature. https://link.springer.com/chapter/10.1007%2F978-3-030-81174-7_28#citeas.

Baeza-Velasco, C., M. C. Gély-Nargeot, A. Bulbena Vilarrasa, and J. F. Bravo. 2011. Joint hypermobility syndrome: Problems that require psychological intervention. *Rheumatology International* 31(9):1131-1136. https://doi.org/10.1007/s00296-011-1839-5.

Bascom, R., R. Dhingra, and C. A. Francomano. 2021a. Respiratory manifestations in the Ehlers–Danlos syndromes. *American Journal of Medical Genetics Part C: Seminars in Medical Genetics* 187(4):533-548. https://doi.org/10.1002/ajmg.c.31953.

Bascom, R., R. Dhingra, C. A. Francomano, and J. R. Schubart. 2021b. A case–control study of respiratory medication and co-occurring gastrointestinal prescription burden among persons with Ehlers–Danlos syndromes. *American Journal of Medical Genetics Part C: Seminars in Medical Genetics* 187(4):549-560. https://doi.org/10.1002/ajmg.c.31947.

Bathen, T., A. B. Hångmann, M. Hoff, L. Andersen, and S. Rand-Hendriksen. 2013. Multidisciplinary treatment of disability in Ehlers-Danlos syndrome hypermobility type/hypermobility syndrome: A pilot study using a combination of physical and cognitive-behavioral therapy on 12 women. *American Journal of Medical Genetics. Part A* 161a(12):3005-3011. https://doi.org/10.1002/ajmg.a.36060.

Baumann, M., C. Giunta, B. Krabichler, F. Rüschendorf, N. Zoppi, M. Colombi, R. E. Bittner, S. Quijano-Roy, F. Muntoni, S. Cirak, G. Schreiber, Y. Zou, Y. Hu, N. B. Romero, R. Y. Carlier, A. Amberger, A. Deutschmann, V. Straub, M. Rohrbach, B. Steinmann, K. Rostásy, D. Karall, C. G. Bönnemann, J. Zschocke, and C. Fauth. 2012. Mutations in *FKBP14* cause a variant of Ehlers-Danlos syndrome with progressive kyphoscoliosis, myopathy, and hearing loss. *American Journal of Human Genetics* 90(2):201-216. https://doi.org/10.1016/j.ajhg.2011.12.004.

Beighton, P. 1970. The Ehlers-Danlos syndrome. *Annals of the Rheumatic Diseases* 29(3):332-333. https://doi.org/10.1136/ard.29.3.332.

Beighton, P. H., and F. T. Horan. 1970. Dominant inheritance in familial generalised articular hypermobility. *Journal of Bone and Joint Surgery (British Volume)* 52(1):145-147. https://doi.org/10.1302/0301-620X.52B1.145.

Beighton, P., L. Solomon, and C. L. Soskolne. 1973. Articular mobility in an African population. *Annals of the Rheumatic Diseases* 32(5):413-418. https://doi.org/10.1136/ard.32.5.413.

Beighton, P., A. de Paepe, D. Danks, G. Finidori, T. Gedde-Dahl, R. Goodman, J. G. Hall, D. W. Hollister, W. Horton, V. A. McKusick, J. M. Opitz, F. M. Pope, R. E. Pyeritz, D. L. Rimoin, D. Sillence, J. W. Spranger, E. Thompson, P. Tsipouras, D. Viljoen, I. Winship, I. Young. 1988. International nosology of heritable disorders of connective tissue, Berlin, 1986. *American Journal of Medical Genetics* 29(3):581-594. https://doi.org/10.1002/ajmg.1320290316.

Beighton, P., A. De Paepe, B. Steinmann, P. Tsipouras, and R. J. Wenstrup. 1998. Ehlers-Danlos syndromes: Revised nosology, Villefranche, 1997. Ehlers-Danlos national foundation (USA) and Ehlers-Danlos support group (UK). *American Journal of Medical Genetics* 77(1):31-37. https://doi.org/10.1002/(sici)1096-8628(19980428)77:1<31::aid-ajmg8>3.0.co;2-o.

Berglund, B., C. Pettersson, M. Pigg, and P. Kristiansson. 2015. Self-reported quality of life, anxiety and depression in individuals with Ehlers-Danlos syndrome (EDS): A questionnaire study. *BMC Musculoskeletal Disorders* 16(1):89. https://doi.org/10.1186/s12891-015-0549-7.

Blackburn, P. R., Z. Xu, K. E. Tumelty, R. W. Zhao, W. J. Monis, K. G. Harris, J. M. Gass, M. A. Cousin, N. J. Boczek, M. V. Mitkov, M. A. Cappel, C. A. Francomano, J. E. Parisi, E. W. Klee, E. Faqeih, F. S. Alkuraya, M. D. Layne, N. B. McDonnell, and P. S. Atwal. 2018. Bi-allelic alterations in *AEBP1* lead to defective collagen assembly and connective tissue structure resulting in a variant of Ehlers-Danlos syndrome. *American Journal of Human Genetics* 102(4):696-705. https://doi.org/10.1016/j.ajhg.2018.02.018.

Bloom, L., P. Byers, C. Francomano, B. Tinkle, and F. Malfait. 2017. The international consortium on the Ehlers–Danlos syndromes. *American Journal of Medical Genetics Part C: Seminars in Medical Genetics* 175(1):5-7. https://doi.org/10.1002/ajmg.c.31547.

Bloom, L., J. Schubart, R. Bascom, A. Hakim, and C. A. Francomano. 2021. The power of patient-led global collaboration. *American Journal of Medical Genetics Part C: Seminars in Medical Genetics* 187(4):425-428. https://doi.org/10.1002/ajmg.c.31942.

Bogni, M., A. Bassotti, G. Leocata, F. Barretta, A. Brunani, P. A. Bertazzi, L. Riboldi, and L. M. Vigna. 2015. Workers with Ehlers-Danlos syndrome: Indications for health surveillance and suitable job assignment. *Medicina del Lavoro* 106(1):23-35. https://mattioli1885journals.com/index.php/lamedicinadellavoro/article/view/2990.

Bonadonna, P., M. Bonifacio, and R. Zanotti. 2016. Mast cell disorders in drug hypersensitivity. *Current Pharmaceutical Design* 22(45):6862-6869. https://doi.org/10.2174/1381612822666160928121857.

Bowen, J. M., G. J. Sobey, N. P. Burrows, M. Colombi, M. E. Lavallee, F. Malfait, and C. A. Francomano. 2017. Ehlers-Danlos syndrome, classical type. *American Journal of Medical Genetics Part C: Seminars in Medical Genetics* 175(1):27-39. https://doi.org/10.1002/ajmg.c.31548.

Brady, A. F., S. Demirdas, S. Fournel-Gigleux, N. Ghali, C. Giunta, I. Kapferer-Seebacher, T. Kosho, R. Mendoza-Londono, M. F. Pope, M. Rohrbach, T. Van Damme, A. Vandersteen, C. van Mourik, N. Voermans, J. Zschocke, and F. Malfait. 2017. The Ehlers-Danlos syndromes, rare types. *American Journal of Medical Genetics Part C: Seminars in Medical Genetics* 175(1):70-115. https://doi.org/10.1002/ajmg.c.31550.

Brock, I., W. Prendergast, and A. Maitland. 2021. Mast cell activation disease and immunoglobulin deficiency in patients with hypermobile Ehlers-Danlos syndrome/hypermobility spectrum disorder. *American Journal of Medical Genetics. Part C: Seminars in Medical Genetics* 187(4):473-481. https://doi.org/10.1002/ajmg.c.31940.

Bulbena, A., J. C. Duro, A. Mateo, M. Porta, and J. Vallejo. 1988. Joint hypermobility syndrome and anxiety disorders. *The Lancet* 332(8612):694. https://doi.org/10.1016/S0140-6736(88)90514-4.

Bulbena, A., J. C. Duró, M. Porta, S. Faus, R. Vallescar, and R. Martín-Santos. 1992. Clinical assessment of hypermobility of joints: Assembling criteria. *Journal of Rheumatology* 19(1):115-122.

Bulbena, A., N. Mallorquí-Bagué, G. Pailhez, S. Rosado, I. González, J. Blanch-Rubió, and J. Carbonell. 2014. Self-reported screening questionnaire for the assessment of joint hypermobility syndrome (SQ-CH), a collagen condition, in Spanish population. *The European Journal of Psychiatry* 28:17-26. https://dx.doi.org/10.4321/S0213-61632014000100002.

Bulbena, A., G. Pailhez, A. Bulbena-Cabré, N. Mallorquí-Bagué, and C. Baeza-Velasco. 2015. Joint hypermobility, anxiety and psychosomatics: Two and a half decades of progress toward a new phenotype. *Advances in Psychosomatic Medicine* 34:143-157. https://doi.org/10.1159/000369113.

Bulbena, A., C. Baeza-Velasco, A. Bulbena-Cabré, G. Pailhez, H. Critchley, P. Chopra, N. Mallorquí-Bagué, C. Frank, and S. Porges. 2017. Psychiatric and psychological aspects in the Ehlers–Danlos syndromes. *American Journal of Medical Genetics Part C: Seminars in Medical Genetics* 175(1):237-245. https://doi.org/10.1002/ajmg.c.31544.

Bulbena-Cabré, A., C. Baeza-Velasco, S. Rosado-Figuerola, and A. Bulbena. 2021. Updates on the psychological and psychiatric aspects of the Ehlers-Danlos syndromes and hypermobility spectrum disorders. *American Journal of Medical Genetics Part C: Seminars in Medical Genetics* 187(4):482-490. https://doi.org/10.1002/ajmg.c.31955.

Burcharth, J., and J. Rosenberg. 2012. Gastrointestinal surgery and related complications in patients with Ehlers-Danlos syndrome: A systematic review. *Digestive Surgery* 29(4):349-357. https://dx.doi.org/10.1159/000343738.

Burkitt Wright, E. M. M., H. L. Spencer, S. B. Daly, F. D. C. Manson, L. A. H. Zeef, J. Urquhart, N. Zoppi, R. Bonshek, I. Tosounidis, M. Mohan, C. Madden, A. Dodds, K. E. Chandler, S. Banka, L. Au, J. Clayton-Smith, N. Khan, L. G. Biesecker, M. Wilson, M. Rohrbach, M. Colombi, C. Giunta, and G. C. M. Black. 2011. Mutations in *PRDM5* in brittle cornea syndrome identify a pathway regulating extracellular matrix development and maintenance. *American Journal of Human Genetics* 88(6):767-777. https://doi.org/10.1016/j.ajhg.2011.05.007.

Byers, P. H. 2019. Vascular Ehlers-Danlos syndrome. In *GeneReviews® [Internet]*, edited by M. P. Adam, H. H. Ardinger, R. A. Pagon, S. E. Wallace, L. J. H. Bean, K. W. Gripp, G. M. Mirzaa, and A. Amemiya. Seattle, WA: University of Washington; 1993-2022. https://www.ncbi.nlm.nih.gov/books/NBK1494/.

Byers, P. H., J. Belmont, J. Black, J. De Backer, M. Frank, X. Jeunemaitre, D. Johnson, M. Pepin, L. Robert, L. Sanders, and N. Wheeldon. 2017. Diagnosis, natural history, and management in vascular Ehlers-Danlos syndrome. *American Journal of Medical Genetics Part C: Seminars in Medical Genetics* 175(1):40-47. https://doi.org/10.1002/ajmg.c.31553.

Carter, C., and J. Wilkinson. 1964. Persistent joint laxity and congenital dislocation of the hip. *Journal of Bone and Joint Surgery (British Volume)* 46:40-45. https://doi.org/10.1302/0301-620X.46B1.40.

Castori, M. 2012. Ehlers-Danlos syndrome, hypermobility type: An underdiagnosed hereditary connective tissue disorder with mucocutaneous, articular, and systemic manifestations. *ISRN Dermatology* 2012:751768. https://doi.org/10.5402/2012/751768.

Castori, M. 2013a. Joint hypermobility syndrome (a.k.a. Ehlers-Danlos syndrome, hypermobility type): An updated critique. *Italian Journal of Dermatology and Venereology* 148(1):13-36.

Castori, M. 2013b. Surgical recommendations in Ehlers-Danlos syndrome(s) need patient classification: The example of Ehlers-Danlos syndrome hypermobility type (a.k.a. joint hypermobility syndrome). *Digestive Surgery* 29(6):453-455. https://doi.org/10.1159/000346068.

Castori, M. 2016. Pain in Ehlers-Danlos syndromes: Manifestations, therapeutic strategies and future perspectives. *Expert Opinion on Orphan Drugs* 4(11):1145-1158. https://doi.org/10.1080/21678707.2016.1238302.

Castori, M., S. Morlino, C. Celletti, M. Celli, A. Morrone, M. Colombi, F. Camerota, and P. Grammatico. 2012a. Management of pain and fatigue in the joint hypermobility syndrome (a.k.a. Ehlers–Danlos syndrome, hypermobility type): Principles and proposal for a multidisciplinary approach. *American Journal of Medical Genetics. Part A* 158A(8):2055-2070. https://doi.org/10.1002/ajmg.a.35483.

Castori, M., S. Morlino, C. Dordoni, C. Celletti, F. Camerota, M. Ritelli, A. Morrone, M. Venturini, P. Grammatico, and M. Colombi. 2012b. Gynecologic and obstetric implications of the joint hypermobility syndrome (a.k.a. Ehlers–Danlos syndrome hypermobility type) in 82 Italian patients. *American Journal of Medical Genetics. Part A* 158A(9):2176-2182. https://doi.org/10.1002/ajmg.a.35506.

Castori, M., S. Morlino, G. Pascolini, C. Blundo, and P. Grammatico. 2015. Gastrointestinal and nutritional issues in joint hypermobility syndrome/Ehlers-Danlos syndrome, hypermobility type. *American Journal of Medical Genetics Part C: Seminars in Medical Genetics* 169C(1):54-75. https://doi.org/10.1002/ajmg.c.31431.

Castori, M., B. Tinkle, H. Levy, R. Grahame, F. Malfait, and A. Hakim. 2017. A framework for the classification of joint hypermobility and related conditions. *American Journal of Medical Genetics Part C: Seminars in Medical Genetics* 175(1):148-157. https://doi.org/10.1002/ajmg.c.31539.

Chelimsky, G., and T. Chelimsky. 2018. The gastrointestinal symptoms present in patients with postural tachycardia syndrome: A review of the literature and overview of treatment. *Autonomic Neuroscience* 215:70-77. https://doi.org/10.1016/j.autneu.2018.09.003.

Chohan, K., N. Mittal, L. McGillis, L. Lopez-Hernandez, E. Camacho, M. Rachinsky, D. S. Mina, W. D. Reid, C. M. Ryan, K. A. Champagne, A. Orchanian-Cheff, H. Clarke, and D. Rozenberg. 2021. A review of respiratory manifestations and their management in Ehlers-Danlos syndromes and hypermobility spectrum disorders. *Chronic Respiratory Disease* 18:14799731211025313. https://doi.org/10.1177/14799731211025313.

Colige, A., A. L. Sieron, S. W. Li, U. Schwarze, E. Petty, W. Wertelecki, W. Wilcox, D. Krakow, D. H. Cohn, W. Reardon, P. H. Byers, C. M. Lapière, D. J. Prockop, and B. V. Nusgens. 1999. Human Ehlers-Danlos syndrome type VII C and bovine dermatosparaxis are caused by mutations in the procollagen I N-proteinase gene. *American Journal of Human Genetics* 65(2):308-317. https://doi.org/10.1086/302504.

Copetti, M., S. Morlino, M. Colombi, P. Grammatico, A. Fontana, and M. Castori. 2019. Severity classes in adults with hypermobile Ehlers–Danlos syndrome/hypermobility spectrum disorders: A pilot study of 105 Italian patients. *Rheumatology* 58(10):1722-1730. https://doi.org/10.1093/rheumatology/kez029.

Coupal, K. E., N. D. Heeney, B. C. D. Hockin, R. Ronsley, K. Armstrong, S. Sanatani, and V. E. Claydon. 2019. Pubertal hormonal changes and the autonomic nervous system: Potential role in pediatric orthostatic intolerance. *Frontiers in Neuroscience* 13:1197. https://doi.org/10.3389/fnins.2019.01197.

D'Hondt, S., T. Van Damme, and F. Malfait. 2018. Vascular phenotypes in nonvascular subtypes of the Ehlers-Danlos syndrome: A systematic review. *Genetics in Medicine* 20(6):562-573. https://doi.org/10.1038/gim.2017.138.

De Baets, S., P. Calders, L. Verhoost, M. Coussens, I. Dewandele, F. Malfait, G. Vanderstraeten, G. Van Hove, and D. Van de Velde. 2021. Patient perspectives on employment participation in the "hypermobile Ehlers-Danlos syndrome." *Disability and Rehabilitation* 43(5):668-677. https://doi.org/10.1080/09638288.2019.1636316.

De Coster, P. J., L. I. Van den Berghe, and L. C. Martens. 2005. Generalized joint hypermobility and temporomandibular disorders: Inherited connective tissue disease as a model with maximum expression. *Journal of Orofacial Pain* 19(1):47-57.

De Wandele, I., P. Calders, W. Peersman, S. Rimbaut, T. De Backer, F. Malfait, A. De Paepe, and L. Rombaut. 2014a. Autonomic symptom burden in the hypermobility type of Ehlers–Danlos syndrome: A comparative study with two other EDS types, fibromyalgia, and healthy controls. *Seminars in Arthritis and Rheumatism* 44(3):353-361. https://doi.org/10.1016/j.semarthrit.2014.05.013.

De Wandele, I., L. Rombaut, L. Leybaert, P. Van de Borne, T. De Backer, F. Malfait, A. De Paepe, and P. Calders. 2014b. Dysautonomia and its underlying mechanisms in the hypermobility type of Ehlers-Danlos syndrome. *Seminars in Arthritis and Rheumatism* 44(1):93-100. https://doi.org/10.1016/j.semarthrit.2013.12.006.

Delbaere, S., T. Dhooge, D. Syx, F. Petit, N. Goemans, A. Destrée, O. Vanakker, R. De Rycke, S. Symoens, and F. Malfait. 2020. Novel defects in collagen XII and VI expand the mixed myopathy/Ehlers-Danlos syndrome spectrum and lead to variant-specific alterations in the extracellular matrix. *Genetics in Medicine* 22(1):112-123. https://doi.org/10.1038/s41436-019-0599-6.

Demmler, J. C., M. D. Atkinson, E. J. Reinhold, E. Choy, R. A. Lyons, and S. T. Brophy. 2019. Diagnosed prevalence of Ehlers-Danlos syndrome and hypermobility spectrum disorder in Wales, UK: A national electronic cohort study and case–control comparison. *BMJ Open* 9(11):e031365. https://doi.org/10.1136/bmjopen-2019-031365.

Dhingra, R., R. Bascom, E. Thompson, C. A. Francomano, and J. R. Schubart. 2021a. Gastrointestinal medication burden among persons with the Ehlers-Danlos syndromes. *Neurogastroenterology and Motility* 33(7):e14077. https://doi.org/10.1111/nmo.14077.

Dhingra, R., A. Hakim, R. Bascom, C. A. Francomano, and J. R. Schubart. 2021b. Prescription claims for immunomodulator and anti-inflammatory drugs among persons with Ehlers-Danlos syndromes. *Arthritis Care & Research*. https://doi.org/10.1002/acr.24819.

Drugs.com. 2021. *What drugs should you avoid with Ehlers-Danlos syndrome?* Medically reviewed by Sally Chao, MD. https://www.drugs.com/medical-answers/drugs-avoid-ehlers-danlos-syndrome-3559403/ (accessed February 14, 2022).

Dündar, M., T. Müller, Q. Zhang, J. Pan, B. Steinmann, J. Vodopiutz, R. Gruber, T. Sonoda, B. Krabichler, G. Utermann, J. U. Baenziger, L. Zhang, and A. R. Janecke. 2009. Loss of dermatan-4-sulfotransferase 1 function results in adducted thumb-clubfoot syndrome. *American Journal of Human Genetics* 85(6):873-882. https://doi.org/10.1016/j.ajhg.2009.11.010.

Eagleton, M. 2016. Arterial complications of vascular Ehlers-Danlos syndrome. *Journal of VascularSurgery* 64(6):1869-1880. https://doi.org/10.1016/j.jvs.2016.06.120.

Ezpeleta, L., J. B. Navarro, N. Osa, E. Penelo, and A. Bulbena. 2018. Joint hypermobility classes in 9-year-old children from the general population and anxiety symptoms. *Journal of Developmental and Behavioral Pediatrics* 39(6):481-488. https://doi.org/10.1097/dbp.0000000000000577.

Feldman, E. C. H., D. P. Hivick, P. M. Slepian, S. T. Tran, P. Chopra, and R. N. Greenley. 2020. Pain symptomatology and management in pediatric Ehlers-Danlos syndrome: A review. *Children (Basel)* 7(9):146. https://doi.org/10.3390/children7090146.

Fikree, A., G. Chelimsky, H. Collins, K. Kovacic, and Q. Aziz. 2017. Gastrointestinal involvement in the Ehlers-Danlos syndromes. *American Journal of Medical Genetics Part C: Seminars in Medical Genetics* 175(1):181-187. https://doi.org/10.1002/ajmg.c.31546.

Gaisl, T., C. Giunta, D. J. Bratton, K. Sutherland, C. Schlatzer, N. Sievi, D. Franzen, P. A. Cistulli, M. Rohrbach, and M. Kohler. 2017. Obstructive sleep apnoea and quality of life in Ehlers-Danlos syndrome: A parallel cohort study. *Thorax* 72(8):729-735. https://doi.org/10.1136/thoraxjnl-2016-209560.

Gilliam, E., J. D. Hoffman, and G. Yeh. 2020. Urogenital and pelvic complications in the Ehlers-Danlos syndromes and associated hypermobility spectrum disorders: A scoping review. *Clinical Genetics* 97(1):168-178. https://doi.org/10.1111/cge.13624.

Giunta, C., N. H. Elçioglu, B. Albrecht, G. Eich, C. Chambaz, A. R. Janecke, H. Yeowell, M. Weis, D. R. Eyre, M. Kraenzlin, and B. Steinmann. 2008. Spondylocheiro dysplastic form of the Ehlers-Danlos syndrome—An autosomal-recessive entity caused by mutations in the zinc transporter gene *SLC39A13*. *American Journal of Human Genetics* 82(6):1290-1305. https://doi.org/10.1016/j.ajhg.2008.05.001.

Gould, G. M., and W. L. Pyle. 1897. *Anomalies and curiosities of medicine*. Philadelphia: W.B. Saunders. https://collections.nlm.nih.gov/catalog/nlm:nlmuid-57221200R-bk.

Guier, C., G. Shi, C. Ledford, M. Taunton, M. Heckman, and B. Wilke. 2020. Primary total hip arthroplasty in patients with Ehlers-Danlos syndrome: A retrospective matched-cohort study. *Arthroplasty Today* 6(3):386-389. https://dx.doi.org/10.1016/j.artd.2020.05.006.

Hakim, A. J., and R. Grahame. 2003. A simple questionnaire to detect hypermobility: An adjunct to the assessment of patients with diffuse musculoskeletal pain. *International Journal of Clinical Practice* 57(3):163-166.

Hakim, A., R. Grahame, P. Norris, and C. Hopper. 2005. Local anaesthetic failure in joint hypermobility syndrome. *Journal of the Royal Society of Medicine* 98(2):84-85. https://www.ncbi.nlm.nih.gov/pmc/articles/PMC1079398/.

Hakim, A., I. De Wandele, C. O'Callaghan, A. Pocinki, and P. Rowe. 2017a. Chronic fatigue in Ehlers-Danlos syndrome-hypermobile type. *American Journal of Medical Genetics Part C: Seminars in Medical Genetics* 175(1):175-180. https://doi.org/10.1002/ajmg.c.31542.

Hakim, A., C. O'Callaghan, I. De Wandele, L. Stiles, A. Pocinki, and P. Rowe. 2017b. Cardiovascular autonomic dysfunction in Ehlers-Danlos syndrome-hypermobile type. *American Journal of Medical Genetics Part C: Seminars in Medical Genetics* 175(1):168-174. https://doi.org/10.1002/ajmg.c.31543.

Hakim, A. J., B. T. Tinkle, and C. A. Francomano. 2021. Ehlers-Danlos syndromes, hypermobility spectrum disorders, and associated co-morbidities: Reports from EDS ECHO. *American Journal of Medical Genetics Part C: Seminars in Medical Genetics* 187(4):413-415. https://doi.org/10.1002/ajmg.c.31954.

Halverson, C. M. E., E. W. Clayton, A. Garcia Sierra, and C. Francomano. 2021. Patients with Ehlers–Danlos syndrome on the diagnostic odyssey: Rethinking complexity and difficulty as a hero's journey. *American Journal of Medical Genetics Part C: Seminars in Medical Genetics* 187(4):416-424. https://doi.org/10.1002/ajmg.c.31935.

Harvard Health Publishing. 2017. *Depression and pain*. https://www.health.harvard.edu/mind-and-mood/depression-and-pain (accessed March 7, 2022).

Hautala, T., J. Heikkinen, K. I. Kivirikko, and R. Myllylä. 1993. A large duplication in the gene for lysyl hydroxylase accounts for the type VI variant of Ehlers-Danlos syndrome in two siblings. *Genomics* 15(2):399-404. https://doi.org/10.1006/geno.1993.1074.

Henderson, F. C., Sr., C. Austin, E. Benzel, P. Bolognese, R. Ellenbogen, C. A. Francomano, C. Ireton, P. Klinge, M. Koby, D. Long, S. Patel, E. L. Singman, and N. C. Voermans. 2017. Neurological and spinal manifestations of the Ehlers-Danlos syndromes. *American Journal of Medical Genetics Part C: Seminars in Medical Genetics* 175(1):195-211. https://doi.org/10.1002/ajmg.c.31549.

Henderson, F. C., C. A. Francomano, M. Koby, K. Tuchman, J. Adcock, and S. Patel. 2019. Cervical medullary syndrome secondary to craniocervical instability and ventral brainstem compression in hereditary hypermobility connective tissue disorders: 5-year follow-up after craniocervical reduction, fusion, and stabilization. *Neurosurgical Review* 42(4):915-936. https://doi.org/10.1007/s10143-018-01070-4.

Hernandez, A. M. C., and J. E. Dietrich. 2020. Gynecologic management of pediatric and adolescent patients with Ehlers-Danlos syndrome. *Journal of Pediatric and Adolescent Gynecology* 33(3):291-295. https://doi.org/10.1016/j.jpag.2019.12.011.

Hicks, D., G. T. Farsani, S. Laval, J. Collins, A. Sarkozy, E. Martoni, A. Shah, Y. Zou, M. Koch, C. G. Bönnemann, M. Roberts, H. Lochmüller, K. Bushby, and V. Straub. 2014. Mutations in the collagen XII gene define a new form of extracellular matrix-related myopathy. *Human Molecular Genetics* 23(9):2353-2363. https://doi.org/10.1093/hmg/ddt637.

Hsieh, F. H. 2018. Gastrointestinal involvement in mast cell activation disorders. *Immunology and Allergy Clinics of North America* 38(3):429-441. https://doi.org/10.1016/j.iac.2018.04.008.

Hugon-Rodin, J., G. Lebègue, S. Becourt, C. Hamonet, and A. Gompel. 2016. Gynecologic symptoms and the influence on reproductive life in 386 women with hypermobility type Ehlers-Danlos syndrome: A cohort study. *Orphanet Journal of Rare Diseases* 11(1):124. https://doi.org/10.1186/s13023-016-0511-2.

Inayet, N., J. O. Hayat, A. Kaul, M. Tome, A. Child, and A. Poullis. 2018. Gastrointestinal symptoms in Marfan syndrome and hypermobile Ehlers-Danlos syndrome. *Gastroenterology Research and Practice* 2018:4854701. https://doi.org/10.1155/2018/4854701.

International Consortium (International Consortium on Ehlers-Danlos Syndromes and Related Disorders). 2017. *Diagnostic criteria for hypermobile Ehlers-Danlos syndrome (hEDS)*. https://www.ehlers-danlos.com/heds-diagnostic-checklist/ (accessed February 14, 2022).

Jackson, S. C., L. Odiaman, R. T. Card, J. G. van der Bom, and M. C. Poon. 2013. Suspected collagen disorders in the bleeding disorder clinic: A case-control study. *Haemophilia* 19(2):246-250. https://doi.org/10.1111/hae.12020.

Jansen, L. H. 1955. Mode of transmission in Ehlers-Danlos disease. *Journal de Génétique Humaine* 4(4):204-218.

Jayarajan, S. N., B. D. Downing, L. A. Sanchez, and J. Jim. 2020. Trends of vascular surgery procedures in Marfan syndrome and Ehlers-Danlos syndrome. *Vascular* 28(6):834-841. https://doi.org/10.1177/1708538120925597.

Johnson, S. A. M., and H. F. Falls. 1949. Ehlers-Danlos syndrome: A clinical and genetic study. *Archives of Dermatology and Syphilology* 60(1):82-105. https://doi.org/10.1001/archderm.1949.01530010085006.

Juul-Kristensen, B., K. Schmedling, L. Rombaut, H. Lund, and R. H. H. Engelbert. 2017. Measurement properties of clinical assessment methods for classifying generalized joint hypermobility—A systematic review. *American Journal of Medical Genetics Part C: Seminars in Medical Genetics* 175(1):116-147. https://doi.org/10.1002/ajmg.c.31540.

Kalisch, L., C. Hamonet, C. Bourdon, L. Montalescot, C. de Cazotte, and C. Baeza-Velasco. 2020. Predictors of pain and mobility disability in the hypermobile Ehlers-Danlos syndrome. *Disability and Rehabilitation* 42(25):3679-3686. https://doi.org/10.1080/09638288.2019.1608595.

Kapferer-Seebacher, I., M. Pepin, R. Werner, T. J. Aitman, A. Nordgren, H. Stoiber, N. Thielens, C. Gaboriaud, A. Amberger, A. Schossig, R. Gruber, C. Giunta, M. Bamshad, E. Björck, C. Chen, D. Chitayat, M. Dorschner, M. Schmitt-Egenolf, C. J. Hale, D. Hanna, H. C. Hennies, I. Heiss-Kisielewsky, A. Lindstrand, P. Lundberg, A. L. Mitchell, D. A. Nickerson, E. Reinstein, M. Rohrbach, N. Romani, M. Schmuth, R. Silver, F. Taylan, A. Vandersteen, J. Vandrovcova, R. Weerakkody, M. Yang, F. M. Pope, P. H. Byers, and J. Zschocke. 2016. Periodontal Ehlers-Danlos syndrome is caused by mutations in *C1R* and *C1S*, which encode subcomponents C1r and C1s of complement. *American Journal of Human Genetics* 99(5):1005-1014. https://doi.org/10.1016/j.ajhg.2016.08.019.

Karthikeyan, A., and N. Venkat-Raman. 2018. Hypermobile Ehlers–Danlos syndrome and pregnancy. *Obstetric Medicine* 11(3):104-109. https://doi.org/10.1177/1753495X18754577.

Kilaru, S. M., K. J. Mukamal, J. W. Nee, S. S. Oza, A. J. Lembo, and J. L. Wolf. 2019. Safety of endoscopy in heritable connective tissue disorders. *American Journal of Gastroenterology* 114(8):1343-1345. doi: 10.14309/ajg.0000000000000189.

Kindgren, E., A. Quiñones Perez, and R. Knez. 2021. Prevalence of ADHD and autism spectrum disorder in children with hypermobility spectrum disorders or hypermobile Ehlers-Danlos syndrome: A retrospective study. *Neuropsychiatric Disease and Treatment* 17:379-388. https://doi.org/10.2147/ndt.S290494.

Klinge, P. M., A. McElroy, J. E. Donahue, T. Brinker, Z. L. Gokaslan, and M. D. Beland. 2021. Abnormal spinal cord motion at the craniocervical junction in hypermobile Ehlers-Danlos patients. *Journal of Neurosurgery* 35(1):18-24. https://doi.org/10.3171/2020.10.Spine201765.

Klinge, P. M., V. Srivastava, A. McElroy, O. P. Leary, Z. Ahmed, J. E. Donahue, T. Brinker, P. De Vloo, and Z. L. Gokaslan. 2022. Diseased filum terminale as a cause of tethered cord syndrome in Ehlers-Danlos syndrome: Histopathology, biomechanics, clinical presentation, and outcome of filum excision. *World Neurosurgery* 162(June):e492–e502. https://doi.org/10.1016/j.wneu.2022.03.038.

Knight, I. 2015. The role of narrative medicine in the management of joint hypermobility syndrome/Ehlers-Danlos syndrome, hypermobility type. *American Journal of Medical Genetics Part C: Seminars in Medical Genetics* 169C(1):123-129. https://doi.org/10.1002/ajmg.c.31428.

Komi, D. E. A, K. Khomtchouk, and P. L. Santa Maria. 2020. A review of the contribution of mast cells in wound healing: Involved molecular and cellular mechanisms. *Clinical Reviews in Allergy & Immunology* 58(3):298-312. https://doi.org/10.1007/s12016-019-08729-w.

Kosashvili, Y., T. Fridman, D. Backstein, O. Safir, and Y. Bar Ziv. 2008. The correlation between pes planus and anterior knee or intermittent low back pain. *Foot & Ankle International* 29(9):910-913. https://doi.org/10.3113/FAI.2008.0910.

Krahe, A. M., R. D. Adams, and L. L. Nicholson. 2018. Features that exacerbate fatigue severity in joint hypermobility syndrome/Ehlers-Danlos syndrome—hypermobility type. *Disability and Rehabilitation* 40(17):1989-1996. https://doi.org/10.1080/09638288.2017.1323022.

Kulas Søborg, M.-L., J. Leganger, J. Rosenberg, and J. Burcharth. 2017. Increased need for gastrointestinal surgery and increased risk of surgery-related complications in patients with Ehlers-Danlos syndrome: A systematic review. *Digestive Surgery* 34(2):161-170. https://dx.doi.org/10.1159/000449106.

Langhinrichsen-Rohling, J., C. L. Lewis, S. McCabe, E. C. Lathan, G. A. Agnew, C. N. Selwyn, and M. E. Gigler. 2021. They've been BITTEN: Reports of institutional and provider betrayal and links with Ehlers-Danlos syndrome patients' current symptoms, unmet needs and healthcare expectations. *Therapeutic Advances in Rare Disease* 2:1-12. https://doi.org/10.1177/26330040211022033.

Last, J. M., ed. 2001. *Dictionary of epidemiology*. Fourth edition. New York: Oxford University Press.

Lam, C. Y., O. S. Palsson, W. E. Whitehead, A. D. Sperber, H. Tornblom, M. Simren, and I. Aziz. 2021. Rome IV functional gastrointestinal disorders and health impairment in subjects with hypermobility spectrum disorders or hypermobile Ehlers-Danlos syndrome. *Clinical Gastroenterology and Hepatology* 19(2):277-287.e273. https://doi.org/10.1016/j.cgh.2020.02.034.

Louie, A., C. Meyerle, C. Francomano, D. Srikumaran, F. Merali, J. J. Doyle, K. Bower, L. Bloom, M. V. Boland, N. Mahoney, Y. Daoud, and E. L. Singman. 2020. Survey of Ehlers-Danlos patients' ophthalmic surgery experiences. *Molecular Genetics & Genomic Medicine* 8(4). https://dx.doi.org/10.1002/mgg3.1155.

Lum, Y. W., B. S. Brooke, and J. H. Black, 3rd. 2011. Contemporary management of vascular Ehlers-Danlos syndrome. *Current Opinion in Cardiology* 26(6):494-501. https://doi.org/10.1097/HCO.0b013e32834ad55a.

Maitland, A. 2020. Mast cell activation syndrome. In *Disjointed: Navigating the diagnosis and management of hypermobile Ehlers-Danlos syndrome and hypermobility spectrum disorders*. 1st ed, edited by D. Jovin. San Francisco: Hidden Stripes Publications. Pp. 217-231.

Malfait, F., C. Francomano, P. Byers, J. Belmont, B. Berglund, J. Black, L. Bloom, J. M. Bowen, A. F. Brady, N. P. Burrows, M. Castori, H. Cohen, M. Colombi, S. Demirdas, J. De Backer, A. De Paepe, S. Fournel-Gigleux, M. Frank, N. Ghali, C. Giunta, R. Grahame, A. Hakim, X. Jeunemaitre, D. Johnson, B. Juul-Kristensen, I. Kapferer-Seebacher, H. Kazkaz, T. Kosho, M. E. Lavallee, H. Levy, R. Mendoza-Londono, M. Pepin, F. M. Pope, E. Reinstein, L. Robert, M. Rohrbach, L. Sanders, G. J. Sobey, T. Van Damme, A. Vandersteen, C. van Mourik, N. Voermans, N. Wheeldon, J. Zschocke, and B. Tinkle. 2017. The 2017 international classification of the Ehlers-Danlos syndromes. *American Journal of Medical Genetics Part C: Seminars in Medical Genetics* 175(1):8-26. https://doi.org/10.1002/ajmg.c.31552.

Mathias, C. J., D. A. Low, V. Iodice, A. P. Owens, M. Kirbis, and R. Grahame. 2011. Postural tachycardia syndrome—Current experience and concepts. *Nature Reviews: Neurology* 8(1):22-34. https://doi.org/10.1038/nrneurol.2011.187.

Mathias, C. J., A. Owens, V. Iodice, and A. Hakim. 2021. Dysautonomia in the Ehlers-Danlos syndromes and hypermobility spectrum disorders—With a focus on the postural tachycardia syndrome. *American Journal of Medical Genetics Part C: Seminars in Medical Genetics* 187(4):510-519. https://doi.org/10.1002/ajmg.c.31951.

Maxwell, A. J. 2020. Dysautonomia. In *Disjointed: Navigating the diagnosis and management of hypermobile Ehlers-Danlos syndrome and hypermobility spectrum disorders*. 1st ed, edited by D. Jovin. San Francisco: Hidden Stripes Publications. Pp. 135-215.

McKusick, V. A. 1956. *Heritable disorders of connective tissue*. 1st ed. St. Louis: C.V. Mosby Company.

McKusick, V. A. 1972. *Heritable disorders of connective tissue*. 4th ed. St. Louis: C.V. Mosby Company.

McNerney, J. E., and W. B. Johnston. 1979. Generalized ligamentous laxity, hallux abducto valgus and the first metatarsocuneiform joint. *Journal of the American Podiatry Association* 69(1):69-82. https://doi.org/10.7547/87507315-69-1-69.

Meester, J., A. Verstraeten, D. Schepers, M. Alaerts, L. Van Laer, and B. L. Loeys. 2017. Differences in manifestations of Marfan syndrome, Ehlers-Danlos syndrome, and Loeys-Dietz syndrome. *Annals of Cardiothoracic Surgery* 6(6):582-594. https://doi.org/10.21037/acs.2017.11.03.

Mehr, S. E., A. Barbul, and C. A. Shibao. 2018. Gastrointestinal symptoms in postural tachycardia syndrome: A systematic review. *Clinical Autonomic Research* 28(4):411-421. https://doi.org/10.1007/s10286-018-0519-x.

Meyer, K. J., C. Chan, L. Hopper, and L. L. Nicholson. 2017. Identifying lower limb specific and generalised joint hypermobility in adults: Validation of the Lower Limb Assessment Score. *BMC Musculoskeletal Disorders* 18(1):514. https://doi.org/10.1186/s12891-017-1875-8.

Miklovic, T., and V. Sieg. 2022. Ehlers Danlos syndrome. In *StatPearls [Internet]*. Treasure Island, FL: StatPearls Publishing. https://www.ncbi.nlm.nih.gov/books/NBK549814/.

Milhorat, T. H., P. A. Bolognese, M. Nishikawa, N. B. McDonnell, and C. A. Francomano. 2007. Syndrome of occipitoatlantoaxial hypermobility, cranial settling, and Chiari malformation type I in patients with hereditary disorders of connective tissue. *Journal of Neurosurgery: Spine* 7(6):601-609. https://doi.org/10.3171/spi-07/12/601.

Mittal, M., D. S. Mina, L. McGillis, A. Weinrib, P. M. Slepian, M. Rachinsky, S. Buryk-Iggers, C. Laflamme, L. Lopez-Hernandez, L. Hussey, J. Katz, L. McLean, D. Rozenberg, L. Liu, Y. Tse, C. Parker, A. Adler, G. Charames, R. Bleakney, C. Veillete, C. J. Nielson, S. Tavares, S. Variano, J. Guzman, H. Faghfoury, and H. Clarke. 2021. The GoodHope Ehlers Danlos Syndrome Clinic: Development and implementation of the first interdisciplinary program for multi-system issues in connective tissue disorders at the Toronto General Hospital. *Orphanet Journal of Rare Diseases* 16(1):357. https://doi.org/10.1186/s13023-021-01962-7.

Moonesinghe, S. R., M. G. Mythen, P. Das, K. M. Rowan, and M. P. Grocott. 2013. Risk stratification tools for predicting morbidity and mortality in adult patients undergoing major surgery: Qualitative systematic review. *Anesthesiology* 119(4):959-981. https://doi.org/10.1097/ALN.0b013e3182a4e94d.

Mu, W., M. Muriello, J. L. Clemens, Y. Wang, C. H. Smith, P. T. Tran, P. C. Rowe, C. A. Francomano, A. D. Kline, and J. Bodurtha. 2019. Factors affecting quality of life in children and adolescents with hypermobile Ehlers-Danlos syndrome/hypermobility spectrum disorders. *American Journal of Medical Genetics. Part A* 179(4):561-569. https://doi.org/10.1002/ajmg.a.61055.

Müller, T., S. Mizumoto, I. Suresh, Y. Komatsu, J. Vodopiutz, M. Dundar, V. Straub, A. Lingenhel, A. Melmer, S. Lechner, J. Zschocke, K. Sugahara, and A. R. Janecke. 2013. Loss of dermatan sulfate epimerase (DSE) function results in musculocontractural Ehlers-Danlos syndrome. *Human Molecular Genetics* 22(18):3761-3772. https://doi.org/10.1093/hmg/ddt227.

Mulvey, M. R., G. J. Macfarlane, M. Beasley, D. P. M. Symmons, K. Lovell, P. Keeley, S. Woby, and J. McBeth. 2013. Modest association of joint hypermobility with disabling and limiting musculoskeletal pain: Results from a large-scale general population–based survey. *Arthritis Care & Research* 65(8):1325-1333. https://doi.org/10.1002/acr.21979.

Murray, B., B. M. Yashar, W. R. Uhlmann, D. J. Clauw, and E. M. Petty. 2013. Ehlers-Danlos syndrome, hypermobility type: A characterization of the patients' lived experience. *American Journal of Medical Genetics. Part A* 161A(12):2981-2988. https://doi.org/10.1002/ajmg.a.36293.

Nakajima, M., S. Mizumoto, N. Miyake, R. Kogawa, A. Iida, H. Ito, H. Kitoh, A. Hirayama, H. Mitsubuchi, O. Miyazaki, R. Kosaki, R. Horikawa, A. Lai, R. Mendoza-Londono, L. Dupuis, D. Chitayat, A. Howard, G. F. Leal, D. Cavalcanti, Y. Tsurusaki, H. Saitsu, S. Watanabe, E. Lausch, S. Unger, L. Bonafé, H. Ohashi, A. Superti-Furga, N. Matsumoto, K. Sugahara, G. Nishimura, and S. Ikegawa. 2013. Mutations in *B3GALT6*, which encodes a glycosaminoglycan linker region enzyme, cause a spectrum of skeletal and connective tissue disorders. *American Journal of Human Genetics* 92(6):927-934. https://doi.org/10.1016/j.ajhg.2013.04.003.

National Institute of Allergy and Infectious Diseases. 2018. *Hereditary alpha tryptasemia and hereditary alpha tryptasemia syndrome FAQ.* https://www.niaid.nih.gov/research/hereditary-alpha-tryptasemia-faq (accessed March 4, 2022).

Nee, J., S. Kilaru, J. Kelley, S. S. Oza, W. Hirsch, S. Ballou, A. Lembo, and J. Wolf. 2019. Prevalence of functional GI diseases and pelvic floor symptoms in Marfan syndrome and Ehlers-Danlos syndrome: A national cohort study. *Journal of Clinical Gastroenterology* 53(9):653-659. https://doi.org/10.1097/MCG.0000000000001173.

Nicholls, A. C., J. Oliver, D. V. Renouf, J. McPheat, A. Palan, and F. M. Pope. 1991. Ehlers-Danlos syndrome type VII: A single base change that causes exon skipping in the type I collagen alpha 2(I) chain. *Human Genetics* 87(2):193-198. https://doi.org/10.1007/bf00204180.

Nicholson, L. L., and C. Chan. 2018. The Upper Limb Hypermobility Assessment Tool: A novel validated measure of adult joint mobility. *Musculoskeletal Science and Practice* 35:38-45. https://doi.org/10.1016/j.msksp.2018.02.006.

NLM (U.S. National Library of Medicine). 2022. *ClinicalTrails.gov.* https://clinicaltrials.gov/ (accessed February 11, 2022).

NORD (National Organization for Rare Disorders). 2017. *Rare disease database: Ehlers-Danlos syndrome.* https://rarediseases.org/rare-diseases/ehlers-danlos-syndrome/ (accessed May 16, 2022).

Okajima, T., S. Fukumoto, K. Furukawa, and T. Urano. 1999. Molecular basis for the progeroid variant of Ehlers-Danlos syndrome. Identification and characterization of two mutations in galactosyltransferase I gene. *Journal of Biological Chemistry* 274(41):28841-28844. https://doi.org/10.1074/jbc.274.41.28841.

Orphanet. 2022a. *Dermatosparaxis Ehlers-Danlos syndrome.* https://www.orpha.net/consor4.01/www/cgi-bin/Disease_Search.php?lng=EN&data_id=4045&Disease_Disease_Search_diseaseGroup=Dermatosparaxis-EDS&Disease_Disease_Search_diseaseType=Pat&Disease(s)/group%20of%20diseases=Dermatosparaxis-Ehlers-Danlos-syndrome&title=Dermatosparaxis%20Ehlers-Danlos%20syndrome&search=Disease_Search_Simple (accessed February 16, 2022).

Orphanet. 2022b. *Musculocontractural Ehlers-Danlos syndrome.* https://www.orpha.net/consor4.01/www/cgi-bin/Disease_Search.php?lng=EN&data_id=3480&Disease_Disease_Search_diseaseGroup=Musculocontractural-EDS&Disease_Disease_Search_diseaseType=Pat&Disease(s)/group%20of%20diseases=Musculocontractural-Ehlers-Danlos-syndrome&title=Musculocontractural%20Ehlers-Danlos%20syndrome&search=Disease_Search_Simple (accessed February 16, 2022).

Pacey, V., L. Tofts, R. D. Adams, C. F. Munns, and L. L. Nicholson. 2015. Quality of life prediction in children with joint hypermobility syndrome. *Journal of Paediatrics and Child Health* 51(7):689-695. https://doi.org/10.1111/jpc.12826.

Palomo-Toucedo, I. C., F. Leon-Larios, M. Reina-Bueno, M. D. C. Vázquez-Bautista, P. V. Munuera-Martínez, and G. Domínguez-Maldonado. 2020. Psychosocial influence of Ehlers-Danlos syndrome in daily life of patients: A qualitative study. *International Journal of Environmental Research and Public Health* 17(17):6425. https://doi.org/10.3390/ijerph17176425.

Parapia, L. A., and C. Jackson. 2008. Ehlers-Danlos syndrome—A historical review. *British Journal of Haematology* 141(1):32-35. https://doi.org/10.1111/j.1365-2141.2008.06994.x.

Patel, M., and V. Khullar. 2021. Urogynaecology and Ehlers-Danlos syndrome. *American Journal of Medical Genetics Part C: Seminars in Medical Genetics* 187(4):579-585. https://doi.org/10.1002/ajmg.c.31959.

Peggs, K. J., H. Nguyen, D. Enayat, N. R. Keller, A. Al-Hendy, and S. R. Raj. 2012. Gynecologic disorders and menstrual cycle lightheadedness in postural tachycardia syndrome. *International Journal of Gynaecology and Obstetrics* 118(3):242-246. https://doi.org/10.1016/j.ijgo.2012.04.014.

Pepin, M., U. Schwarze, A. Superti-Furga, and P. H. Byers. 2000. Clinical and genetic features of Ehlers-Danlos syndrome type IV, the vascular type. *New England Journal of Medicine* 342(10):673-680. https://doi.org/10.1056/nejm200003093421001.

Pepin, M. G., U. Schwarze, K. M. Rice, M. Liu, D. Leistritz, and P. H. Byers. 2014. Survival is affected by mutation type and molecular mechanism in vascular Ehlers-Danlos syndrome (EDS type IV). *Genetics in Medicine* 16(12):881-888. https://doi.org/10.1038/gim.2014.72.

Pezaro, S., G. Pearce, and E. Reinhold. 2018. Hypermobile Ehlers-Danlos syndrome during pregnancy, birth and beyond. *British Journal of Midwifery* 26(4):217-223. https://doi.org/10.12968/bjom.2018.26.4.217.

Pinnell, S. R., S. M. Krane, J. E. Kenzora, and M. J. Glimcher. 1972. A heritable disorder of connective tissue. Hydroxylysine-deficient collagen disease. *New England Journal of Medicine* 286(19):1013-1020. https://doi.org/10.1056/nejm197205112861901.

Puledda, F., A. Viganò, C. Celletti, B. Petolicchio, M. Toscano, E. Vicenzini, M. Castori, G. Laudani, D. Valente, F. Camerota, and V. Di Piero. 2015. A study of migraine characteristics in joint hypermobility syndrome a.k.a. Ehlers-Danlos syndrome, hypermobility type. *Neurological Sciences* 36(8):1417-1424. https://doi.org/10.1007/s10072-015-2173-6.

Pyeritz, R. E. 2000. Ehlers-Danlos syndromes. In *Cecil Textbook of Medicine*. 21st ed. Vol. 1, edited by L. Goldman and J. C. Bennett. Philadelphia: W.B. Saunders. Pp. 1119-1120.

Quatman, C. E., K. R. Ford, G. D. Myer, M. V. Paterno, and T. E. Hewett. 2008. The effects of gender and pubertal status on generalized joint laxity in young athletes. *Journal of Science and Medicine in Sport* 11(3):257-263. https://doi.org/10.1016/j.jsams.2007.05.005.

Ramírez-Paesano, C., A. Juanola Galceran, C. Rodiera Clarens, V. Gilete Garcsía, B. Oliver Abadal, V. Vilchez Cobo, B. Ros Nebot, S. Julián González, L. Cao López, J. Santaliestra Fierro, and J. Rodiera Olivé. 2021. Opioid-free anesthesia for patients with joint hypermobility syndrome undergoing craneo-cervical fixation: A case-series study focused on anti-hyperalgesic approach. *Orphanet Journal of Rare Diseases* 16(1):172. https://doi.org/10.1186/s13023-021-01795-4.

Roma, M., C. L. Marden, I. De Wandele, C. A. Francomano, and P. C. Rowe. 2018. Postural tachycardia syndrome and other forms of orthostatic intolerance in Ehlers-Danlos syndrome. *Autonomic Neuroscience* 215:89-96. https://doi.org/10.1016/j.autneu.2018.02.006.

Rombaut, L., F. Malfait, I. De Wandele, A. Cools, Y. Thijs, A. De Paepe, and P. Calders. 2011. Medication, surgery, and physiotherapy among patients with the hypermobility type of Ehlers-Danlos syndrome. *Archives of Physical Medicine and Rehabilitation* 92(7):1106-1112. https://doi.org/10.1016/j.apmr.2011.01.016.

Ronchese, F. 1936. Dermatorrhexis: With dermatochalasis and arthrochalasis (the so-called Ehlers-Danlos syndrome). *American Journal of Diseases of Children* 51(6):1403-1414. https://doi.org/10.1001/archpedi.1936.01970180149012.

Rotés Querol, J. 1983. *Reumatología clínica*. Barcelona: Espaxs.

Rowe, P. 2022. *The functional impact of orthostatic intolerance in Ehlers-Danlos syndrome.* Paper commissioned by the Committee on Heritable Disorders of Connective Tissue and Disability, National Academies of Sciences, Engineering, and Medicine, Washington, DC.

Rowe, P. C., D. F. Barron, H. Calkins, I. H. Maumenee, P. Y. Tong, and M. T. Geraghty. 1999. Orthostatic intolerance and chronic fatigue syndrome associated with Ehlers-Danlos syndrome. *Journal of Pediatrics* 135(4):494-499. https://doi.org/10.1016/s0022-3476(99)70173-3.

Schalkwijk, J., M. C. Zweers, P. M. Steijlen, W. B. Dean, G. Taylor, I. M. van Vlijmen, B. van Haren, W. L. Miller, and J. Bristow. 2001. A recessive form of the Ehlers-Danlos syndrome caused by tenascin-X deficiency. *New England Journal of Medicine* 345(16):1167-1175. https://doi.org/10.1056/NEJMoa002939.

Schubart, J. R., E. Schaefer, A. J. Hakim, C. A. Francomano, and R. Bascom. 2019a. Use of cluster analysis to delineate symptom profiles in an Ehlers-Danlos syndrome patient population. *Journal of Pain and Symptom Management* 58(3):427-436. https://doi.org/10.1016/j.jpainsymman.2019.05.013.

Schubart, J. R., E. Schaefer, P. Janicki, S. D. Adhikary, A. Schilling, A. J. Hakim, R. Bascom, C. A. Francomano, and S. R. Raj. 2019b. Resistance to local anesthesia in people with the Ehlers-Danlos syndromes presenting for dental surgery. *Journal of Dental Anesthesia and Pain Medicine* 19(5):261. https://dx.doi.org/10.17245/jdapm.2019.19.5.261.

Schubart, J. R., S. E. Mills, E. W. Schaefer, R. Bascom, and C. A. Francomano. 2022. Longitudinal analysis of symptoms in the Ehlers-Danlos syndromes. *American Journal of Medical Genetics. Part A.* 188(4):1204-1213. https://doi.org/10.1002/ajmg.a.62640.

Schwarze, U., R. Hata, V. A. McKusick, H. Shinkai, H. E. Hoyme, R. E. Pyeritz, and P. H. Byers. 2004. Rare autosomal recessive cardiac valvular form of Ehlers-Danlos syndrome results from mutations in the *COL1A2* gene that activate the nonsense-mediated RNA decay pathway. *American Journal of Human Genetics* 74(5):917-930. https://doi.org/10.1086/420794.

Seneviratne, S. L., A. Maitland, and L. Afrin. 2017. Mast cell disorders in Ehlers-Danlos syndrome. *American Journal of Medical Genetics Part C: Seminars in Medical Genetics* 175(1):226-236. https://doi.org/10.1002/ajmg.c.31555.

Sestak, Z. 1962. Ehlers-Danlos syndrome and cutis laxa: An account of families in the Oxford area. *Annals of Human Genetics* 25(4):313-321. https://doi.org/10.1111/j.1469-1809.1962.tb01768.x.

Shalhub, S., P. H. Byers, K. L. Hicks, K. Charlton-Ouw, D. Zarkowsky, D. M. Coleman, F. M. Davis, E. S. Regalado, G. De Caridi, K. N. Weaver, E. M. Miller, M. L. Schermerhorn, K. Shean, G. Oderich, M. Ribeiro, C. Nishikawa, C. A. Behrendt, E. S. Debus, Y. von Kodolitsch, R. J. Powell, M. Pepin, D. M. Milewicz, P. F. Lawrence, and K. Woo. 2019. A multi-institutional experience in the aortic and arterial pathology in individuals with genetically confirmed vascular Ehlers-Danlos syndrome. *Journal of Vascular Surgery* 70(5):1543-1554. https://doi.org/10.1016/j.jvs.2019.01.069.

Song, B., P. Yeh, D. Nguyen, U. Ikpeama, M. Epstein, and J. Harrell. 2020. Ehlers-Danlos syndrome: An analysis of the current treatment options. *Pain Physician* 23(4):429-438.

Sordet, C., A. Cantagrel, T. Schaeverbeke, and J. Sibilia. 2005. Bone and joint disease associated with primary immune deficiencies. *Joint, Bone, Spine: Revue du Rhumatisme* 72(6):503-514. https://doi.org/10.1016/j.jbspin.2004.07.012.

Steinmann, B., P. M. Royce, and A. Superti-Furga. 2002. The Ehlers-Danlos syndrome. In *Connective tissue and its heritable disorders: Molecular, genetic, and medical aspects.* 2nd ed., edited by B. Steinmann and P. M. Royce. New York: Wiley-Liss, Inc. https://doi.org/10.1002/0471221929.ch9.

Tahir, F., T. Bin Arif, Z. Majid, J. Ahmed, and M. Khalid. 2020. Ivabradine in postural orthostatic tachycardia syndrome: A review of the literature. *Cureus* 12(4):e7868. https://doi.org/10.7759/cureus.7868.

Tai, F. W. D., O. S. Palsson, C. Y. Lam, W. E. Whitehead, A. D. Sperber, H. Tornblom, M. Simren, and I. Aziz. 2020. Functional gastrointestinal disorders are increased in joint hypermobility-related disorders with concomitant postural orthostatic tachycardia syndrome. *Neurogastroenterology and Motility* 32(12):e13975. https://doi.org/10.1111/nmo.13975.

Terry, R. H., S. T. Palmer, K. A. Rimes, C. J. Clark, J. V. Simmonds, and J. P. Horwood. 2015. Living with joint hypermobility syndrome: Patient experiences of diagnosis, referral and self-care. *Family Practice* 32(3):354-358. https://doi.org/10.1093/fampra/cmv026.

Tinkle, B. T. 2020. Symptomatic joint hypermobility. *Best Practice & Research: Clinical Rheumatology* 34(3):101508. https://doi.org/10.1016/j.berh.2020.101508.

Tinkle, B., M. Castori, B. Berglund, H. Cohen, R. Grahame, H. Kazkaz, and H. Levy. 2017. Hypermobile Ehlers-Danlos syndrome (a.k.a. Ehlers-Danlos syndrome type III and Ehlers-Danlos syndrome hypermobility type): Clinical description and natural history. *American Journal of Medical Genetics Part C: Seminars in Medical Genetics* 175(1):48-69. https://doi.org/10.1002/ajmg.c.31538.

Tobias, N. 1934. Danlos syndrome associated with congenital lipomatosis. *Archives of Dermatology and Syphilology* 30(4):540-551. https://doi/0.1001/archderm.1934.01460160054008.

Tran, S. T., A. Jagpal, M. L. Koven, C. E. Turek, J. S. Golden, and B. T. Tinkle. 2020. Symptom complaints and impact on functioning in youth with hypermobile Ehlers-Danlos syndrome. *Journal of Child Health Care* 24(3):444-457. https://doi.org/10.1177/1367493519867174.

Tschernogobow, A. 1892. Cutis laxa (presentation at first meeting of Moscow). Dermatologic and Venereology Society, November 13, 1891. *Monatshefte für Praktische Dermatologie* 14:76.

Vernino, S., K. M. Bourne, L. E. Stiles, B. P. Grubb, A. Fedorowski, J. M. Stewart, A. C. Arnold, L. A. Pace, J. Axelsson, J. R. Boris, J. P. Moak, B. P. Goodman, K. R. Chémali, T. H. Chung, D. S. Goldstein, A. Diedrich, M. G. Miglis, M. M. Cortez, A. J. Miller, R. Freeman, I. Biaggioni, P. C. Rowe, R. S. Sheldon, C. A. Shibao, D. M. Systrom, G. A. Cook, T. A. Doherty, H. I. Abdallah, A. Darbari, and S. R. Raj. 2021. Postural orthostatic tachycardia syndrome (POTS): State of the science and clinical care from a 2019 National Institutes of Health expert consensus meeting—part 1. *Autonomic Neuroscience* 235:102828. https://doi.org/10.1016/j.autneu.2021.102828.

Voermans, N. C., H. Knoop, G. Bleijenberg, and B. G. van Engelen. 2010a. Pain in Ehlers-Danlos syndrome is common, severe, and associated with functional impairment. *Journal of Pain and Symptom Management* 40(3):370-378. https://doi.org/10.1016/j.jpainsymman.2009.12.026.

Voermans, N. C., H. Knoop, N. van de Kamp, B. C. Hamel, G. Bleijenberg, and B. G. van Engelen. 2010b. Fatigue is a frequent and clinically relevant problem in Ehlers-Danlos syndrome. *Seminars in Arthritis and Rheumatism* 40(3):267-274. https://doi.org/10.1016/j.semarthrit.2009.08.003.

Warnink-Kavelaars, J., L. E. de Koning, L. Rombaut, L. A. Menke, M. W. Alsem, H. A. van Oers, A. I. Buizer, R. H. H. Engelbert, J. Oosterlaan, and Pediatric Heritable Connective Tissue Disorder Study Group. 2022. Heritable connective tissue disorders in childhood: Decreased health-related quality of life and mental health. *American Journal of Medical Genetics. Part A.* 188(7):2096-2109. https://doi.org/10.1002/ajmg.a.62750.

Weil, D., M. D'Alessio, F. Ramirez, W. de Wet, W. G. Cole, D. Chan, and J. F. Bateman. 1989. A base substitution in the exon of a collagen gene causes alternative splicing and generates a structurally abnormal polypeptide in a patient with Ehlers-Danlos syndrome type VII. *EMBO Journal* 8(6):1705-1710. https://doi.org/10.1002/j.1460-2075.1989.tb03562.x.

Wilder-Smith, C. H., A. M. Drewes, A. Materna, and S. S. Olesen. 2019. Symptoms of mast cell activation syndrome in functional gastrointestinal disorders. *Scandinavian Journal of Gastroenterology* 54(11):1322-1325. https://doi.org/10.1080/00365521.2019.1686059.

Wile, H. 1883. The elastic skin man. *Medical News (NY)* 43:705.

Yonko, E. A., H. M. Loturco, E. M. Carter, and C. L. Raggio. 2021. Orthopedic considerations and surgical outcomes in Ehlers–Danlos syndromes. *American Journal of Medical Genetics Part C: Seminars in Medical Genetics* 187(4):458-465. https://dx.doi.org/10.1002/ajmg.c.31958.

Zierau, O., A. C. Zenclussen, and F. Jensen. 2012. Role of female sex hormones, estradiol and progesterone, in mast cell behavior. *Frontiers in Immunology* 3:169. https://doi.org/10.3389/fimmu.2012.00169.

ANNEX TABLE 4-1
Overview of Ehlers-Danlos Syndromes and Hypermobility Spectrum Disorders

Selected HDCTs	Description	Documentation (e.g., laboratory tests, diagnostic criteria)
Hypermobile EDS (hEDS)	The hypermobile type of EDS is an autosomal-dominant disorder that presents with phenotypic variability. Common signs and symptoms include joint hypermobility, affecting large and small joints; soft, smooth skin that may be slightly elastic, with easy bruising and unexplained striae; piezogenic papules of the heel; chronic musculoskeletal pain (as differentiated from acute due to injury); early-onset osteoarthritis; osteopenia; gastrointestinal issues (dysmotility, bloating, nausea, vomiting, heartburn, constipation); migraine headaches; dysfunction of the nervous system, including pain and postural orthostatic tachycardia syndrome. Rapid labor and delivery, psychological dysfunction, and psychosocial impairments are common.	**Diagnostic criteria** Simultaneous presence of three criteria: 1. Generalized joint hypermobility 2. Evidence of syndrome features, musculoskeletal complications, and/or family history 3. Exclusion of alternative diagnoses **Laboratory** genetic (mutation) testing Genetic etiology remains unresolved
Classical EDS	The classical type of EDS is an autosomal-dominant connective tissue disorder associated with skin hyperextensibility, articular hypermobility, and tissue fragility with peculiar "cigarette-paper" scars. Clinical findings include mild short stature; narrow maxilla; myopia; ectopia lentis; small, irregularly placed teeth; mitral valve prolapse; aortic root dilatation; inguinal or umbilical hernia; spontaneous bowel rupture; bowel diverticula; osteoarthritis; joint hypermobility and dislocations (hip, shoulder, elbow, knee, or clavicle); pes planus; fragile skin; cigarette-paper scars; dystrophic scarring; poor wound healing; molluscoid pseudotumors; skin hyperextensibility; hypotonia in infancy; muscle fatigue and cramps; and premature birth following premature rupture of fetal membranes.	**Diagnostic criteria** International EDS Consortium **Laboratory** genetic (mutation) testing *COL5A1*

Classical-like EDS type 1	Classical-like EDS type 1 is either an autosomal-recessive disorder due to mutations in the gene encoding *TNXB* or a contiguous gene-deletion syndrome that includes *TNXB* and *CYP21A2*. Characteristic findings include childhood onset, mitral valve prolapse and quadricuspid aortic valve (deletion syndrome), hiatal hernia and other gastrointestinal issues, urogenital anomalies in the deletion syndrome (ambiguous genitalia, bicornuate uterus, renal agenesis, urethral prolapse), joint hypermobility and subluxations, arthralgia, piezogenic papules and brachydactyly of the feet, leg edema, hyperextensible skin with no scarring, proximal muscle weakness and atrophy, and chronic fatigue.	**Diagnostic criteria** Similar to classical form of EDS but lacks skin scarring and has autosomal-recessive inheritance **Laboratory** genetic (mutation) testing *TNXB* Contiguous deletion that includes *TNXB* and *CYP21A2* **Other laboratory findings** Serum, absence of TNX Electromyogram with myopathic pattern Elevated serum 17-hydroxyprogesterone level (seen in patients with contiguous gene defect)
Classical-like EDS type 2	Classical-like EDS type 2 is an autosomal-recessive disorder that falls in the EDS spectrum, associated with joint hypermobility, skin laxity, delayed wound healing, abnormal scarring, and aortic dilation. Clinical findings include joint laxity with dislocations, redundant and hyperextensible skin, poor wound healing with abnormal scarring, piezogenic papules, osteoporosis, micrognathia, ptosis, mitral valve prolapse and aortic dilation, bowel rupture, gut dysmotility, hernias, pes planus, and hallux valgus.	**Diagnostic criteria** Similar to classical form of EDS but with autosomal-recessive inheritance **Laboratory** genetic (mutation) testing AE-Binding Protein 1 (*AEBP1*) **Other laboratory findings** Transmission electron microscopy of skin shows irregular disrupted collagen fibrils with moderate variation in collagen size

continued

ANNEX TABLE 4-1 Continued

Selected HDCTs	Description	Documentation (e.g., laboratory tests, diagnostic criteria)
Cardiac-valvular EDS	The cardiac-valvular type of EDS is an ultrarare autosomal-recessive disorder characterized by generalized peripheral joint hypermobility, moderate to severe cardiac valvular disease (particularly the mitral valve), skin hyperextensibility, variable atrophic scarring, easy bruising, lower-eyelid ptosis, inguinal hernias, bilateral flatfeet with hindfoot pronation, genu recurvata, and hypoplasia of the interphalangeal creases.	**Diagnostic criteria** Findings of EDS Suspected if patient presents with severe cardiovascular involvement that is progressive **Laboratory** genetic (mutation) testing Recessively inherited *COL1A2* nonsense (null mutations)
Vascular EDS (vEDS)	The vascular form of EDS is an autosomal-dominant disorder defined by the major complications of arterial and bowel rupture, and uterine rupture during pregnancy. Clinical features include short stature; thin lips; lobeless ears; keratoconus; pinched-appearing, thin nose; periodontal disease and early loss of teeth; mitral valve prolapse; intracranial aneurysms; spontaneous pneumothorax and hemoptysis; inguinal hernias; spontaneous rupture of bowel; uterine rupture during pregnancy; uterine and bladder prolapse; joint laxity of the distal phalanges with acro-osteolysis; hip dislocations; clubfeet; fragile skin with paper-thin scars and prominent vascular markings, poor wound healing, molluscoid pseudotumors and acrogeria; and scalp alopecia. Death often occurs before the fifth decade.	**Diagnostic criteria** Suspected if patient, particularly younger than age 40, presents with one of the following: arterial aneurysms, dissection, or rupture; intestinal rupture; uterine rupture during pregnancy; family history of vEDS **Laboratory** genetic (mutation) testing *COL3A1*

Arthrochalasia EDS	The arthrochalasia type of EDS, formerly EDS type 7A and 7B, is an autosomal-dominant disorder that is distinguished from other types of EDS by the markedly increased frequency of congenital hip dislocation and extreme joint laxity with recurrent joint subluxations and minimal skin involvement. Clinical findings include mild to moderate short stature; midface hypoplasia; severe joint dislocations with recurrent joint subluxations; early-onset osteoarthritis; osteopenia with increased risk for fractures; kyphoscoliosis and scoliosis; congenital hip dislocations; thin, hyperextensible, atrophic scars; hypotonia with gross-motor developmental delay.	**Diagnostic criteria** Severe joint hypermobility, congenital hip dislocation, facial dysmorphism, osteopenia, kyphoscoliosis **Laboratory** genetic (mutation) testing *COL1A1* *COL1A2*
Dermatosparaxis EDS	Dermatosparaxis EDS is an autosomal-recessive disorder of connective tissue resulting from deficiency of procollagen peptidase. Characteristic findings include extreme skin fragility with congenital and postnatal skin tears, soft and doughy skin with hyperextensibility and atrophic scars, excessive skin at joints with increased palmar creases, and severe bruisability with risk for hematomas and hemorrhage. Facial findings include delayed closure of the anterior fontanel, blue sclera, epicanthal folds, blepharochalasis, prominent lips, hypodontia, and discolored teeth. Other findings include umbilical and inguinal hernias, short stature, joint laxity, osteopenia, delayed motor milestones, organ system abnormalities due to visceral fragility (diaphragmatic and bladder rupture, rectal prolapse), and prematurity.	**Diagnostic criteria** Autosomal-recessive inheritance Minimal criteria for diagnosis include extreme skin fragility and characteristic facial findings **Laboratory** genetic (mutation) testing *ADAMTS2* **Other laboratory findings** Collagen fibrils demonstrate hieroglyphic pattern

continued

ANNEX TABLE 4-1
Continued

Selected HDCTs	Description	Documentation (e.g., laboratory tests, diagnostic criteria)
Kyphoscoliotic EDS type 1	Kyphoscoliotic EDS type 1 is an autosomal-recessive disorder resultant from mutations in the gene *PLOD1*. Characteristic findings include marfanoid habitus, keratoconus, microcornea, myopia, retinal detachment, ocular rupture, glaucoma, blindness, tooth crowding, gastrointestinal hemorrhage, bladder prolapse, joint laxity with dislocations, osteoporosis, congenital scoliosis and progressive kyphosis, arachnodactyly, pes planus, talipes equinovarus, thin skin, moderate scarring, molluscoid pseudotumors, decreased fetal movements, and premature rupture of membranes. Risks include rupture of medium-size arteries, cardiac failure, decreased pulmonary function, recurrent pneumonias, and respiratory insufficiency secondary to chest deformity.	**Diagnostic criteria** Autosomal-recessive inheritance Major criteria: Congenital muscular hypotonia (progressive or early-onset kyphoscoliosis) Generalized joint hypermobility with dislocations/subluxations (shoulders, hips, and knees in particular) **Laboratory** genetic (*mutation*) *testing* *PLOD1* **Other laboratory findings** Increased ratio of deoxypyridinoline to pyridinoline crosslinks in urine measured by high-performance liquid chromatography
Kyphoscoliotic EDS type 2	Kyphoscoliotic EDS type 2 is an autosomal-recessive disorder caused by mutations in the gene encoding *FKBP14*. Characteristic findings include hearing loss, myopia, occasional cleft palate, tricuspid valve insufficiency, aortic rupture and arterial dissection, subdural hygroma, insufficiency of cardiac valves, restrictive lung disease due to severe scoliosis, hernias, bladder diverticulum, progressive kyphoscoliosis, hypermobility of large and small joints, pes planus, equinovarus, hyperelastic skin, easy bruising, follicular hyperkeratosis, muscular atrophy, and myopathy.	**Diagnostic criteria** Autosomal-recessive inheritance Major criteria: Congenital muscular hypotonia Congenital or early-onset kyphoscoliosis Generalized joint hypermobility **Laboratory** genetic (mutation) testing *FKBP14* **Other laboratory findings** Normal pyridinoline excretion in urine Electromyography: myopathic pattern in adulthood

Brittle cornea syndrome type 1	Brittle cornea syndrome type 1, one of the EDS, is an autosomal-recessive disorder due to mutations in the gene *ZNF469*. Characteristic findings include marfanoid habitus, macrocephaly, hearing loss, myopia, brittle cornea (extreme thinning of the cornea, with risk of tearing or rupture leading to blindness), keratoconus, keratoglobus, blue sclera, dentinogenesis imperfecta, mitral valve prolapse, joint laxity, hip dislocations and dysplasia, scoliosis, skin scarring, molluscoid pseudotumor, excessively wrinkled skin (particularly palms and soles), and red hair.	**Diagnostic criteria** Corneal topography, anterior segment optical coherence tomography, corneal pachymetry Ocular manifestations with extraocular findings of deafness, developmental hip dysplasia, and joint hypermobility **Laboratory** genetic (mutation) testing *ZFN469* **Other laboratory findings** Normal lysyl hydroxylase activity Normal dermal hydroxylysine content
Brittle cornea syndrome type 2	Brittle cornea syndrome type 2, one of the EDS, is an autosomal-recessive disorder due to mutations in the gene *PDRM5*. Characteristic findings include hearing loss due to hypercompliant tympanic membranes, myopia, brittle cornea with corneal thinning and risk of rupture, blue sclera, keratoconus, megalocornea, sclerocornea, cornea plana, keratoglobus, hernias, small-joint hypermobility, increased fracture incidence, hip dysplasia, myalgias, skin hyperelasticity, and poor wound healing.	**Diagnostic criteria** Corneal topography, anterior segment optical coherence tomography, corneal pachymetry Ocular manifestations with extraocular findings of deafness, developmental hip dysplasia, and joint hypermobility **Laboratory** genetic (mutation) testing *PDRM5*

continued

ANNEX TABLE 4-1 Continued

Selected HDCTs	Description	Documentation (e.g., laboratory tests, diagnostic criteria)
Spondylodysplastic EDS 1 type	Spondylodysplastic EDS type 1 is an autosomal-recessive disorder caused by mutations in the *B4GALT7* gene. Characteristic findings include dysmorphic features, sparse hair, blue sclera, occasional pectus excavatum, large-joint laxity, kyphoscoliosis, spatulate fingers, talipes equinovarus, hypotonia, hyperextensible skin, cutis laxa, mild developmental delay (occasional), and multiple radiographic abnormalities.	**Diagnostic criteria** Progressive short stature Poor muscle tone Bowing of lower extremities Characteristic facial features Radiographic findings **Laboratory** genetic (mutation) testing *B3GALT7* **Other laboratory findings** Galactosyltransferase I deficiency in fibroblasts
Spondylodysplastic EDS type 2	Spondylodysplastic EDS type 2 is an autosomal-recessive disorder caused by mutations in the *B3GALT6* gene. Characteristic findings include dysmorphic features, sparse hair, blue sclera, occasional pectus excavatum, large-joint laxity, kyphoscoliosis, spatulate fingers, talipes equinovarus, hypotonia, hyperextensible skin, cutis laxa, and multiple radiographic abnormalities.	**Diagnostic criteria** Progressive short stature Poor muscle tone Bowing of lower extremities Characteristic facial features Radiographic findings **Laboratory** genetic (mutation) testing *B3GALT6*

Spondylodysplastic EDS type 3	Spondylodysplastic EDS type 3 is an autosomal-recessive disorder caused by mutations in the zinc transporter gene *SLC39A13*. The disorder is characterized by moderate short stature; protuberant eyes; high-arched palate with bifid uvula; hypodontia; sparse hair; joint laxity; finger contractures; fine-wrinkled palms; hypothenar muscle atrophy; inability to adduct thumbs; short fingers; pes planus; thin, hyperelastic skin; abnormal scars with poor healing; delayed wound healing; muscle weakness; osteopenia; mild intellectual disability; and radiographic abnormalities.	**Diagnostic criteria** Progressive short stature Poor muscle tone Bowing of lower extremities Characteristic facial features Radiographic findings **Laboratory** genetic (mutation) testing *SLC39A13* **Other laboratory findings** Lysyl pyridinoline/hydroxylysyl pyridinoline (LP/HP) ratio approximately 1 (nl LP/HP: 0.2 + 0.03)
Musculocontractural EDS type 1	Musculocontractural EDS type 1 is an autosomal-recessive disorder caused by mutations in the *CHST14* gene. Characteristic findings include wasted body build; dysmorphic facies with prominent ears; hearing impairment; blue sclera; strabismus; myopia; glaucoma; microcornea; retinal detachment; anterior chamber abnormality; cleft palate; cardiac valvular anomalies; atrial septal defect; hemopneumothorax; pectus excavatum; hernias; constipation; duodenal obstruction; hydronephrosis; recurrent cystitis; congenital contractures that include adducted thumbs and distal arthrogryposis; joint laxity and dislocations; tendon abnormalities; scoliosis; progressive talipes valgus and planus; hyperextensible, fragile, transparent skin with atrophic scarring; delayed wound healing; hyperalgesia; recurrent subcutaneous infections; low muscle mass and gross motor delay; and developmental delay in some.	**Diagnostic criteria** Congenital malformations Contractures of hands and feet Dysmorphic features **Laboratory** genetic (mutation) testing *CHST14*

continued

ANNEX TABLE 4-1 Continued

Selected HDCTs	Description	Documentation (e.g., laboratory tests, diagnostic criteria)
Musculocontractural EDS type 2	Musculocontractural EDS type 2 is an autosomal-recessive disorder caused by mutations in the *DSE* gene. Characteristic findings include hypotonic facies with prominent and abnormally shaped ears, hypertelorism, blue sclera, mitral valve prolapse and regurgitation, mixomatous degeneration of mitral valve, eventration of abdominal wall after surgery, hernia, uterine and bladder prolapse in females, arachnodactyly, camptodactyly, talipes equinovarus, delayed wound healing with atrophic scars, recurrent large subcutaneous hematomas, postecchymotic calcifications, generalized muscle weakness, pain, and occasional cerebral atrophy.	**Diagnostic criteria** Clinical findings **Laboratory** genetic (*mutation*) *testing* *DSE* **Other laboratory findings** Adulthood, abnormal muscle fiber pattern in histology
Myopathic EDS	The myopathic type of EDS, also known as Bethlem myopathy-2, is an autosomal-dominant disorder due to mutations in the gene that encodes type XII collagen (*COL12A1*) and recessive mutations in the gene *COL6A1*. Characteristic findings include muscle weakness present in childhood that improves with age but is followed by some deterioration, distal hyperlaxity and flexion contractures, joint hypermobility, and hypertrophic scars.	**Diagnostic criteria** Clinical findings **Laboratory** genetic (mutation) testing *COL12A1* (autosomal-dominant) *COL6A1* (autosomal-recessive) **Other laboratory findings** Increased serum creatine kinase Fibroblasts show a reduction of and disorganization in type XII collagen in the extracellular matrix

Periodontal EDS type 1	Periodontal EDS type 1 is an autosomal-dominant disorder caused by heterozygous mutations in the *C1R* gene, with the defining feature of severe periodontal inflammation. Characteristic findings include significant gingivitis with gum inflammatory destruction of dental attachments and premature loss of teeth; tall stature; acrogeric facies; cerebral and aortic aneurysm; scoliosis; joint laxity; hypermobility; and thin, atrophic skin with easy tearing and bruisability, pretibial hyperpigmentation, and pretibial plaques.	**Diagnostic criteria** Early-onset severe periodontitis Generalized lack of attached gingiva Pretibial plaques Family history in a first-degree relative **Laboratory** genetic (mutation) testing *C1R* **Other laboratory findings** Electron microscopy: Abnormally enlarged endoplasmic reticulum cisterna Abnormal variation in collagen fibril diameter
Periodontal EDS type 2	Periodontal EDS type 2 is an autosomal-dominant disorder caused by heterozygous mutation in the *C1S* gene. Characteristic findings include aggressive periodontitis with gingival recession, tooth loss, hernias, prominent subcutaneous vasculature, irritable bowel and gastrointestinal symptoms, scoliosis, spinal osteoarthritis, joint hypermobility and pain, skin fragility, pretibial hyperpigmentation, abnormal scarring, and increased incidence of cancer.	**Diagnostic criteria** Early-onset severe periodontitis Generalized lack of attached gingiva Pretibial plaques Family history in a first-degree relative **Laboratory** genetic (mutation) testing *C1S*

continued

ANNEX TABLE 4-1 Continued

Selected HDCTs	Description	Documentation (e.g., laboratory tests, diagnostic criteria)
Hypermobility spectrum disorders (HSD)	Hypermobility spectrum disorders are a wide spectrum of related disorders with joint hypermobility (JH) of unknown molecular etiology. HSD is used as a diagnosis after other well-defined types of EDS, including hEDS, are excluded. Joint hypermobility is defined as the ability of a joint or group of joints to move passively or actively beyond normal physiologic limits. It can be an isolated finding in some individuals. There are four types of JH: generalized (joint) HSD (G-HSD), peripheral (joint) HSD, localized (joint) HSD, and historical (joint) HSD. Individuals with HSD are predisposed to joint trauma, including dislocations, subluxations, and damage to joint tissues; increased occasional and recurrent musculoskeletal pain; decreased muscle mass; and decreased proprioception. G-HSD can be also associated with extra-articular complications that include anxiety disorders, orthostatic tachycardia, a variety of functional gastrointestinal disorders, and pelvic and bladder dysfunction often similar to what is seen in hEDS.	**Diagnostic Criteria** Ability of a joint or group of joints to move beyond physiologic limits Exclusion of other well-defined etiologies for joint hypermobility

NOTE: HDCT = heritable disorder of connective tissue and disability.

SOURCES: Bertoli-Avella et al., 2015; Callewaert, 2019; Doyle et al., 2012; Frischmeyer-Guerrerio et al., 2013; Greally, 2020; Gupta et al., 2002; Lindsay et al., 2012; Loeys and Dietz, 2018; Loeys et al., 2005, 2010; Matyas et al., 2014; Regalado et al., 2011; Rienhoff et al., 2013; Tan et al., 2013; Van Hemelrijk et al., 2010.

5

Heritable Disorders of Connective Tissue and Effects on Function

As discussed in previous chapters, heritable disorders of connective tissue (HDCTs) manifest as physical and mental secondary impairments, potentially in many different body systems. The severity of the disease process varies among individuals and relates to the type, number, and severity of the secondary impairments, as well as the combined effects of multiple "less severe" impairments.

As described in Chapter 1, the International Classification of Functioning, Disability and Health (ICF) model of disability identifies three domains of functioning: (1) body function and structure (i.e., physiological functions of the body, including psychological functions, and functioning of body structures); (2) activities (i.e., actions or tasks); and (3) participation (i.e., performance of tasks in a societal context, such as school or work (WHO, 2001). "Impairments" are deficits in body function and structure; "limitations" refer to deficits in completing activities; and "restrictions" refer to reductions in participation (WHO, 2001). Personal and environmental factors act on the ICF domains to either enhance or diminish an individual's activity and participation.

Some effects of HDCTs, and in some cases their treatment, manifest as impairments in body structures and physical and psychological functions, with resulting activity limitations and restrictions on participation. The impairments associated with HDCTs affect mental (e.g., cognitive, psychosocial, emotional) functioning as well as physical functioning.

Moreover, these areas of functioning interact such that impairments in one area (e.g., physical) may precipitate or exacerbate impairments in one or more of the others (cognitive, psychosocial, and/or emotional). Chronic pain, for example, is reported to have a bidirectional relationship with depression (Vadivelu et al., 2017), and an association between gastrointestinal and psychological disorders has also been reported (Stasi et al., 2017). Similarly, physical conditions such as pain and fatigue can adversely affect cognitive functioning (Higgins et al., 2018; Moriarty et al., 2011; Vadivelu et al., 2017).

This chapter first describes the relationship between secondary impairments associated with HDCTs and functioning, and then provides an overview of the potential effects on global (full-body); physical; vision, hearing, and speech; and mental functioning. The chapter also reviews selected listings from the U.S. Social Security Administration's (SSA's) Listing of Impairments that may be particularly applicable to individuals with specific HDCTs.

SECONDARY IMPAIRMENTS

The statement of task for this study asks the committee "to describe to the degree possible" the "secondary impairments that result from either the [selected HDCTs] or their treatments (if applicable)." As defined in Chapter 1, the committee understands "secondary impairments" to mean physical and mental manifestations (medical diagnoses, syndromes, or health conditions) that are associated with and may also result from an HDCT, although they may occur independently in individuals without an HDCT. Annex Tables 5-3–5-12 at the end of this chapter present selected manifestations (organized by body system) and some of the HDCTs with which they are associated, as well as common diagnostic techniques and potential treatments.

The number, type, and severity of the secondary impairments experienced by an individual with an HDCT drive the person's functioning and potential disability. Annex Tables 5-13–5-16 summarize the potential implications of secondary impairments for global functioning; physical functioning; vision, hearing, and speech functioning; and mental functioning in individuals with HDCTs. The tables list physical and mental activities the committee determined to be of particular interest to SSA,[1] the potential reasons for limitations in those activities for individuals with HDCTs, selected measures for assessing function in the relevant areas, and selected assistive technologies and reasonable accommodations that could help mitigate the effects of the impairment(s) on an individual's ability to work, participate in school, and the like. The assessment measures are categorized primarily as performance-based or self-reported. Performance-based measures require that the individual being assessed perform a set of physical or mental activities or tasks so that his or her ability to execute them can be ascertained. Self-reported (or proxy-reported) measures require the individual being assessed or a third party to complete a questionnaire asking about symptoms (e.g., pain, fatigue, anxiety) or the individual's ability to perform a specific set of mental or physical tasks. Patient-reported outcome or experience measures, questionnaires regarding activities of daily living (ADLs) and instrumental activities of daily living (IADLs), and some types of psychological tests are examples of such measures.

The medical tables (Annex Tables 5-3–5-12) and the function tables (Annex Tables 5-13–5-16) in this chapter can be used together to understand how secondary impairments associated with different HDCTs may affect an individual's functioning in various areas. The "potential reasons" column in the function tables provides information and cross-references that allow the reader to identify the relevant medical tables (e.g., musculoskeletal, neurological), which include information about specific diagnoses.

As discussed in the final section of the chapter, the secondary impairments identified in the medical tables can also serve as an interface with

---

[1] SSA classifies jobs as sedentary, light, medium, heavy, and very heavy based on the level of physical exertion requirements of the work (CFR § 416.967). Annex Table 5-1 provides the definitions for each level of work. When a person applies for disability benefits, SSA collects information about the applicant's physical and mental impairment(s) and functioning from a variety of sources, including the applicant, medical providers, employers, teachers, and other third parties with knowledge of the applicant. Information collected about physical functioning includes information about such activities as sitting, standing, walking, lifting, carrying, reaching, handling large objects, writing, typing, handling small objects, and low work (stooping, kneeling, crouching, crawling) (SSA, 2020). Information is collected as well about the applicant's ability to perform various daily activities, such as dressing, bathing, self-feeding, and using the toilet, as well as preparing meals, doing house- and yardwork, getting around, shopping, and the like. SSA also must consider information about the physical and mental demands of different jobs, such as the amount of time an employee is required to stand or walk and whether a job requires driving, using a keyboard, or reaching overhead (SSA, n.d.-a). The physical; vision, hearing, and speech; and mental activities addressed in this chapter (Annex Table 5-2) are those the committee determined to be most relevant to SSA based on the information SSA collects about applicants and the information the U.S. Bureau of Labor Statistics collects about the physical and mental demands of jobs for inclusion in the Occupational Information System, which is being developed to serve as the main source of occupational information for SSA's disability adjudication process (SSA, 2022).

existing SSA listings. For example, some individuals with HDCTs applying for SSA disability benefits might qualify at the listing level step in the determination process on the basis of the secondary impairment(s) they are experiencing rather than the HDCT itself.

ENVIRONMENTAL FACTORS AND FUNCTIONING

Environmental factors can adversely affect functioning in some people. Environmental factors that can impair an individual's functioning include extreme heat and cold; noise; vibration; wetness; humidity; and atmospheric conditions that can affect the respiratory system, nervous system, eyes, or skin (e.g., scents, allergens, fumes, noxious odors, dusts, mists, gases, and poor ventilation) (BLS, 2020). SSA recognizes this and takes an individual's environmental restrictions into account. "A nonexertional impairment is one which is medically determinable and causes a nonexertional limitation of function or an *environmental restriction*" (SSR 85-15, emphasis added; SSA, n.d.-f). Accordingly, SSA takes into account the relative availability of jobs that would not expose an affected individual to the relevant environmental factors. For example, a restriction on exposure to excessive amounts of noise, vibration, or dust would have little effect "because most job environments do not involve great noise, [vibration, or] amounts of dust" (SSA, n.d.-f). But "where an individual can tolerate very little noise, [vibration, or] dust, …the impact on the ability to work would be considerable because very few job environments are entirely free of [such] irritants…" (SSA, n.d.-f).

Environmental factors can significantly affect functioning in some individuals with HDCTs. For example, patients with the Ehlers-Danlos syndromes (EDS) and hypermobility spectrum disorders (HSD) are at increased risk of mast cell activation disease (MCAD), a condition that can be triggered by environmental substances (Frieri, 2018). Humidity and changes in atmospheric pressure appear to have a negative effect on functioning in EDS/HSD patients, which causes psychosocial distress (Palomo-Toucedo et al., 2020). There may be a number of reasons for this effect on functioning. First, patients with EDS/HSD have lowered cold and heat pain thresholds (Di Stefano et al., 2016). In addition, migraine, known to be more common in patients with either Marfan syndrome (MFS) (von Kodolitsch et al., 2019) or EDS/HSD (Puledda et al., 2015) relative to the general population, are triggered by environmental substances and weather changes (Marmura, 2018). Furthermore, cardiovascular autonomic dysfunction in EDS/HSD patients appears to have environmental triggers (Hakim et al., 2017b), and changes in temperature and barometric pressure can exacerbate joint problems and symptoms of dysautonomia and affect intracranial pressure (Herbowski, 2017, 2019; Palomo-Toucedo et al., 2020). Likewise, sound, odors, light, and foods can trigger or exacerbate manifestations in individuals with EDS/HSD (Syx et al., 2017).

GLOBAL FUNCTIONING

Chronic pain, chronic fatigue, and a type of cognitive dysfunction or mild cognitive impairment sometimes referred to as "brain fog" are some of the most common and potentially disabling manifestations of EDS/HSD, especially hypermobile EDS (hEDS)/HSD (Arnold et al., 2015; Chopra et al., 2017; Ocon, 2013; Raj et al., 2018; Rombaut et al., 2011; Ross et al., 2013; Sacheti et al., 1997; Voermans et al., 2010a; Wells et al., 2020). Chronic pain and fatigue are also common among individuals with MFS (Nelson et al., 2015b; Peters et al., 2001; Ratiu et al., 2018).

This section begins with a discussion of the effect of chronic pain and chronic fatigue on global functioning and selected measures for assessing their severity. It then reviews the roles of two global modulators of function (orthostatic intolerance and MCAD) in individuals with EDS/HSD, particularly hEDS/HSD. The section concludes with a discussion of two categories of measures for assessment of global functioning.

Chronic Pain

Pain can be characterized in two broad ways. The first is by its cause. *Neuropathic pain* is caused by damage to or irritation of the nerves themselves. *Nociceptive pain* is caused by stimulation of pain receptors, which send signals to the brain leading to the experience of pain. Depending on the location of the pain receptors, nociceptive pain may be somatic (surface of the body or musculoskeletal system) or visceral (stemming from pain receptors within the body cavity). *Nociplastic pain* arises from altered nociception in the absence of damage to the somatosensory system or stimulation of pain receptors in response to an assault (IASP, 2021). Most EDS/HSD patients experience all three types of pain.

Pain also may be classified by its duration. Typically, *acute pain* is a time-limited response to an injury (e.g., pulled muscle, broken bone) or warning of potential injury (e.g., from a hot stove or sharp object). *Chronic pain* has been defined as "persistent or recurrent pain lasting longer than 3 months" (Treede et al., 2015; WHO, 2021). *Breakthrough pain* occurs when an episode of acute pain "breaks through" otherwise well-controlled chronic pain.

Everyone experiences acute pain from time to time. While estimates indicate that 20 percent of individuals worldwide experience chronic pain (Treede et al., 2015), studies have found that 80–100 percent of individuals with EDS, especially hEDS/HSD, and MFS experience chronic pain (Chopra et al., 2017; Nelson et al., 2015a; Peters et al., 2001; Ratiu et al., 2018; Rombaut et al., 2011; Speed et al., 2017; Voermans et al., 2010a).

The *International Classification of Diseases, Eleventh Edition* (ICD-11) (WHO, 2021) identifies seven categories of chronic pain, five of which are most relevant to individuals with HDCTs such as EDS/HSD and MFS: (1) chronic primary pain, (2) chronic secondary musculoskeletal pain (Voermans et al., 2010a), (3) chronic secondary visceral pain (Fikree et al., 2017), (4) chronic neuropathic pain (Camerota et al., 2011; Rombaut et al., 2015), and (5) chronic secondary headache or orofacial pain (Mitakides and Tinkle, 2017). Individuals with EDS/HSD may also appear to be more predisposed to chronic postsurgical or posttraumatic pain (Chopra et al., 2017; Voermans et al., 2010a), perhaps because of increased difficulty with healing. The seventh pain category, chronic cancer-related pain, does not apply to pain secondary to an HDCT.

Potential Reasons

Individuals with hEDS/HSD may experience neuropathic or nociceptive pain (Camerota et al., 2011; Rombaut et al., 2015; Voermans et al., 2010a), and some individuals also experience central sensitization, stemming from "a generalized hyperexcitability of central nociceptive pathways" (Rombaut et al., 2015, p. 1126). Pain is most frequently reported in the neck, shoulders, hips, and legs (Voermans et al., 2010a).

Chronic pain and hypersensitivity are explained by peripheral and central sensitization. Persistent nociceptive input from musculoskeletal and visceral sources can lead to peripheral and central sensitization, which often perpetuates chronic pain through processes involving neuroplasticity (Ji et al., 2018; Matsuda et al., 2019). In response to persistent nociceptive signaling from peripheral sensitized tissue, a number of synapse-to-nucleus messengers are recruited. As peripheral sensitization persists, it leads to central sensitization. Peripheral sensitization is accompanied by a reduction in threshold and increase in magnitude of response at the peripheral end of sensory nerve fibers (Gangadharan and Kuner, 2013). Chemical inflammatory mediators (e.g., mast cells, platelets, neutrophils, basophils, endothelial cells) are released by nociceptors and non-neuronal tissue. This release of inflammatory mediators can exacerbate local connective tissue dysfunction and local tissue damage (Chiu et al., 2012). Furthermore, since histamine is a key mediator in neurogenic inflammation (Rosa and Fantozzi, 2013), the prevalent comorbidity of MCAD with HCDTs suggests that neurogenic inflammation may contribute to the link between peripheral or central sensitization and connective tissue involvement in HDCTs.

Under normal circumstances, the spinal cord sends modulatory signals to suppress pain signals. When a constant barrage of pain signals reaches the spinal cord, it causes sensitization of the dorsal horn cells; as a result, the central nervous system (CNS) switches from suppressing signals to enhancing its response to stimuli. The persistent barrage of pain signals to and increased modulatory signals from the CNS lead to central sensitization. Central sensitization explains why chronic pain persists and even increases.

Pain may be caused by secondary impairments in virtually every body system, including musculoskeletal disorders, such as joint subluxations or dislocations and myofascial disorders (see Annex Table 5-3); neurological disorders, such as neuropathies, and nerve compression disorders (see Annex Tables 5-3 and 5-4); gastrointestinal disorders, such as gastroenteritis, mast cell disorders, and inflammatory bowel disease (see Annex Table 5-8); and genitourinary disorders, such as chronic pelvic pain and dysmenorrhea (see Annex Table 5-10). MCAD (see Annex Table 5-7) contributes to pain through the role of mast cells in neurogenic inflammation, which causes pain as well as itching (Gupta and Harvima, 2018), and in immune-mediated disorders that cause pain (see, e.g., Annex Tables 5-4 and 5-8). In addition, individuals with chronic pain have a higher risk of developing symptoms of anxiety or depression, and individuals with anxiety or depression are more likely to experience chronic or intensified pain (Anxiety & Depression Association of America, 2021; Harvard Health Publishing, 2017; Vadivelu et al., 2017). Poor sleep quality, experienced by many individuals with EDS/HSD, also contributes to the experience of pain (Voermans et al., 2010a).

Interventions

Management of chronic pain depends on the type of pain (nociceptive, neuropathic, or nociplastic) and its location. Notably, individuals with HDCTs may experience multiple root causes of pain and related loss of function, necessitating a comprehensive approach to their evaluation and treatment. Treatment often is multimodal, involving physical therapy, occupational therapy, medication, psychological interventions, surgical co-management, good sleep hygiene, education, and taking care of one's overall health. Although analgesics and other treatments (e.g., braces) may be used to mitigate pain and improve functionality, it is important to identify and address the root cause(s) of the pain and, when applicable, implement preventive measures to reduce the risk of recurrence (Chopra, 2020). For example, pain caused by a dislocation would be treated by fixing the dislocation (underlying cause), potentially treating the acute pain with analgesics until it had resolved, and prescribing physical therapy and exercises to reduce the risk of another dislocation. Although anti-inflammatory and nerve pain medications may be used to treat pain, opioids typically are not helpful for individuals with EDS/HSD and may exacerbate other symptoms, such as those associated with certain gastrointestinal disorders and MCAD (Chopra, 2020). Use or overuse of steroids can lead to increased instability in joints, as well as increased risk for glaucoma and cataracts (Liu et al., 2103).

Selected Assessment Measures

Because the experience of pain differs from individual to individual, the gold standard of pain assessment is self-report. Annex Table 5-13 (on global functioning) includes a list of several common self-reported pain measures.

Effects on Functioning

Chronic pain in particular can adversely affect individuals' functioning. Voermans and colleagues (2010a) found that pain severity among individuals with EDS/HSD was independently related to functional impairment. Children with chronic pain may experience significant adverse effects on participation in academic, athletic, and social activities (Rabin et al., 2017).

Pain can interfere with all types of physical activities that may be involved in work or school, including such sedentary activities as sitting at a desk, writing, or working on a computer. Chronic pain also has an effect on cognitive functioning, including such areas as long-term memory, selective attention, processing speed, and executive functioning (Berryman et al., 2013, 2014; Khera and Rangasamy, 2021; Lee et al., 2010; Ratiu et al., 2018).

Chronic Fatigue

Chronic fatigue has been defined as persistent or recurrent tiredness or exhaustion that typically persists for 6 months or more, cannot be explained by other diagnoses, does not result from ongoing exertion, is not alleviated by rest or sleep, and prevents patients from carrying out normal activities (Hakim et al., 2017a). EDS/HSD has long been associated with a high prevalence of chronic fatigue, which, together with pain, is an important determinant of impaired health-related quality of life in this condition (Ritelli et al., 2020; Rombaut et al., 2010). It has been estimated that more than 75 percent of patients with EDS/HSD suffer from severe fatigue, which appears to be more common in hEDS/HSD than in the classic type of EDS (Ritelli et al., 2020; Voermans et al., 2010b). Fatigue in patients with hEDS/HSD is different from tiredness and has several symptoms that overlap with a condition called myalgic encephalomyelitis (ME), or chronic fatigue syndrome (CFS) (ME/CFS) (Hakim et al., 2017a). Chronic fatigue may be a major presenting symptom of hEDS/HSD, and an appropriate diagnostic workup should distinguish between hEDS/HSD and ME/CFS (Hakim et al., 2017a). Fatigue also has been reported in as many as 89 percent of individuals with MFS (Bathen et al., 2014; Peters et al., 2001; van Dijk et al., 2008).

Potential Reasons

Common causes of fatigue in patients with EDS/HSD include the following:

- **Ligament laxity.** People with EDS/HSD have ligament laxity, or loose ligaments, which can require muscles, including those in the proprioceptive system responsible for balance, to work harder to compensate for the laxity and joint instability. People with ligament laxity resulting from EDS/HSD may experience postural instability and rely on muscles to maintain postural control (Galli et al., 2011). However, these muscles are affected by weak connective tissue, resulting in extra work for them to maintain posture, and this excess demand on muscles can cause fatigue.
- **Dysautonomia.** Many people with EDS/HSD experience orthostatic intolerance (described later in this chapter), or dysautonomia (dysfunction of the autonomic nervous system that controls involuntary bodily functions). Patients with secondary dysautonomia—that is, dysautonomia associated with a disease such as EDS/HSD—may experience a variety of symptoms including fatigue, balance problems, mild cognitive impairment, weakness, and exercise intolerance (De Wandele et al., 2016). Postural orthostatic tachycardia syndrome (POTS; discussed in the section on orthostatic intolerance) is one form of dysautonomia, as is pure autonomic failure, which is characterized by tiredness, dizziness, and fainting (Cleveland Clinic, 2020).
- **Medication.** Some medications, such as benzodiazepines and antidepressants, have sedative side effects that can contribute to fatigue (Voermans et al., 2010b). People with EDS/HSD are often prescribed multiple medications for pain, MCAD, POTS, or other forms of dysautonomia, and some or all of these medications can contribute to lethargy, which adds to fatigue.
- **Nonrestorative sleep.** People with EDS/HSD and dysautonomia experience either decreased parasympathetic tone or an excessively high sympathetic activity that essentially keeps one's brain active when sleeping. These patients often present with nonrestorative sleep that may be the result of pain, nocturnal tachycardia, or

sleep-disordered breathing (sleep apnea) (Hakim et al., 2017a; Ritelli et al., 2020).
- **Nutritional.** Gastrointestinal issues, including bowel dysfunction, are common in EDS/HSD (Fikree et al., 2017; Ritelli et al., 2020). They vary from slowing of intestinal motility to chronic nausea, constipation, and/or diarrhea. Malabsorption and poor nutritional status can result in nutritional deficiencies, including low iron storage levels that may result in decreased blood oxygen levels with concomitant fatigue.
- **Physical deconditioning.** Chronic pain, poor physical activity, and exercise intolerance can result in fatigue upon exertion (Hakim et al., 2017a; Ritelli et al., 2020).

Other manifestations of EDS/HSD associated with chronic fatigue include chronic pain, anxiety and depression, nocturnal micturition (possibly contributing to nonrestorative sleep), and headaches and migraines (Hakim et al., 2017a; Ritelli et al., 2020).

Interventions

Treatment of the fatigue associated with EDS/HSD is multimodal and may require a team of health care experts. Medications, such as antidepressants, pain medications, anti-anxiety drugs, sleep aids, and medications for orthostatic intolerance, may be used to address the underlying causes of the fatigue. Nutritional supplements and dietary modification, preferably based on recommendations from a dietician, may help with nutritional deficiencies. Lifestyle modifications, such as rest and relaxation techniques and good sleep hygiene, can also help alleviate some aspects of fatigue. Graded exercise therapy may be appropriate for some patients with joint hypermobility. Relaxation techniques (e.g., yoga, mindfulness, progressive muscle relaxation), other exercise regimens, physical therapy, and planned management of daily activities are also important therapeutic approaches to fatigue, but all of them must be tailored to the individual patient's needs. Finally, cognitive-behavioral therapy may be beneficial for encouraging exercise and adherence to the lifestyle modifications necessary to control the underlying causes of the fatigue, including anxiety, depression, and chronic pain (Hakim et al., 2017a). In some more severe cases, assistive devices, such as wheelchairs and reachers, may be necessary.

One important aspect of chronic fatigue associated with HDCTs is that it is often unpredictable. Patients report that they may be functioning well one day and completely unable to perform job-related activities and ADLs the next. This variability in performance capability may lead to frequent absences from work and difficulty in maintaining employment.

Selected Assessment Measures

Assessment of chronic fatigue is based on self-reports, and a number of self-report instruments are available to provide a consistent measure of the impact and severity of fatigue. These instruments include the Brief Fatigue Inventory, the Fatigue Impact Scale, the Fatigue Severity Scale, the Fatigue Symptom Inventory, the Multidimensional Assessment of Fatigue scale, and the Multidimensional Fatigue Symptom Inventory. It must be noted, however, that these instruments are used most often in research and are not typically used in the clinical setting. The Wood Mental Fatigue Inventory is one instrument that can be used in the clinic to assess the cognitive symptoms of fatigue (Hakim et al., 2017a). The CRESTA Fatigue Clinic booklet (Newcastle upon Tyne Hospitals: NHS Foundation Trust, 2020), developed by the UK National Health Service Foundation Trust, uses a patient-oriented approach to help patients identify what daily tasks and activities result in fatigue and how often, and encourages them to keep an activity log. Such self-report measures may assist both the patient and clinician in developing an exercise program and a symptom management plan to minimize fatigue on an ongoing basis.

Effects on Functioning

Chronic fatigue associated with HDCTs can result in a number of functional impairments that affect daily activities; the more severe the fatigue, the greater is the impairment (Voermans et al., 2010b). These impairments can include an inability to remain upright for even short periods of time, difficulty with concentration (De Wandele et al., 2016), difficulty in moving from standing to sitting and back to standing, and decreased executive functioning resulting from poor sleep; planning and sequencing, memory, and attention may also be affected (Capuron et al., 2006; Dobbs et al., 2001; Joyce et al., 1996; Ratiu et al., 2018). Many patients with EDS/HSD rest or sleep during the day as a result of their fatigue, which can impact social functioning, work, and other activities (Voermans et al., 2010b). The inability to remain upright or standing in particular can negatively affect the performance of many normal activities for both children and adults. In one study, parents of children aged 4–12 years reported that their children were unable to "keep up with peers" because of fatigue and other factors (Warnink-Kavelaars et al., 2019). Fatigue also can prevent people with EDS/HSD from working at jobs that are physically demanding (De Baets et al., 2021). One study found that fatigue was the major reason people with hEDS did not work (De Baets et al., 2021). And a Norwegian study of individuals with MFS found severe fatigue to be "significantly associated with low work participation" (Velvin et al., 2015; see also Bathen et al., 2014).

Orthostatic Intolerance[2]

Orthostatic intolerance refers to a condition in which individuals develop symptoms upon assuming and maintaining upright posture, with symptoms improving (although not necessarily resolving completely) after they return to a recumbent position (Low et al., 2009). Symptoms, many of which overlap with those of EDS/HSD, include rapid heart rate (tachycardia) or palpitations, feeling faint or fainting, lightheadedness or dizziness upon standing, vertigo, blurred vision, weakness, fatigue, pain, headaches, anxiety, exercise intolerance, difficulty regulating body temperature, sensitivity to auditory or visual stimuli, nutrient imbalance, and cognitive difficulties (Goodman, 2018; Rich et al., 2020).

Hemodynamic abnormalities in orthostatic intolerance can include classical or delayed orthostatic hypotension, neurally mediated hypotension, and POTS (Freeman et al., 2011; Goldstein et al., 2002; Low et al., 2009; Rosen and Cryer, 1982; Schondorf and Low, 1993; Sheldon et al., 2015; Stewart et al., 2018). Classical orthostatic hypotension, common in particular in older adults, is defined by a sustained blood pressure reduction of at least 20 mm Hg systolic or 10 mm Hg diastolic during the first 3 min after assuming an upright posture (Freeman et al., 2011). POTS is increasingly being recognized as a common form of orthostatic intolerance in individuals with EDS/HSD, and is diagnosed (1) in the absence of orthostatic hypotension in the first 3 minutes of standing or tilt testing, and (2) upon an increase in heart rate of ≥ 30 beats per minute (bpm) in adults (≥ 40 bpm in those under age 20 years) in the first 10 minutes after going from recumbent to standing or passive upright tilt; a heart rate of > 120 bpm during the first 10 minutes upright may be an additional criterion (Roma et al., 2018; Rowe, 2022). Inappropriate sinus tachycardia, which has symptoms similar to those of POTS, is characterized by a sinus rhythm with a heart rate greater than 100 bpm at rest (Sheldon et al., 2015). Neurally mediated hypotension, which occurs in both adults and children, is a reflex form of hypotension, and is defined by at least a 25 mm Hg reduction in systolic blood pressure, often accompanied by a relative slowing of the heart rate at the time of presyncope or hypotension (Rowe, 2022).

The true prevalence of orthostatic intolerance in EDS/HSD is not known. In clinical studies, however, 41–100 percent of people with joint hypermobility or EDS have reported orthostatic symptoms on a regular basis (Rowe, 2022).

---

[2]This section draws heavily on a paper by Peter Rowe (2022) commissioned by the committee (see Appendix B).

Potential Reasons

Orthostatic intolerance results primarily from two physiological changes in response to upright posture: (1) a reduction in cerebral blood flow, and (2) an exaggerated compensatory adrenergic response to the reduction in cerebral blood flow (Low et al., 2009). Other potential causes of orthostatic intolerance in persons with HDCTs include the development of autoantibodies to adrenergic receptors and rarely Chiari I malformation (Hakim et al., 2017b). The reduction in cerebral blood flow may result from excessive gravitational pooling of blood, low blood volume, and an increased sympathetic nervous system and adrenal catecholamine response (Rowe, 2022). Increased peripheral pooling of blood or decreased vasoconstriction is affected by the duration of quiet upright posture, increased compliance of the blood vessel wall in response to hydrostatic pressure, the presence of venous varicosities, obstruction of venous return, and vasodilating substances. Low blood volume occurs with a variety of conditions of orthostatic intolerance, including POTS and ME/CFS (Hurwitz et al., 2009; Okamoto et al., 2012; Streeten and Bell, 1998). Low blood volume has been associated with lower renin:aldosterone ratios and lower levels of antidiuretic hormone (Okamoto et al., 2012; Wyller et al., 2010). Physical inactivity can result in reductions in plasma volume, thereby aggravating symptoms of orthostatic intolerance and interfering with daily function (Rowe, 2022).

Interventions

Management of orthostatic intolerance requires a comprehensive care program beginning with nonpharmacologic interventions. These interventions include (1) avoiding conditions that increase dependent pooling of blood, such as prolonged standing or sitting; (2) improving venous return to the heart by using the muscle pump of the lower limbs, such as by crossing the legs while standing or shifting weight from one leg to the other and using compression garments; (3) avoiding depletion of salt and water and other causes of low blood volume; and (4) avoiding increasing catecholamines beyond their baseline levels (which may be elevated) by minimizing stress and in some patients reducing caffeine consumption (Rowe et al., 2017). Further care focuses on managing migraine headaches; allergies; mast cell activation syndrome; anxiety; depression; menstrual dysfunction; and areas of biomechanical dysfunction, which can be managed with physical therapy or osteopathic manual therapy, as well as occupational therapy and environmental modifications (Levine et al., 2021; Rowe, 2016). Individuals with POTS and fatigue may need to lie down during the day to avoid flares of their condition.

Most individuals with more than a minor degree of functional impairment from orthostatic intolerance will need medication. Pharmacologic treatments, such as low-dose beta blockers, fludrocortisone, or midodrine, may ameliorate some of the effects of the condition. Those with neutrally mediated hypotension (NMH) may benefit from selective serotonin reuptake inhibitors. Adolescent girls and women may benefit from hormone therapy (Rowe, 2022, citing Boehm et al., 1997). And individuals with POTS with fatigue and tachycardia may be treated with ivabradine (Rowe, 2022).

Assessment

Clinical assessment of orthostatic intolerance is based on two main tests—standing tests and head-up tilt tests. There is no gold standard for such assessments, and techniques for these tests vary (Rowe, 2022). The impact of orthostatic intolerance on overall function is best assessed with self-reported health-related quality of life questionnaires, such as the SF-36, Euro QOL, or PROMIS measures in adults (Cook et al., 2012; EuroQol Group, 1990; Ware and Sherbourne, 1992) and the age-specific Functional Disability Inventory of Pediatric Quality of Life (PedsQL) for children (Varni et al., 2001). Brief self-reported measures of general or cognitive fatigue include the PedsQL Mutidimensional Fatigue Inventory (MFI), the Wood Mental Fatigue Inventory, and the Fatigue Severity Scale, among others. The SF-36 physical functioning scale can distinguish between diseased and nondiseased individuals. However, it is less useful for ascertaining the degree of disability in individual patients (van Campen et al., 2020). This may be the case for those with EDS/HSD, as function can be affected not just by orthostatic intolerance and fatigue but also by joint stability and pain.

Effects on Functioning

The symptoms of orthostatic intolerance and ME/CFS and their severity can be unpredictable. They are influenced by the level of activity or degree of orthostatic and other physiologic stressors in the preceding days, which can provoke postexertional malaise (PEM). PEM denotes an exacerbation of any of a variety of symptoms—fatigue, lightheadedness, cognitive dysfunction, headache, sensitivity to sensory stimuli, and generalized pain—after people have increased their usually tolerated physical, cognitive, or orthostatic stress (Rowe, 2022).

In a study by Ross and colleagues (2013), 96 percent of patients with POTS self-reported cognitive deficits, referred to as "brain fog." Blurred or double vision can impact reading, driving, and mobility, and acute sensitivity to smells, temperatures, sounds, and lights can affect socialization, child care, bathing, and participation in such activities as grocery shopping and doctor's appointments (Rich et al., 2020). A consistent finding among people with orthostatic intolerance is exacerbation of symptoms in the morning (Rich et al., 2020).

Mast Cell Activation Disease

Mast cells reside throughout the connective tissues, but tend to cluster in the skin and at the epithelial borders of the gastrointestinal, respiratory, and urogenital tracts, which interact with the external world. Mast cells have a variety of functions, including phagocytosis, antigen presentation, cytokine and chemokine production, and the release of vasoactive substances; they also play a role in local tissue homeostasis (tissue repair, angiogenesis) and coordination of immune responses to numerous pathogens (Seneviratne et al., 2017). MCAD is an immune syndrome that can be localized; localized mast cell disorders include, for example, rhinitis, hypersensitivity gastroenteritis, asthma, and urticaria. Systemic mast cell activation, called mast cell activation syndrome, presents with symptoms involving two or more organ systems (skin: urticaria [hives], angioedema [swelling under the skin], and flushing; gastrointestinal: nausea, vomiting, diarrhea, and abdominal cramping; cardiovascular: hypotensive syncope [fainting] or near syncope and tachycardia; respiratory: wheezing; naso-ocular: conjunctival injection, pruritus [itching], and nasal congestion) (Akin, 2017).

Mast cell activation syndrome can result from abnormal production of progenitor mast cells with genetic mutations or mast cell activation events triggered by comorbid disorders (Akin, 2017). The former etiology reflects clonal mast cell disorders with a neoplastic gain of function leading to production of abnormal mast cells; an example of this type of disorder is systemic mastocytosis. The latter etiology reflects mast cell activation that is disproportionate to that required to protect the body from the perceived assault (Akin, 2017). This second form of mast cell activation syndrome, termed nonclonal or secondary mast cell activation syndrome, is the more prevalent and reflects inappropriate activation of the cells to stimuli that otherwise would be tolerated if the individual were in a nonreactive state (Akin, 2017; Hamilton, 2018).

Mast cell dysregulation appears to play a role in EDS/HSD, as well as neuropathies and hypersensitivity syndromes, both immediate and delayed (Seneviratne et al., 2017). Co-occurrence of MCAD and EDS, particularly hEDS/HSD, has been linked to primary immunodeficiency disorders in these patients (Brock et al., 2021). In a study of 974 patients attending an allergy/immunology clinic, Brock and colleagues (2021) sought to identify those with the diagnostic codes for immunoglobulin deficiency, MCAD, and hEDS/HSD. They found that 46 percent of the 974 patients had MCAD but no codes for immunoglobulin deficiency or hEDS/HSD, 10 percent had a diagnosis of both MCAD and hEDS/HSD, and 19 percent had a diagnosis of all three disorders. The authors point out that HDCTs may increase susceptibility to aberrant mast cell activation (Brock et al., 2021).

Potential Reasons

Mast cells are closely associated with the epithelium of internal organs and the endothelium lining blood vessels and the lymphatic system and play a central role in the detection of and response to tissue injury. As described by Brock and colleagues (2021), mast cells are activated by factors derived from injured connective tissue, as well as activated inflammatory cascades. Following detection of danger or inflammatory signals, mast cells use an array of pathogen receptors to determine the nature of the impending danger, which may include infectious agents, toxins, and physical insults. Mast cells are thereby primed to release their cache of chemical mediators to recruit and activate other components of the innate and adaptive immune systems, as well as release chemicals that play a role in regulating angiogenesis, tissue remodeling, and wound healing (Brock et al., 2021).

Interventions

Treatment for MCAD is typically based on the etiology of mast cell reactivity, clonal versus nonclonal MCAD, triggers of mast cell activation events, and symptoms (see Annex Table 5-7). Therapy starts with identification and avoidance of triggers, such as foods, physical environmental factors, and medications. The latter category of triggers is important in the setting of pain management and surgeries, since several antibiotics, anesthetic agents, and pain relievers, including opioids and nonsteroidal anti-inflammatory agents, are known to be direct mast cell secretagogues. Patients with mast cell activation syndrome should receive premedication recommendations and treatment recommendations for anaphylaxis. Premedication and treatment recommendations consist of histamine and leukotriene blockade, as well as mast cell membrane–stabilizing compounds, such as ketotifen and cromolyn (Hamilton, 2018; Weiler et al., 2019). In addition to medications and foods, patients with EDS/HSD and comorbid MCAD need to identify and reduce exposure to nonimmunologic triggers, such as chemicals, stress, pollen, heat/cold, and exercise (Seneviratne et al., 2017). For patients with more recalcitrant MCAD, desensitization therapy may be appropriate, as well as use of nonsteroidal immunosuppressants and some biologic therapies, including omalizumab and possibly supplemental gamma globulin (Molderings et al., 2016; Seneviratne et al., 2017).

Glucocorticoid therapy is not recommended for patients with both EDS/HSD and MCAD (Seneviratne et al., 2017). Regular exercise to the patient's usual limit of tolerance is recommended; however, strenuous exercise may trigger a mast cell activation flare (Seneviratne et al., 2017).

Assessment

Three criteria have been proposed for diagnosing mast cell activation syndrome: (1) typical signs and symptoms of mast cell mediator release (affecting at least two organ systems); (2) specific symptoms in six organ systems (skin, cardiovascular, gastrointestinal, respiratory, naso-ocular, and anaphalyxis); and (3) objective evidence of mast cell–derived mediator release or chronically activated mast cells, typically obtained with laboratory testing (Seneviratne et al., 2017). Elevated serum tryptase is often used in the diagnosis of mast cell activation syndrome, although symptoms of MCAD may occur without elevated tryptase. Annex Table 5-7 summarizes common methods used to diagnose MCAD.

Effects on Functioning

Patients with MCAD and EDS/HSD may experience fatigue and malaise. Both physical and psychological stress can activate mast cells. Pain is a common characteristic of MCAD that can be treated with nonsteroidal anti-inflammatory drugs, although their use needs to be tailored to the individual patient. Among the many symptoms of MCAD that may affect function are urticaria, angioedema, asthma, neurocognitive impairment, throat swelling, diarrhea, and cramping (Seneviratne et al., 2017).

Full-Body Functioning

One of the challenges of assessment of functioning, especially as it relates to SSA disability determinations, is capturing the full effect of an individual's impairment(s) on daily activities (see NASEM, 2019). This is particularly true when a person has multiple impairments that individually do not rise to the level of severity required by SSA but collectively may do so. Given that individuals with HDCTs typically experience secondary impairments in multiple body systems, it is important to assess the collective effect of all their physical and mental impairments on their ability to function in daily life, including at work and in school. In addition, as discussed previously, some frequently experienced conditions, such as chronic pain, fatigue, mild cognitive impairment, anxiety, and depression, can affect individuals' overall functioning. As described in Chapter 1, SSA's disability determination process for children includes a concept called functional equivalence.

The technique for determining functional equivalence is a "whole child" approach that "accounts for all of the effects of a child's impairments singly and in combination—the interactive and cumulative effects of the impairments—because it starts with a consideration of actual functioning in all settings" (SSA, 2009). This approach is particularly well suited to evaluating the combined effects on functioning of the many and varied impairments that often manifest in HDCTs and other multisystem disorders.

Potential Reasons

Annex Table 5-13 lists some of the potential reasons for limitations in full-body functioning among individuals with HDCTs. These include pain; weakness; fatigue; deconditioning; joint instability throughout the body; dysautonomia, including POTS; balance dysfunction; and cardiovascular, respiratory, and gastrointestinal impairments.

Assessment

A number of performance-based and self-reported measures for assessing overall physical functioning are included in Annex Table 5-13. The Bruininks-Oseretsky Test of Motor Proficiency, 2nd Edition (BOT-2) is an established performance-based measure for assessing gross and fine motor function in children and young adults (ages 4–21) (Bruininks and Bruininks, 2005). BOT-2 comprises eight subtests: fine motor precision, fine motor integration, manual dexterity, bilateral coordination, balance, running speed and agility, upper-limb coordination, and strength (Bruininks and Bruininks, 2005). A small Swedish study of children aged 8–16 years found that children with joint hypermobility scored lower on the BOT-2 balance subtest compared with the control group (Schubert-Hjalmarsson et al., 2012). The Bruininks Motor Ability Test (BMAT) is an adaptation of the BOT-2 for adults aged 40 and older (Bruininks and Bruininks, 2012). BMAT subtests include fine motor integration, manual dexterity, coordination, balance and mobility, and strength and flexibility (Bruininks and Bruininks, 2012). A small study of healthy adults aged 65–92 living in the community in Australia found scores on the fine motor integration and manual dexterity subtests of BMAT to be predictive of the participants' level of activity and participation as assessed on several measures, while scores on the coordination, balance, and mobility subtests were not (Seaton and Brown, 2018). Similar research using validated measures for working-age adults would be informative. Other performance-based assessments that provide information about individuals' overall physical functioning include functional capacity evaluation (Chen, 2007; Fore et al., 2015; Genovese and Galper, 2009; Jahn et al., 2004; Kuijer et al., 2012; Soer et al., 2008) and exercise testing that includes assessment of aerobic capacity and neuromuscular performance (Liguori and American College of Sports Medicine, 2021).

The Composite Autonomic Symptom Score-31 (COMPASS-31) is a 31-item self-report questionnaire about individuals' experience of symptoms related to dysautonomia (Sletten et al., 2012). A study aimed at differentiating severity groups among individuals with hEDS/HSD using a set of validated self-report questionnaires found that COMPASS-31 accurately differentiated individuals with more from those with less severely involved hEDS/HSD (Copetti et al., 2019).

Selected Assistive Technologies and Relevant Accommodations

The assistive technologies and accommodations that are relevant to individuals with limitations in full-body functioning will depend on the specific impairments or conditions that are affecting their physical functioning. Annex Tables 5-14 (physical functioning) and 5-15 (vision, hearing, and speech functioning) list selected assistive technologies and reasonable accommodations for specific areas of physical functioning.

Work-Related Functioning, Activities of Daily Living, and Instrumental Activities of Daily Living

Potential Reasons

Potential reasons for limitations in work activities, ADLs, and IADLs are listed in Annex Table 5-13 and are similar to those for full-body functioning.

Assessment

A number of measures can be used to perform an integrated assessment of overall physical and mental functioning (see NASEM, 2019, Chapter 4). Five such measures that provide information on work-related functioning are the Work Disability Functional Assessment Battery (WD-FAB), the Work Ability Index (WAI), the Sheehan Disability Scale (SDS), the Social and Occupational Functioning Assessment Scale (SOFAS), and the Mental Illness Research, Education, and Clinical Center version of the Global Assessment of Functioning scale (MIRECC GAF).

WD-FAB is a computerized self-report measure designed to assess work-related functioning in two domains: physical and mental health (Brandt and Smalligan, 2019; Meterko et al., 2019). WD-FAB consists of eight scales: basic mobility, upper-body function, fine motor function, community mobility, resilience and sociability, self-regulation, communication and cognition, and mood and emotions (Marfeo et al., 2019). Content relating to physical functioning includes such activities as sitting, standing, walking, and using a wheelchair/device to move around, as well as driving; using transportation; and pushing, pulling, lifting, and carrying (Marfeo et al., 2019). Content related to mental functioning includes cognitive functioning; communication; and management of mood, emotions, and behaviors (Marfeo et al., 2019).

The WAI is a seven-item self-report questionnaire designed to measure the work capacity of individuals in an occupational health clinic environment (Ilmarinen, 2007; NASEM, 2019; Tuomi et al., 1998, p. 90). It asks respondents about their "current work ability compared with the lifetime best," their "work ability in relation to the demands of the job," the "number of current diseases diagnosed by a physician," their "estimated work impairment due to diseases," the amount of "sick leave during the past year (12 months)," their "own prognosis of work ability 2 years from now," and "mental resources" (Ilmarinen, 2007). The responses are used to calculate a score categorizing the individual's work capability as poor, moderate, good, or excellent. The WAI can be used to predict early retirement, work disability, absence due to sickness, and mortality relatively well (NASEM, 2019). It also can be used to identify individuals who need supportive intervention (Adel et al., 2019). Repeated administration of the WAI over time may be particularly informative.

The SDS is a five-item self-report questionnaire designed to measure the effect of symptoms due to a physical or mental health condition on an individual's functioning in three areas: work or school, social life, and family life or home responsibilities (Sheehan, 1983). It can be used to assess change in functioning over time and has been shown to be sensitive to treatment effects in a selected group of mental health conditions, including anxiety disorders and depression (Sheehan and Sheehan, 2008).

The SOFAS provides a rating of social and occupational functioning on a scale from 0 to 100: lower scores indicate lower functioning (Rybarczyk, 2011). In contrast to the Global Assessment of Functioning scale, the SOFAS focuses on functioning independent of the severity of the person's psychological symptoms, and it includes impairments caused by physical as well as mental disorders (Rybarczyk, 2011).

The MIRECC GAF measures occupational, social, and psychological functioning separately on three different subscales—occupational, social, and symptom—that use ratings of 0 to 100, with lower scores indicating worse functioning and greater symptom burden (Niv et al., 2007).

ADLs and IADLs are tasks typically performed by individuals in the course of everyday life. ADLs include such basic self-care tasks as "personal care and hygiene, dressing, feeding, continence management, and mobility"

(NASEM, 2019, p. 77). IADLs are "more complex tasks related to independent living in the community, such as navigating transportation options and shopping, preparing meals, managing one's household, managing finances and medications, communicating with others, and providing companionship and mental support" (NASEM, 2019, p. 77). ADLs and IADLs can be assessed through self report, third-party report (e.g., caretaker, family member), direct observation, and/or specific assessment measures, a number of which are listed in Annex Table 5-13. The assessment of ADLs and IADLs and their relevance to work disability are discussed in detail in *Functional Assessment for Adults with Disability* (NASEM, 2019, pp. 76–82). Although information about individuals' ability to perform ADLs and IADLs may help inform determinations about their ability to work, there is no evidence to support a direct correlation between ADL and IADL assessments and the ability to perform work (NASEM, 2019).

Selected Assistive Technologies and Relevant Accommodations

Annex Table 5-13 lists a number of assistive technologies and accommodations that may improve individuals' ability to perform ADLs and IADLs, as well as work-related functioning. These include devices to improve mobility, reachers, built-up handles on home or work tools, and reorganization of or modifications to the home and workplace. The specific types of devices and accommodations needed depend on individuals' specific impairments and the activities affected.

PHYSICAL FUNCTIONING

The physical activities addressed in Annex Tables 5-2 and 5-14 are sitting, standing, walking, strenuous physical activity, lifting (floor to waist and overhead), carrying (which usually requires the ability to stand, lift, and walk), pushing or pulling, reaching, overhead reaching, at or below the shoulder reaching, gross manipulation, fine manipulation, foot and leg controls, climbing (which may include stairs, ramps, ladders, scaffolding, ropes, etc.), and low work (including stooping, crouching, kneeling, crawling, or lying on the ground). As previously mentioned, the committee identified these activities as most relevant to SSA based on the information SSA collects about applicants and the information the U.S. Bureau of Labor and Statistics collects about the physical demands of jobs for inclusion in the Occupational Information System. The committee added "strenuous physical activity" to the list and modified the grouping of some of the other activities on the basis of their functional similarities or dissimilarities. Annex Table 5-2 provides definitions of the various physical activities along with explanations for deviations from the definitions of relevant physical job demands provided in the *ORS* [Occupational Requirements Survey] *Collection Manual* (BLS, 2020).

Potential Reasons

The committee identified seven potential reasons for limitations in any of the physical activities listed above: (1) pain, (2) joint instability, (3) weakness, (4) balance dysfunction, (5) fatigue and deconditioning, (6) neurological compromise, and (7) orthostatic intolerance and dysautonomia (see Annex Table 5-14). The specific activities affected depend on the location of the pain, the affected joints, weakness, and/or neurological compromise experienced by the individual. For example, instability in the cervical or lumbar spine, pelvis, and knees, as well as weakness and balance dysfunction affecting the trunk, can limit an individual's ability to sit, especially uninterrupted for prolonged periods of time. Instability in the cervical or upper-extremity joints and weakness in the arms and hands can limit an individual's ability to perform activities requiring fine manipulation, including keyboarding. Gross and fine manipulation may also be affected by coordination deficits. In addition to the effects of musculoskeletal and neurological impairments, such activities as walking and strenuous physical activity can be limited by cardiac and/or respiratory dysfunction and exercise intolerance. Recovery from major aortic surgery can take up to a year depending on extent of aortic replacement, further restricting participation during that time. Cardiac and aortic dysfunction also can restrict an individual's ability to lift objects from floor to waist or overhead.

Physical activity guidelines and restrictions for individuals with MFS and related disorders must be tailored to the specific person. However, general guidelines include avoidance of intense isometric exercise, such as occurs when straining to lift a heavy weight; contact sports that can lead to blows to the head; activities that involve rapid acceleration and deceleration over short distances (sprinting); activities that involve rapid changes in pressure (e.g., scuba diving); and exercise to the point of exhaustion (Paris and Brigham and Women's Hospital, 2008; Marfan Foundation, 2017). Metabolic equivalent of task (MET), or simply metabolic equivalent, is a physiological measure expressing the energy cost (or calories expended) of physical activities as a multiple of resting energy consumption. Generally, it is recommended that individuals with MFS and related disorders keep the intensity of their physical activity in the low to moderate range (i.e., < 6 METs) (Marfan Foundation, 2017). The physical activity guidelines from The Marfan Foundation (2017, p. 3) include a table of common physical and recreational activities that fall into light (< 3 METs), moderate (3–6 METs), and vigorous (> 6 METs) categories of intensity. Also included is a table of competitive sports and athletic activities organized by risk of contact and intensity (Marfan Foundation, 2017, p. 7). The mental and physical health benefits of exercise are well known, but it is important to tailor the type and intensity of physical activity to the specific needs of individuals with HDCTs. Especially for children and adolescents, the benefits of physical activities often extend beyond the physical. Participation in spontaneous and organized physical activities, from playing tag and climbing trees to engaging in contact sports, gymnastics, and dance, is often the center of social interaction and central to the psychosocial and emotional well-being of many children and adolescents. Research on the relative benefits versus risks of participation in common physical activities is therefore important to better inform disease management in these age groups.

Maintaining a static position uninterrupted, such as sitting (especially the prolonged sitting often required to perform sedentary work or participate in a classroom) or standing for a prolonged period of time can be particularly problematic for individuals with HDCTs. Weak connective tissue and limited functionality of primary stabilizers (ligaments and tendons) can limit the ability to be erect in sitting or standing or for travel, and POTS can limit the ability to stand for extended periods. Jobs that might be considered sedentary but require an employee to move frequently between a seated and standing position may also be difficult for individuals with orthostatic intolerance. The freedom to move about and change position as needed (e.g., sitting to standing, walking in place) is important for these individuals to maintain function and reduce impairment. Conditions such as POTS, discussed earlier, can limit an individual's ability to remain in a seated position for even a few minutes or to function effectively while sitting or standing because of mild cognitive impairment. Individuals with EDS/HSD and other HDCTs may be unable to perform repetitive motions, including the fine manipulations, writing, and, in some cases, keyboarding that are often integral to sedentary work and school activities, over an extended period of time.

It is important to remember that the performance of a specific physical activity rarely if ever occurs independently of other physical activities. Annex Table 5-14 notes some of the overlaps among physical activities. Also, as previously mentioned, the committee includes lying down on the ground under "low work," along with stooping, crouching, kneeling, and crawling. This contrasts with the collection of occupational data on "sitting," which includes "active lying down. For example, a mechanic lying on a dolly working underneath a vehicle is sitting" (BLS, 2020, p. 112). Although lying on a raised surface (e.g., a bed) may be grouped with sitting, sitting is distinct from lying down on the ground (e.g., lying on a dolly underneath a vehicle). From a functional perspective, lying on the ground has more in common with other low work activities in that it includes the need to get up and down from the ground and potentially squirming around to do work while on the ground. These are difficult tasks that are equivalent to the other low work activities.

Assessment

Annex Table 5-14 lists performance-based and self-reported outcome measures that provide information relevant to an individual's ability to perform specific physical activities. Because of the importance of matching an individual's functional capacities to specific job requirements, a functional capacity evaluation is advised for individuals with hEDS/HSD (De Baets et al., 2021). Alternatively, specific function testing performed by a trained clinician (e.g., physical therapist, occupational therapist, exercise physiologist), directed at an individual's ability to perform the activities of interest, provides information about the person's ability to sustain those activities for the length of time required to perform a specific job or participate in classroom or other activities. When extrapolating from the testing environment to the workplace or school, it is important to remember that environmental conditions can affect individuals' symptoms and functioning. Performance at work and school, where physical, cognitive, and emotional stressors are often greater than in the testing environment, may be affected in ways not observed during testing.

Selected Assistive Technologies and Relevant Accommodations

Annex Table 5-14 lists a variety of assistive technologies and accommodations that can assist individuals in performing specific physical activities. Braces and other supports can assist with sitting, and allowing students or employees to alternate between sitting and other positions and to take rest breaks as needed can help them participate successfully in school and work. Specialized pencil/pen grips and alternative keyboards may facilitate handwriting and keyboarding. Students may benefit from a number of other school-based accommodations as well (SchoolToolkit, 2022), which can be formalized in a 504 plan or individualized education program. The use of certain assistive devices, in particular mobility devices to assist with standing and walking, including wheelchairs, can be very stressful for upper-extremity joints and may interfere with those activities requiring use of the upper extremities (e.g., lifting or carrying while using crutches). Similarly, ambulation devices that allow one to move well on a level or sloped surface may not be usable for climbing or ascending steep inclines.

VISION, HEARING, AND SPEECH FUNCTIONING

To a greater or lesser extent, vision, hearing, and speech functions may be affected in people with HDCTs (see Annex Tables 5-11 and 5-15).

Vision

Near visual acuity is defined as "clarity of vision at approximately 20 inches or less, as when working with small objects or reading small print" (BLS, 2020, p. 154). Close work, such as reading, writing, computer use, and manipulation of small objects, requires not only near visual acuity but also the ability of the eyes to work together as a team (binocular vision). When one's eyes do not work together because of accommodative or vergence dysfunction, one's ability to perform tasks requiring near vision (close work) may be impaired even when vision is normal in each eye independently (monocular vision). Difficulties performing close work can affect performance in school, recreational activities (sports, riding a bicycle), and jobs requiring close work.

Far visual acuity is defined as "clarity of vision at a distance of 20 feet or more, involving the ability to distinguish features of a person or objects at a distance" (BLS, 2020, p. 154). Peripheral vision refers to "what is seen above, below, to the left or right by the eye while staring straight ahead" (BLS, 2020, p. 154). Such tasks as driving, reading a blackboard, or participating in certain sports require far visual acuity. Driving and participating in certain sports are examples of tasks that also require peripheral vision.

Potential Reasons

A number of potential reasons for limitations in near and far visual acuity and peripheral vision are listed in Annex Table 5-15. They range from uncorrected refractive error to lens dislocation, retinal detachment or scarring, and cataract formation.

Assessment

Assessment of near and far visual acuity is performed using eye charts (e.g., Snellen, Bailey-Lovie) at a distance and handheld charts, respectively. Convergence (the ability of the eyes to work together) is assessed through orthoptic evaluation. One test of convergence asks the subject to maintain focus on a near target at a fixed distance while passing progressively stronger base-out prisms in front of one eye until the person experiences double vision or the examiner sees one of the eyes drift outward. Peripheral vision is assessed using kinetic or semiautomated kinetic perimetry to create maps of an individual's visual field. *Functional Assessment for Adults with Disabilities* includes a more detailed discussion of visual functioning and assessment (NASEM, 2019, pp. 128-133).

Selected Assistive Technologies and Relevant Accommodations

Assistive technologies for individuals with vision impairments include low-vision devices (refractive lenses), over-the-counter reading glasses to help with accommodative insufficiency, and base-in prism glasses to help with double vision during near work when impairment is related to convergence insufficiency. Other interventions include auditory replacements for vision tasks, glare-reducing equipment, orientation and mobility training (for impaired far and peripheral vision), and such modifications as sitting closer to the blackboard/screen in a classroom.

Hearing

Hearing is defined as the "ability to hear, understand, and distinguish speech and/or other sounds" (BLS, 2020, p. 149). Hearing is typically needed for jobs and schooling requiring communication, one-on-one and in group settings, in person or through video conferencing. It also is needed when a job requires use of a telephone or similar device, such as a radio, walkie-talkie, intercom, or public address system, or the ability to hear such sounds as machinery alarms and equipment sounds (BLS, 2020).

Potential Reasons

Hearing loss generally is classified as sensorineural, conductive, or a mix of the two, all of which may be seen in individuals with EDS/HSD, MFS, and Loeys-Dietz syndrome (LDS). People with EDS/HSD also may experience tinnitus, which refers to hearing sounds (e.g., ringing, clicking) in the absence of a corresponding external noise. Some people with tinnitus experience a muffling or distortion of external sounds (Møller, 2007).

Assessment

Performance-based measures for assessing hearing include pure tone audiometry (McBride et al., 1994; Yueh et al., 2003), speech recognition in noise testing (Giguère et al., 2008; Laroche et al., 2003), and internet- and telephone-based screening (Smits et al., 2004; Watson et al., 2012). Self-reported outcome measures for individuals with hearing impairments include the Hearing Handicap Inventory for Adults (Newman et al., 1990) and the Speech, Spatial, and Qualities of Hearing Scale (Gatehouse and

Noble, 2004). Assessment of hearing impairments and their effects on individuals' functioning are discussed in *Functional Assessment for Adults with Disabilities* (NASEM, 2019, pp. 133–143).

Selected Assistive Technologies and Relevant Accommodations

A 2017 National Academies report provides an analysis of selected assistive technologies and devices, including products and technologies pertaining to hearing (NASEM, 2017). Such technologies include hearing aids, personal sound amplification products, remote microphone hearing assistive technology, captioning, and telecommunications relay services. Environmental modifications (e.g., to improve acoustics) are also helpful.

Speech

Speech is defined as the expression or exchange of "ideas by means of the spoken word to impart oral information…accurately, loudly, or quickly" (BLS, 2020, p. 149). Although functional communication need not involve speech (but may involve, for example, alternative expressive modalities, nonverbal interactions, written language, and social communication), speech is necessary for certain jobs and is important if children are to be able to participate fully in school, including interaction with their peers. Language is another component of functional communication. Whereas speech comprises the physical processes of forming word sounds to convey a message, language is defined as the use of words, grammar rules, and the like to construct the content of the message.

Potential Reasons

Many factors contribute to communication, including the skills of the individual and the communication partner(s), as well as environmental conditions (e.g., background noise). With respect to the individual, "physical factors specific to communication (articulation accuracy, speaking rate, voice quality, loudness, fluency, effort, and fatigue) affect the intelligibility and comprehensibility of speech production" (NASEM, 2019, p. 144). Functional speech among individuals with HDCTs may be affected by temporomandibular joint dysfunction, laryngeal dysfunction, oral and dental pain, and vocal fatigue. Individuals with EDS/HSD may experience "painless dysphonia, fluctuating hoarseness, weak voice, dysphagia, recurrent episodes of laryngospasm, and subglottic stenosis" (Chohan et al., 2021, citing Arulanandam et al., 2017). Dysphonia among individuals with EDS/HSD may be attributable, at least in part, to "laxity, hypotonia, discoordination or decreased movement of the vocal cords, as well as reduced mobility of the cricoarytenoid joint" (Chohan et al., 2021, citing Arulanandam et al., 2017; Castori et al., 2010; Hunter et al., 1998). Individuals with cervical medullary syndrome and Chiari malformation may also experience dysarthria (Henderson et al., 2019).

With respect to language, "mental factors specific to communication at the individual level (receptive, expressive, and pragmatic language skills) affect message comprehension" (NASEM, 2019, p. 144). For example, difficulties with word finding, experienced by some individuals with mild cognitive impairment, affect language.

Assessment

Annex Table 5-15 lists a selection of measures of speech function, including measures of intelligibility, dysarthria, and apraxia, as well as several communication scales. A more complete discussion of speech functioning in the context of work, along with assessment measures, is included in *Functional Assessment for Adults with Disabilities* (NASEM, 2019, pp. 143–157).

Selected Assistive Technologies and Relevant Accommodations

A number of technologies can assist individuals with functional communication when speech is impaired. Personal voice amplification devices may be used to increase the volume of one's natural speech, and a wide variety of augmentative and alternative communication devices can replace oral communication if necessary (see NASEM, 2017, Chapter 6). Environmental modifications may help as well. For example, dry or dusty environments can exacerbate speech difficulties among individuals with EDS/HSD.

MENTAL FUNCTIONING

The committee focused on the mental activities included in Annex Table 5-16 because they are areas of mental functioning of particular interest to SSA for adults and children aged 3–18 years. The following mental activities are found in Paragraph B of SSA's Listing of Impairments for mental disorders (SSA, n.d.-c, n.d.-d): understand, remember, and apply information; concentrate, persist, or maintain pace; problem solve; interact with others; and adapt or manage oneself. Annex Table 5-2 provides definitions for each of these areas of mental functioning. Difficulties in these areas can affect quality of life in individuals with HDCTs.

A study of executive functioning and quality of life in adults with MFS found that "mental fatigue, commitment, instructions, problem solving, prospective memory, impulsivity, and flexibility" were all reliable predictors of satisfaction with quality of life (Ratiu et al., 2018). Cognitive dysfunction also has been reported in patient populations with conditions associated with HDCTs, including POTS (Raj et al., 2018; Ross et al., 2013; Wells et al., 2020) and CFS (Ocon, 2013). Such patients often complain of "brain fog," a type of cognitive dysfunction involving mild cognitive impairment. Patient-reported descriptors of "brain fog" include forgetfulness, difficulty thinking, difficulty focusing, feeling cloudy, difficulty finding the right words/communicating, mental fatigue, slowness, mind going blank, feeling "spacey," and difficulty processing what others say (Ross et al., 2013). Individuals reporting "brain fog" have shown mild to moderate cognitive impairment (Raj et al., 2018). Specific deficits have been found in short-term and working memory, selective attention, cognitive processing, reaction times, and executive functioning, although specific results vary among studies (Arnold et al., 2015; Ocon, 2013; Wells et al., 2020). Chapman (2020) reports effects on verbal recall and ability to do basic math, as well as short-term memory and concentration; word choice and language may also be affected.

Ross and colleagues (2013) found that 96 percent of respondents (aged 14–29) with POTS reported "brain fog," with 67 percent experiencing it daily. The majority of respondents said their symptoms adversely affected "their ability to complete schoolwork (86%), be productive at work (80%), and participate in social activities (67%)." These findings are consistent with other reports that individuals with "brain fog" "often complain of an inability to perform day-to-day tasks, organize thoughts, or hold a conversation," as well as difficulty with focus, learning and retaining information, and maintaining employment (Chapman, 2020).

A recent review of literature on the psychological burden associated with EDS/HSD found the highest prevalence for "language disorders (63.2%), attention-deficit/hyperactivity disorder (ADHD) (52.4%), anxiety (51.2%), learning disabilities (42.4%), and depression (30.2%)," although there often is great variability among studies in the prevalence reported (Kennedy et al., 2022). The reported prevalence for depression, for example, ranged from 11.1 to 30.2 percent, while that for anxiety ranged from 9.0 to 51.2 percent (Kennedy et al., 2022). Anxiety can manifest as feeling nervous, restless, or tense; worry; brooding—trouble concentrating or thinking about anything except the present worry; anticipatory anxiety; a sense of dread; task avoidance; and irritability, as well as physical symptoms (Mayo Clinic, 2022a; NLM, 2020). Depressive episodes manifest in symptoms (sadness, irritability, and emptiness; loss of pleasure or interest in activities) that persist for most of the day, almost every day, for at least 2 weeks (WHO, 2022). Other symptoms may include trouble concentrating, a feeling of excessive guilt or low self-worth, and hopelessness, in addition to physical symptoms (Mayo Clinic, 2022b; WHO, 2022). Anxiety and depression, which may coexist, can significantly interfere with daily activities, including participation in school and work; personal and social activities; and relationships with family, friends, teachers, coworkers, and others (Mayo Clinic 2022b; WHO, 2022).

Potential Reasons

Importantly, both physical and psychiatric conditions contribute to decrements in mental functioning. Chronic pain, fatigue, cognitive impairments, depression, mood disorders, anxiety, and impulsivity, individually and collectively, can affect mental functioning in the areas identified (see Annex Table 5-16).

Impaired cerebral blood flow associated with POTS (Ross et al., 2013; Wells et al., 2020); chronic inflammatory processes, which may disrupt the normal neuroimmune communication that is important to learning and memory (Mackay, 2015); and fatigue and poor sleep quality (Ross et al., 2013) may play a role in the cognitive dysfunction experienced by patients. Orthostatic and cognitive stressors, such as prolonged standing and prolonged concentration, have been reported to trigger or worsen cognitive dysfunction (Ocon, 2013; Ross et al., 2013), although some patients have reported that symptoms continue even after they return to a supine position, and others have reported that cognitive stressors (e.g., prolonged concentration) trigger symptoms while they are lying down (Ross et al., 2013).

Research on the effects of anxiety and depression on work and school performance in populations without HDCTs shows that both conditions can adversely affect performance (Beck et al. 2019; Jaycox et al., 2009; Mazzone et al., 2007; Plaisier et al., 2010), although depression may have a larger effect than anxiety (Plaisier et al., 2010). Plaisier and colleagues (2010) found that the risk of absenteeism and decreased work performance was greater among individuals who had more severe anxiety and depression. Beck and colleagues (2019) also found a relationship between productivity loss and severity of depression based on PHQ-9 scores, with even minor levels of depression being associated with decreased work function. In another study, teenagers with versus those without depression reported significantly greater impairment in academic, peer, and family functioning and physical health-related quality of life, as well as more days of impairment (Jaycox et al., 2009). Anxiety also adversely affects school performance and is associated with impaired memory and cognitive functions (Mazzone et al., 2007). Anxiety may interfere as well with the development of social skills, social life, and overall well-being (Mazzone et al., 2007).

Assessment

Annex Table 5-16 lists a variety of psychological and neuropsychological measures for assessing individuals' functioning in each of the areas of interest. More generally, as discussed in the section on work-related functioning, ADLs, and IADLs, the SDS has been widely used to assess the effects of symptoms of different mental health conditions on an individual's functioning at work or in school, in social life, and in family or home responsibilities (Sheehan, 1983). In addition, the WD-FAB is designed to assess cognitive functioning; communication; and management of mood, emotions, and behaviors relevant to work (Marfeo et al., 2019).

Selected Assistive Technologies and Relevant Accommodations

Annex Table 5-16 lists a number of accommodations that may support or improve individuals' mental functioning in the specified areas. Providing short, step-by-step instructions and breaking work tasks down into sequential steps is helpful, along with providing a written summary of the steps or recording them for playback by the individual as needed. Arranging for work to be performed in a quiet area without distractions and allowing individuals to sit or stand at will and take breaks as needed can also improve functioning.

HERITABLE DISORDERS OF CONNECTIVE TISSUE AND THE U.S. SOCIAL SECURITY ADMINISTRATION'S LISTING OF IMPAIRMENTS

The statement of task for this study asked the committee to "identify [for the selected HDCTs] non-exertional physical limitations (e.g., balancing or using the upper extremities for fine or gross movements) and mental limitations (e.g., cognitive or behavioral) that are equivalent in severity to the standard represented in the listings (i.e., that would prevent any gainful activity) but are not captured by currently existing listings and are not currently reflected in SSA's disability grid rules."

For SSA, nonexertional limitations occur when "limitations and restrictions imposed by [an individual's] impairment(s) and related symptoms, such as pain, affect only [their] ability to meet the demands of jobs other than the strength demands."[3] Examples include "difficulty functioning because [one is] nervous, anxious, or depressed"; "difficulty maintaining attention or concentrating"; "difficulty understanding or remembering detailed instructions"; "difficulty in seeing or hearing"; "difficulty tolerating

---

[3] 20 CFR 404.1569a.

some physical feature(s) of certain work settings, e.g., one cannot tolerate dust or fumes"; and "difficulty performing the manipulative or postural functions of some work such as reaching, handling, stooping, climbing, crawling, or crouching."[4]

It is clear from the variety of physical and mental secondary impairments throughout all body systems, related symptoms (e.g., pain, fatigue), and potential environmental triggers experienced by individuals with HDCTs that they can experience nonexertional limitations in any of the above areas. In some cases, the limitations may be sufficiently severe as to preclude the individual's participation in any gainful activity. In other cases, the combined effects of an individual's qualifying physical and/or mental secondary impairments may limit function sufficiently to preclude participation in work "in an ordinary work setting, on a regular and continuing basis, and for 8 hours a day, 5 days a week, or an equivalent work schedule" (SSA, 2021) or, for children, to cause "marked and severe functional limitations."[5]

Some individuals with HDCTs may qualify for SSA disability benefits at the listing-level step in the determination process on the basis of the secondary impairment(s) they are experiencing, rather than the HDCT itself. With the exception of MFS, which is identified under the cardiovascular listing 4.10 (aneurysm of aorta or major branches), HDCTs are not currently specified in the listings; for both adults and children, SSA disability claims related to HDCTs are evaluated under listings for the affected body system. Annex Table 5-17 includes some of the listings that may apply to certain individuals with HDCTs, as well as notes indicating special considerations. Examples of musculoskeletal SSA listings that could apply directly to some applicants with an HDCT include

1.15 Disorders of the skeletal spine resulting in compromise of a nerve root(s);
1.16 Lumbar spinal stenosis resulting in compromise of the cauda equina;
1.17 Reconstructive surgery or surgical arthrodesis of a major weight-bearing joint;
1.18 Abnormality of a major joint(s) in any extremity; and
1.21 Soft tissue injury or abnormality under continuing surgical management (see SSA, n.d.-b).

Joint and soft-tissue injury or abnormalities and pain are very common in individuals with HDCTs and hypermobility, resulting in significant functional limitations. It is important to note that certain abnormalities

---

[4] 20 CFR 404.1569a.
[5] 20 CFR 416.906.

may not be seen on standard imaging, necessitating the use of specialized imaging (e.g., flexion or extension imaging; magnetic resonance imaging [MRI], potentially upright, if tolerated; dynamic or soft-tissue imaging). In addition, as discussed previously, individuals with versus those without HDCTs are more likely to have poor outcomes with major surgery, especially if their HCDT was not previously recognized or taken into account in performing the surgery and providing aftercare. Wound healing is slow in many HDCTs, and wound dehiscence may occur despite excellent surgical and postoperative care. Some patients are unable to engage fully in postoperative therapy because of such HDCT-associated problems as fatigue, orthostatic intolerance, MCAD, depression, mild cognitive impairment, gastrointestinal disorders, or other musculoskeletal issues, which may further comprise surgical outcomes. As a result, surgical intervention, especially repeated surgery, for soft-tissue injuries or abnormalities may be contraindicated in some people with HDCTs even if it would be standard treatment for someone without an HDCT. The absence of surgery therefore need not imply that the person's functional limitations are any less severe. Further, individuals with significant upper-extremity involvement may not be candidates for assistive technology to aid mobility because they would not be able to use it effectively and therefore may not have been prescribed such a device.

Listings in other body systems that may apply directly to some individuals with HDCTs include

2.02	Loss of central visual acuity;
2.03	Contraction of the visual field in the better eye (meeting the specified criteria);
2.04	Loss of visual efficiency, or visual impairment, in the better eye (meeting the specified criteria);
3.03	Asthma;
3.07	Bronchiectasis;
3.14	Respiratory failure;
4.10	Aneurysm of aorta or major branches;
5.08	Weight loss due to any digestive disorder (meeting the specified criteria);
11.08	Spinal cord disorders;
12.04	Depressive, bipolar and related disorders;
12.06	Anxiety and obsessive-compulsive disorders; and
14.09	Inflammatory arthritis (SSA, n.d.-b).

The relationship between HDCTs and immune system dysfunction is a subject of ongoing research. It is clear that immune system dysfunction (e.g., MCAD) mediates HDCT-related secondary impairments in multiple body systems. Criteria in two of the listings for immune system disorders are especially relevant to the multisystem presentation and symptoms of HDCTs. The specific disorders listed—systemic lupus erythematosus and Sjogren's syndrome—are central to each set of criteria but are not common to HDCTs. The criteria listed for these disorders include

A. Involvement of two or more organs/body systems, with:
   1. One of the organs/body systems involved to at least a moderate level of severity; and
   2. At least two of the constitutional symptoms or signs (severe fatigue, fever, malaise, or involuntary weight loss).
OR
B. Repeated manifestations of [the listed disorder], with at least two of the constitutional symptoms or signs (severe fatigue, fever, malaise, or involuntary weight loss) and one of the following at the marked level:
   1. Limitation of activities of daily living.
   2. Limitation in maintaining social functioning.
   3. Limitation in completing tasks in a timely manner due to deficiencies in concentration, persistence, or pace. (SSA, n.d.-b, 14.02, 14.10)

Given that individuals with HDCTs typically experience physical and mental secondary impairments in multiple body systems, it is important to assess the collective effect of all their physical and mental impairments on their ability to function in daily life, including at work and in school. This is particularly true when a person has multiple impairments that individually do not rise to the level of severity required by SSA but collectively may do so. The concept of functional equivalence used by SSA in some disability determinations in children is particularly well suited to evaluating the combined effects on an applicant's functioning of the many and varied impairments that often manifest in HDCTs and other multisystem disorders.

FINDINGS AND CONCLUSIONS

Findings

5-1. The number, type, and severity of the physical and mental secondary impairments experienced by an individual with a heritable disorder of connective tissue (HDCT) drive the person's functioning and potential disability.

5-2. Environmental factors (e.g., temperature extremes, noise, vibration, atmospheric conditions, inhaled or skin irritants) can have significant adverse effects on function for some individuals with HDCTs.

5-3. Both physical and mental conditions can precipitate or exacerbate decrements in physical and mental functioning in individuals with HDCTs.

5-4. Chronic pain, chronic fatigue, and mild cognitive impairment are some of the most common and potentially disabling manifestations of the Ehlers-Danlos syndromes (EDS), especially hypermobile EDS (hEDS), hypermobility spectrum disorders (HSD), and Marfan syndrome (MFS).

5-5. A complex relationship exists among pain, fatigue, postural orthostatic tachycardia syndrome, and mast cell activation disease.

5-6. Pain can interfere with all types of physical activities that may be entailed in work or school, including sedentary activities. Pain also has an effect on cognitive functioning.

5-7. Fatigue associated with EDS/HSD and MFS can result in a number of physical and mental functional impairments that affect daily activities, including participation in work and physical activities.

5-8. Mild cognitive impairment can adversely affect participation in school, work, and social activities.

5-9. A challenge in assessment of functioning is capturing the full effect of individuals' impairments on their daily activities, including at work and in school. This is particularly true when a person has multiple impairments.

5-10. Numerous validated performance-based and self-reported measures are available for assessing physical and mental functioning, including several that can be used to perform an integrated assessment of an individual's overall physical and mental functioning.

5-11. Performance of a specific physical activity rarely if ever occurs independently of other physical activities.

5-12. Performance at work and in school, where physical, cognitive, and emotional stressors are often greater than in the testing environment, may be affected in ways not observed during testing.

5-13. Physical activity guidelines and restrictions for individuals with HDCTs need to be tailored to the specific person.

5-14. General physical activity guidelines exist for people with MFS and related disorders, such as avoidance of intense isometric exercise, contact sports that can lead to blows to the head, activities that involve rapid acceleration and deceleration over short distances (sprinting) or rapid changes in pressure (e.g., scuba diving), and exercise to the point of exhaustion.

5-15. Depending on a person's underlying impairment(s), assistive technologies and relevant accommodations can improve physical and mental functioning in some cases.

5-16. Some of the listings in SSA's Listing of Impairments—Adult Listings include severity criteria for some of the secondary impairments that may be experienced by individuals with HDCTs such as MFS, EDS, and related disorders.

5-17. Individuals with HDCTs may experience significant variability in their physical and/or mental secondary impairments from day to day or even within a single day. This variability is often unpredictable and may limit the ability to sustain gainful employment.

Conclusions

5-1. Given that individuals with HDCTs typically experience physical and mental secondary impairments in multiple body systems, it is important to assess the collective effect of all their physical and mental impairments on their ability to function in daily life, including at work and in school.

5-2. Accurately assessing the full effect of an individual's impairment(s) is especially important for SSA disability determinations. This is particularly true when a person has multiple impairments that individually do not rise to the level of severity required by SSA but collectively may do so. The concept of functional equivalence used by SSA in some disability determinations in children is particularly well suited to evaluating the combined effects on an applicant's functioning of the many and varied impairments that often manifest in HDCTs and other multisystem disorders.

5-3. Because of the importance of matching an individual's functional capacities to specific job requirements, functional capacity evaluation or specific function testing, performed by a trained clinician and directed at an individual's ability to perform the activities of interest, is suggested to provide information about the person's ability to sustain those activities for the length of time required to perform a specific job or participate in classroom or other activities.

5-4. When extrapolating from the testing environment to the workplace or school, it is important to take into account specific environmental conditions that can affect the individual's symptoms and functioning.

5-5. Some of SSA's Listing of Impairments—Adult Listings apply directly to secondary impairments experienced by individuals with HDCT syndromes and could be used to evaluate disability in those individuals. Other listings, with some modification, could apply to individuals with certain secondary impairments associated with their HDCTs.

5-6. The combined effects of an individual's physical and/or mental secondary impairments may limit function with a degree of severity sufficient to preclude the ability to participate in work on a "regular and continuing basis" (8 hours per day, 5 days per week, or an equivalent work schedule) or, for children, to cause "marked and severe functional limitations."

REFERENCES

Aasheim, T., and V. Finsen. 2013. The DASH and the QuickDASH instruments. Normative values in the general population in Norway. *Journal of Hand Surgery (European Volume)* 39(2):140-144. https://doi.org/10.1177/1753193413481302.

Abishek, K., S. S. Bakshi, and A. B. Bhavanani. 2019. The efficacy of yogic breathing exercise Bhramari pranayama in relieving symptoms of chronic rhinosinusitis. *International Journal of Yoga* 12(2):120-123. https://doi.org/10.4103/ijoy.IJOY_32_18.

Abonia, J. P., T. Wen, E. M. Stucke, T. Grotjan, M. S. Griffith, K. A. Kemme, M. H. Collins, P. E. Putnam, J. P. Franciosi, K. F. von Tiehl, B. T. Tinkle, K. A. Marsolo, L. J. Martin, S. M. Ware, and M. E. Rothenberg. 2013. High prevalence of eosinophilic esophagitis in patients with inherited connective tissue disorders. *Journal of Allergy and Clinical Immunology* 132(2):378-386. https://doi.org/10.1016/j.jaci.2013.02.030.

Adel, M., R. Akbar, and G. Ehsan. 2019. Validity and reliability of Work Ability Index (WAI) questionnaire among Iranian workers: A study in petrochemical and car manufacturing industries. *Journal of Occupational Health* 61(2):165-174. https://doi.org/10.1002/1348-9585.12028.

Akin, C. 2017. Mast cell activation syndromes. *Journal of Allergy and Clinical Immunology* 140(2):349-355. https://doi.org/10.1016/j.jaci.2017.06.007.

American Academy of Dermatology Association. 2022. *Hyperhidrosis: Diagnosis and treatment.* https://www.aad.org/public/diseases/a-z/hyperhidrosis-treatment (accessed March 3, 2022).

American Thoracic Society, and European Respiratory Society. 2002. ATS/ERS statement on respiratory muscle testing. *American Journal of Respiratory and Critical Care Medicine* 166(4):518-624. https://doi.org/10.1164/rccm.166.4.518.

Anxiety & Depression Association of America. 2021. *Chronic pain.* https://adaa.org/understanding-anxiety/related-illnesses/other-related-conditions/chronic-pain (accessed March 7, 2022).

Arkwright, P. D., and A. R. Gennery. 2011. Ten warning signs of primary immunodeficiency: A new paradigm is needed for the 21st century. *Annals of the New York Academy of Sciences* 1238:7-14. https://doi.org/10.1111/j.1749-6632.2011.06206.x.

Arnold, A. C., K. Haman, E. M. Garland, V. Raj, W. D. Dupont, I. Biaggioni, D. Robertson, and S. R. Raj. 2015. Cognitive dysfunction in postural tachycardia syndrome. *Clinical Science (London, England: 1979)* 128(1):39-45. https://doi.org/10.1042/cs20140251.

Arulanandam, S., A. J. Hakim, Q. Aziz, G. Sandhu, and M. A. Birchall. 2017. Laryngological presentations of Ehlers-Danlos syndrome: Case series of nine patients from two London tertiary referral centres. *Clinical Otolaryngology* 42(4):860-863. https://doi.org/10.1111/coa.12708.

ASHA (American Speech-Language-Hearing Association). 2005. *Guidelines for manual pure-tone threshold audiometry.* www.asha.org/policy (accessed May 26, 2022).

Baeza-Velasco, C., T. Van den Bossche, D. Grossin, and C. Hamonet. 2016. Difficulty eating and significant weight loss in joint hypermobility syndrome/Ehlers–Danlos syndrome, hypermobility type. *Eating and Weight Disorders—Studies on Anorexia, Bulimia and Obesity* 21(2):175-183. https://doi.org/10.1007/s40519-015-0232-x.

Baeza-Velasco, C., C. Bourdon, R. Polanco-Carrasco, M. de Jouvencel, M. C. Gely-Nargeot, A. Gompel, and C. Hamonet. 2017. Cognitive impairment in women with joint hypermobility syndrome/Ehlers-Danlos syndrome hypermobility type. *Rheumatology International* 37(6):937-939. https://doi.org/10.1007/s00296-017-3659-8.

Baeza-Velasco, C., D. Cohen, C. Hamonet, E. Vlamynck, L. Diaz, C. Cravero, E. Cappe, and V. Guinchat. 2018. Autism, joint hypermobility-related disorders and pain. *Frontiers in Psychiatry* 9(December):656. https://doi.org/10.3389/fpsyt.2018.00656.

Baeza-Velasco, C., S. Lorente, E. Tasa-Vinyals, S. Guillaume, M. S. Mora, and P. Espinoza. 2021. Gastrointestinal and eating problems in women with Ehlers–Danlos syndromes. *Eating and Weight Disorders—Studies on Anorexia, Bulimia and Obesity* 26(8):2645-2656. https://doi.org/10.1007/s40519-021-01146-z.

Baeza-Velasco, C., P. Espinoza, A. Bulbena, A. Bulbena-Cabré, M. Seneque, and S. Guillaume. 2022a. Hypermobility spectrum disorders/Ehlers–Danlos syndrome and disordered eating behavior. In *Hidden and Lesser-known Disordered Eating Behaviors in Medical and Psychiatric Conditions*, edited by E. Manzato, M. Cuzzolaro, and L. M. Donini. Switzerland: Springer Nature. https://link.springer.com/chapter/10.1007%2F978-3-030-81174-7_28#citeas.

Baeza-Velasco, C., M. Seneque, P. Courtet, É. Olié, C. Chatenet, P. Espinoza, G. Dorard, and S. Guillaume. 2022b. Joint hypermobility and clinical correlates in a group of patients with eating disorders. *Frontiers in Psychiatry* 12(January):803614. https://doi.org/10.3389/fpsyt.2021.803614.

Bandelow, B. 1999. *Panic and agoraphobia scale (PAS)*. Ashland, OH: Hogrefe & Huber Publishers.

Barrett, E., L. Larkin, S. Caulfield, N. de Burca, A. Flanagan, C. Gilsenan, M. Kelleher, E. McCarthy, R. Murtagh, and K. McCreesh. 2021. Physical therapy management of non-traumatic shoulder problems lacks high-quality clinical practice guidelines: A systematic review with quality assessment using the AGREE II checklist. *Journal of Orthopaedic and Sports Physical Therapy* 51(2):63-71. https://doi.org/10.2519/jospt.2021.9397.

Bas, O., I. Nalbant, N. Can Sener, H. Firat, S. Yeşil, K. Zengin, F. Yalcınkaya, and A. Imamoglu. 2015. Management of renal cysts. *JSLS: Journal of the Society of Laparoendoscopic Surgeons* 19(1):e2014.00097. https://doi.org/10.4293/jsls.2014.00097.

Bascom, R., R. Dhingra, and C. A. Francomano. 2021. Respiratory manifestations in the Ehlers–Danlos syndromes. *American Journal of Medical Genetics Part C: Seminars in Medical Genetics* 187(4):533-548. https://doi.org/10.1002/ajmg.c.31953.

Bathen, T., G. Velvin, S. Rand-Hendriksen, and H. S. Robinson. 2014. Fatigue in adults with Marfan syndrome, occurrence and associations to pain and other factors. *American Journal of Medical Genetics Part A* 164(8):1931-1939. https://doi.org/10.1002/ajmg.a.36574.

Baum, C. M., L. T. Connor, T. Morrison, M. Hahn, A. W. Dromerick, and D. F. Edwards. 2008. Reliability, validity, and clinical utility of the Executive Function Performance Test: A measure of executive function in a sample of people with stroke. *American Journal of Occupational Therapy* 62(4):446-455. https://doi.org/10.5014/ajot.62.4.446.

Baylor, C., K. Yorkston, T. Eadie, R. Miller, and D. Amtmann. 2008. Levels of speech usage: A self-report scale for describing how people use speech. *Journal of Medical Speech-Language Pathology* 16(4):191-198. https://www.ncbi.nlm.nih.gov/pmc/articles/PMC3130613/.

Baylor, C., K. Yorkston, T. Eadie, J. Kim, H. Chung, and D. Amtmann. 2013. The Communicative Participation Item Bank (CPIB): Item bank calibration and development of a disorder-generic short form. *Journal of Speech, Language, and Hearing Research* 56(4):1190-1208. https://doi.org/10.1044/1092-4388(2012/12-0140).

Beaton, D. E., A. M. Davis, P. Hudak, and S. McConnell. 2001. The DASH (disabilities of the arm, shoulder and hand) outcome measure: What do we know about it now? *The British Journal of Hand Therapy* 6(4):109-118. https://doi.org/10.1177/175899830100600401.

Bechara, F. G., T. Gambichler, A. Bader, M. Sand, P. Altmeyer, and K. Hoffmann. 2007. Assessment of quality of life in patients with primary axillary hyperhidrosis before and after suction-curettage. *Journal of the American Academy of Dermatology* 57(2):207-212. https://doi.org/10.1016/j.jaad.2007.01.035.

Beck, A., A. L. Crain, L. I. Solberg, J. Unützer, R. E. Glasgow, M. V. Maciosek, and R. Whitebird. 2011. Severity of depression and magnitude of productivity loss. *Annals of Family Medicine* 9(4):305-311. https://doi.org/10.1370/afm.1260.

Becker, J. H., J. J. Lin, M. Doernberg, K. Stone, A. Navis, J. R. Festa, and J. P. Wisnivesky. 2021. Assessment of cognitive function in patients after COVID-19 infection. *JAMA Network Open* 4(10):e2130645. https://doi.org/10.1001/jamanetworkopen.2021.30645.

Beighton, P. 1969. Obstetric aspects of the Ehlers-Danlos syndrome. *Journal of Obstetrics and Gynaecology of the British Commonwealth* 76(2):97-101. https://doi.org/10.1111/j.1471-0528.1969.tb05801.x.

Berglund, B., and E. Björck. 2012. Women with Ehlers-Danlos syndrome experience low oral health-related quality of life. *Journal of Oral & Facial Pain and Headache* 26(4):307-314.

Berglund, B., C. Pettersson, M. Pigg, and P. Kristiansson. 2015. Self-reported quality of life, anxiety and depression in individuals with Ehlers-Danlos syndrome (EDS): A questionnaire study. *BMC Musculoskeletal Disorders* 16(1):89. https://doi.org/10.1186/s12891-015-0549-7.

Berryman, C., T. R. Stanton, K. J. Bowering, A. Tabor, A. McFarlane, and G. L. Moseley. 2013. Evidence for working memory deficits in chronic pain: A systematic review and meta-analysis. *Pain* 154(8):1181-1196. https://doi.org/10.1016/j.pain.2013.03.002.

Berryman, C., T. R. Stanton, K. J. Bowering, A. Tabor, A. McFarlane, and G. L. Moseley. 2014. Do people with chronic pain have impaired executive function? A meta-analytical review. *Clinical Psychology Review* 34(7):563-579. https://doi.org/10.1016/j.cpr.2014.08.003.

Bezerra, L. A., H. F. de Melo, A. P. Garay, V. M. Reis, F. J. Aidar, A. R. Bodas, N. D. Garrido, and R. J. de Oliveira. 2014. Do 12-week yoga program influence respiratory function of elderly women? *Journal of Human Kinetics* 43(November):177-184. https://doi.org/10.2478/hukin-2014-0103.

Bier, J. D., W. G. M. Scholten-Peeters, J. B. Staal, J. Pool, M. W. van Tulder, E. Beekman, J. Knoop, G. Meerhoff, and A. P. Verhagen. 2018. Clinical practice guideline for physical therapy assessment and treatment in patients with nonspecific neck pain. *Physical Therapy* 98(3):162-171. https://doi.org/10.1093/ptj/pzx118.

Bijur, P. E., W. Silver, and E. J. Gallagher. 2001. Reliability of the visual analog scale for measurement of acute pain. *Academic Emergency Medicine* 8(12):1153-1157. https://doi.org/10.1111/j.1553-2712.2001.tb01132.x.

Bilberg, A., T. Bremell, and K. Mannerkorpi. 2012. Disability of the Arm, Shoulder and Hand questionnaire in Swedish patients with rheumatoid arthritis: A validity study. *Journal of Rehabilitation Medicine* 44(1):7-11. https://doi.org/10.2340/16501977-0887.

Birchall, M. A., C. M. Lam, and G. Wood. 2021. Throat and voice problems in Ehlers–Danlos syndromes and hypermobility spectrum disorders. *American Journal of Medical Genetics Part C: Seminars in Medical Genetics* 187(4):527-532. https://doi.org/10.1002/ajmg.c.31956.

Blagowidow, N. 2021. Obstetrics and gynecology in Ehlers-Danlos syndrome: A brief review and update. *American Journal of Medical Genetics Part C: Seminars in Medical Genetics* 187(4):593-598. https://doi.org/10.1002/ajmg.c.31945.

Blanpied, P. R., A. R. Gross, J. M. Elliott, L. L. Devaney, D. Clewley, D. M. Walton, C. Sparks, and E. K. Robertson. 2017. Neck pain: Revision 2017. *Journal of Orthopaedic and Sports Physical Therapy* 47(7):a1-a83. https://doi.org/10.2519/jospt.2017.0302.

BLS (Bureau of Labor Statistics). 2020. *ORS collection manual*. https://www.bls.gov/ors/information-for-survey-participants/pdf/occupational-requirements-survey-collection-manual-082020.pdf (accessed February 27, 2022).

Boehm, K., K. Kip, B. Grubb, and D. Kosinski. 1997. Neurocardiogenic syncope: Response to hormonal therapy. *Pediatrics* 99(4):623-25. https://doi.org/10.1542/peds.99.4.623.

Boone, P. M., R. M. Scott, S. J. Marciniak, E. P. Henske, and B. A. Raby. 2019. The genetics of pneumothorax. *American Journal of Respiratory and Critical Care Medicine* 199(11):1344-1357. https://doi.org/10.1164/rccm.201807-1212CI.

Bozkurt, S., G. Kayalar, N. Tezel, T. Güler, B. Kesikburun, M. Denizli, S. Tan, and H. Yilmaz. 2018. Hypermobility frequency in school children: Relationship with idiopathic scoliosis, age, sex and musculoskeletal problems. *Archives of Rheumatology* 34(3):268-273. https://doi.org/10.5606/ArchRheumatol.2019.7181.

Bragée, B., A. Michos, B. Drum, M. Fahlgren, R. Szulkin, and B. C. Bertilson. 2020. Signs of intracranial hypertension, hypermobility, and craniocervical obstructions in patients with myalgic encephalomyelitis/chronic fatigue syndrome. *Frontiers in Neurology* 11(August):828. https://doi.org/10.3389/fneur.2020.00828.

Brandt, D., and J. Smalligan. 2019. *A new approach to examining disability: How the WD-FAB could improve SSA's processes and help people with disabilities stay employed.* Washington, DC: Urban Institute. https://www.urban.org/research/publication/new-approach-examining-disability (accessed March 7, 2022).

Braverman, A. C., K. J. Blinder, S. Khanna, and M. Willing. 2020. Ectopia lentis in Loeys-Dietz syndrome type 4. *American Journal of Medical Genetics Part A* 182(8):1957-1959. https://doi.org/10.1002/ajmg.a.61633.

Brock, I., W. Prendergast, and A. Maitland. 2021. Mast cell activation disease and immunoglobulin deficiency in patients with hypermobile Ehlers-Danlos syndrome/hypermobility spectrum disorder. *American Journal of Medical Genetics Part C: Seminars in Medical Genetics* 187(4):473-481. https://doi.org/10.1002/ajmg.c.31940.

Brooks, R. S., J. Grady, T. W. Lowder, and S. Blitshteyn. 2021. Prevalence of gastrointestinal, cardiovascular, autonomic and allergic manifestations in hospitalized patients with Ehlers-Danlos syndrome: A case-control study. *Rheumatology (Oxford, England)* 60(9):4272-4280. https://doi.org/10.1093/rheumatology/keaa926.

Bruininks, B. D., and R. H. Bruininks. 2012. *Bruininks motor ability test.* https://www.pearsonassessments.com/store/usassessments/en/Store/Professional-Assessments/Cognition-%26-Neuro/Bruininks-Motor-Ability-Test/p/100000324.html (accessed January 3, 2022).

Bruininks, R. H., and B. D. Bruininks. 2005. *Bruininks-Oseretsky test of motor proficiency*, 2nd ed. https://www.pearsonassessments.com/store/usassessments/en/Store/Professional-Assessments/Motor-Sensory/Bruininks-Oseretsky-Test-of-Motor-Proficiency-%7C-Second-Edition/p/100000648.html (accessed January 3, 2022).

Bulbena-Cabré, A., C. Baeza-Velasco, S. Rosado-Figuerola, and A. Bulbena. 2021. Updates on the psychological and psychiatric aspects of the Ehlers–Danlos syndromes and hypermobility spectrum disorders. *American Journal of Medical Genetics Part C: Seminars in Medical Genetics* 187(4):482-490. https://doi.org/10.1002/ajmg.c.31955.

Burnett, J., C. B. Dyer, and A. D. Naik. 2009. Convergent validation of the Kohlman Evaluation of Living Skills as a screening tool of older adults' ability to live safely and independently in the community. *Archives of Physical Medicine and Rehabilitation* 90(11):1948-1952. https://doi.org/10.1016/j.apmr.2009.05.021.

Butts, R., J. Dunning, R. Pavkovich, J. Mettille, and F. Mourad. 2017. Conservative management of temporomandibular dysfunction: A literature review with implications for clinical practice guidelines (narrative review part 2). *Journal of Bodywork and Movement Therapies* 21(3):541-548. https://doi.org/10.1016/j.jbmt.2017.05.021.

Buysse, D. J., C. F. Reynolds, 3rd, T. H. Monk, S. R. Berman, and D. J. Kupfer. 1989. The Pittsburgh Sleep Quality Index: A new instrument for psychiatric practice and research. *Psychiatry Research* 28(2):193-213. https://doi.org/10.1016/0165-1781(89)90047-4.

Camacho, M., V. Certal, J. Abdullatif, S. Zaghi, C. M. Ruoff, R. Capasso, and C. A. Kushida. 2015. Myofunctional therapy to treat obstructive sleep apnea: A systematic review and meta-analysis. *Sleep* 38(5):669-675. https://doi.org/10.5665/sleep.4652.

Camerota, F., C. Celletti, M. Castori, P. Grammatico, and L. Padua. 2011. Neuropathic pain is a common feature in Ehlers-Danlos syndrome. *Journal of Pain and Symptom Management* 41(1):e2-e4. https://doi.org/10.1016/j.jpainsymman.2010.09.012.

Capuron, L., L. Welberg, C. Heim, D. Wagner, L. Solomon, D. A. Papanicolaou, R. C. Craddock, A. H. Miller, and W. C. Reeves. 2006. Cognitive dysfunction relates to subjective report of mental fatigue in patients with chronic fatigue syndrome. *Neuropsychopharmacology* 31(8):1777-1784. https://doi.org/10.1038/sj.npp.1301005.

Carley, M. E., and J. Schaffer. 2000. Urinary incontinence and pelvic organ prolapse in women with Marfan or Ehlers Danlos syndrome. *American Journal of Obstetrics and Gynecology* 182(5):1021-1023. https://doi.org/10.1067/mob.2000.105410.

Carpal tunnel syndrome: A summary of clinical practice guideline recommendations—Using the evidence to guide physical therapist practice. 2019. *Journal of Orthopaedic and Sports Physical Therapy* 49(5):359-360. https://www.jospt.org/doi/abs/10.2519/jospt.2019.0501.

Carr, A. J., A. A. Chiodo, J. M. Hilton, C. W. Chow, A. Hockey, and W. G. Cole. 1994. The clinical features of Ehlers-Danlos syndrome type VIIB resulting from a base substitution at the splice acceptor site of intron 5 of the *COL1A2* gene. *Journal of Medical Genetics* 31(4):306-311. https://doi.org/10.1136/jmg.31.4.306.

Carvalho, G. F., A. Schwarz, T. M. Szikszay, W. M. Adamczyk, D. Bevilaqua-Grossi, and K. Luedtke. 2020. Physical therapy and migraine: Musculoskeletal and balance dysfunctions and their relevance for clinical practice. *Brazilian Journal of Physical Therapy* 24(4):306-317. https://doi.org/10.1016/j.bjpt.2019.11.001.

Castori, M. 2012. Ehlers-Danlos syndrome, hypermobility type: An underdiagnosed hereditary connective tissue disorder with mucocutaneous, articular, and systemic manifestations. *ISRN Dermatology* 2012:751768. https://doi.org/10.5402/2012/751768.

Castori, M., and N. C. Voermans. 2014. Neurological manifestations of Ehlers-Danlos syndrome(s): A review. *Iranian Journal of Neurology* 13(4):190-208. https://www.ncbi.nlm.nih.gov/pmc/articles/PMC4300794/?report=classic.

Castori, M., F. Camerota, C. Celletti, C. Danese, V. Santilli, V. M. Saraceni, and P. Grammatico. 2010. Natural history and manifestations of the hypermobility type Ehlers-Danlos syndrome: A pilot study on 21 patients. *American Journal of Medical Genetics Part A* 152(3):556-564. https://doi.org/10.1002/ajmg.a.33231.

Castori, M., S. Morlino, C. Dordoni, C. Celletti, F. Camerota, M. Ritelli, A. Morrone, M. Venturini, P. Grammatico, and M. Colombi. 2012. Gynecologic and obstetric implications of the joint hypermobility syndrome (a.k.a. Ehlers–Danlos syndrome hypermobility type) in 82 Italian patients. *American Journal of Medical Genetics Part A* 158(9):2176-2182. https://doi.org/10.1002/ajmg.a.35506.

Castori, M., S. Morlino, G. Ghibellini, C. Celletti, F. Camerota, and P. Grammatico. 2015a. Connective tissue, Ehlers-Danlos syndrome(s), and head and cervical pain. *American Journal of Medical Genetics Part C: Seminars in Medical Genetics* 169(1):84-96. https://doi.org/10.1002/ajmg.c.31426.

Castori, M., S. Morlino, G. Pascolini, C. Blundo, and P. Grammatico. 2015b. Gastrointestinal and nutritional issues in joint hypermobility syndrome/Ehlers-Danlos syndrome, hypermobility type. *American Journal of Medical Genetics Part C: Seminars in Medical Genetics* 169(1):54-75. https://doi.org/10.1002/ajmg.c.31431.

Catala-Pétavy, C., L. Machet, G. Georgesco, F. Pétavy, A. Maruani, and L. Vaillant. 2009. Contribution of skin biometrology to the diagnosis of the Ehlers-Danlos syndrome in a prospective series of 41 patients. *Skin Research and Technology* 15(4):412-417. https://doi.org/10.1111/j.1600-0846.2009.00379.x.

Cauldwell, M., P. J. Steer, S. Curtis, A. R. Mohan, S. Dockree, L. Mackillop, H. Parry, J. Oliver, M. Sterrenburg, A. Bolger, F. Siddiqui, M. Simpson, N. Walker, F. Bredaki, F. Walker, and M. R. Johnson. 2019a. Maternal and fetal outcomes in pregnancies complicated by the inherited aortopathy Loeys-Dietz syndrome. *BJOG: An International Journal of Obstetrics and Gynaecology* 126(8):1025-1031. https://doi.org/10.1111/1471-0528.15670.

Cauldwell, M., P. J. Steer, S. L. Curtis, A. Mohan, S. Dockree, L. Mackillop, H. M. Parry, J. Oliver, M. Sterrenburg, S. Wallace, G. Malin, G. Partridge, L. J. Freeman, A. P. Bolger, F. Siddiqui, D. Wilson, M. Simpson, N. Walker, K. Hodson, K. Thomas, F. Bredaki, R. Mercaldi, F. Walker, and M. R. Johnson. 2019b. Maternal and fetal outcomes in pregnancies complicated by Marfan syndrome. *Heart* 105(22):1725-1731. https://doi.org/10.1136/heartjnl-2019-314817.

Cazzato, D., M. Castori, R. Lombardi, F. Caravello, E. D. Bella, A. Petrucci, P. Grammatico, C. Dordoni, M. Colombi, and G. Lauria. 2016. Small fiber neuropathy is a common feature of Ehlers-Danlos syndromes. *Neurology* 87(2):155-159. https://doi.org/10.1212/WNL.0000000000002847.

Cederlöf, M., H. Larsson, P. Lichtenstein, C. Almqvist, E. Serlachius, and J. F. Ludvigsson. 2016. Nationwide population-based cohort study of psychiatric disorders in individuals with Ehlers–Danlos syndrome or hypermobility syndrome and their siblings. *BMC Psychiatry* 16(1):207. https://doi.org/10.1186/s12888-016-0922-6.

Celletti, C., T. Paolucci, L. Maggi, G. Volpi, M. Billi, R. Mollica, and F. Camerota. 2021. Pain management through neurocognitive therapeutic exercises in hypermobile Ehlers–Danlos syndrome patients with chronic low back pain. *BioMed Research International* 2021:1-7. https://doi.org/10.1155/2021/6664864.

Chan, C., A. Krahe, Y. T. Lee, and L. L. Nicholson. 2019. Prevalence and frequency of self-perceived systemic features in people with joint hypermobility syndrome/Ehlers-Danlos syndrome hypermobility type. *Clinical Rheumatology* 38(2):503-511. https://doi.org/10.1007/s10067-018-4296-7.

Chansirinukor, W., C. G. Maher, J. Latimer, and J. Hush. 2005. Comparison of the Functional Rating Index and the 18-item Roland-Morris Disability Questionnaire: Responsiveness and reliability. *Spine* 30(1):141-145. https://doi.org/10.1097/00007632-200501010-00023.

Chapman, M. 2020. *How to manage brain fog when you have EDS.* https://ehlersdanlosnews.com/2020/06/17/manage-brain-fog/ (accessed October 14, 2021).

Chen, C. C., and R. K. Bode. 2010. Psychometric validation of the Manual Ability Measure-36 (MAM-36) in patients with neurologic and musculoskeletal disorders. *Archives of Physical Medicine and Rehabilitation* 91(3):414-420. https://doi.org/10.1016/j.apmr.2009.11.012.

Chen, J. J. 2007. Functional capacity evaluation & disability. *The Iowa Orthopaedic Journal* 27:121-127. https://www.ncbi.nlm.nih.gov/pmc/articles/PMC2150654/.

Cheung, I., and P. Vadas. 2015. A new disease cluster: Mast cell activation syndrome, postural orthostatic tachycardia syndrome, and Ehlers-Danlos syndrome. *Journal of Allergy and Clinical Immunology* 135(2, Supplement):AB65. https://doi.org/10.1016/j.jaci.2014.12.1146.

Chisholm, D., P. Toto, K. Raina, M. Holm, and J. Rogers. 2014. Evaluating capacity to live independently and safely in the community: Performance assessment of self-care skills. *British Journal of Occupational Therapy* 77(2):59-63. https://doi.org/10.4276/030802214X13916969447038.

Chiu, I. M., C. A. von Hehn, and C. J. Woolf. 2012. Neurogenic inflammation and the peripheral nervous system in host defense and immunopathology. *Nature Neuroscience* 15(8):1063-1067. https://doi.org/10.1038/nn.3144.

Chohan, K., N. Mittal, L. McGillis, L. Lopez-Hernandez, E. Camacho, M. Rachinsky, D. S. Mina, W. D. Reid, C. M. Ryan, K. A. Champagne, A. Orchanian-Cheff, H. Clarke, and D. Rozenberg. 2021. A review of respiratory manifestations and their management in Ehlers-Danlos syndromes and hypermobility spectrum disorders. *Chronic Respiratory Disease* 18:14799731211025313. https://doi.org/10.1177/14799731211025313.

Chopra, P. 2020. Pain management. In *Disjointed: Navigating the diagnosis and management of hypermobile Ehlers-Danlos syndrome and hypermobility spectrum disorders*. 1st ed., edited by D. Jovin. San Francisco: Hidden Stripes Publications. Pp. 365-419.

Chopra, P., B. Tinkle, C. Hamonet, I. Brock, A. Gompel, A. Bulbena, and C. Francomano. 2017. Pain management in the Ehlers–Danlos syndromes. *American Journal of Medical Genetics Part C: Seminars in Medical Genetics* 175(1):212-219. https://doi.org/10.1002/ajmg.c.31554.

Chow, K., R. E. Pyeritz, and H. I. Litt. 2007. Abdominal visceral findings in patients with Marfan syndrome. *Genetics in Medicine* 9(4):208-212. https://doi.org/10.1097/GIM.0b013e3180423cb3.

Chung, K. C., M. S. Pillsbury, M. R. Walters, and R. A. Hayward. 1998. Reliability and validity testing of the Michigan Hand Outcomes Questionnaire. *Journal of Hand Surgery* 23(4):575-587. https://doi.org/10.1016/s0363-5023(98)80042-7.

Cicerone, K. D., Y. Goldin, K. Ganci, A. Rosenbaum, J. V. Wethe, D. M. Langenbahn, J. F. Malec, T. F. Bergquist, K. Kingsley, D. Nagele, L. Trexler, M. Fraas, Y. Bogdanova, and J. P. Harley. 2019. Evidence-based cognitive rehabilitation: Systematic review of the literature from 2009 through 2014. *Archives of Physical Medicine and Rehabilitation* 100(8):1515-1533. https://doi.org/10.1016/j.apmr.2019.02.011.

Claar, R. L., and L. S. Walker. 2006. Functional assessment of pediatric pain patients: Psychometric properties of the Functional Disability Inventory. *Pain* 121(1-2):77-84. https://doi.org/10.1016/j.pain.2005.12.002.

Cleveland Clinic. 2020. *Dysautonomia*. https://my.clevelandclinic.org/health/diseases/6004-dysautonomia (accessed February 10, 2022).

Clinical guidance to optimize work participation after injury or illness: Using the evidence to guide physical therapist practice. 2021. *Journal of Orthopaedic and Sports Physical Therapy* 51(8):380-381. https://www.jospt.org/doi/abs/10.2519/jospt.2021.0505.

Cloutier, M. M., A. P. Baptist, K. V. Blake, E. G. Brooks, T. Bryant-Stephens, E. DiMango, A. E. Dixon, K. S. Elward, T. Hartert, J. A. Krishnan, R. F. Lemanske, D. R. Ouellette, W. D. Pace, M. Schatz, N. S. Skolnik, J. W. Stout, S. J. Teach, C. A. Umscheid, and C. G. Walsh. 2020. 2020 focused updates to the asthma management guidelines: A report from the National Asthma Education and Prevention Program Coordinating Committee Expert Panel Working Group. *Journal of Allergy and Clinical Immunology* 146(6):1217-1270. https://doi.org/10.1016/j.jaci.2020.10.003.

Collins, E., and M. Orpin. 2021. Physical therapy management of neurogenic thoracic outlet syndrome. *Thoracic Surgery Clinics* 31(1):61-69. https://doi.org/10.1016/j.thorsurg.2020.09.003.

Collins, N. J., D. Misra, D. T. Felson, K. M. Crossley, and E. M. Roos. 2011. Measures of knee function: International Knee Documentation Committee (IKDC) Subjective Knee Evaluation Form, Knee Injury and Osteoarthritis Outcome Score (KOOS), Knee Injury and Osteoarthritis Outcome Score Physical Function Short Form (KOOS-PS), Knee Outcome Survey Activities of Daily Living Scale (KOS-ADL), Lysholm Knee Scoring Scale, Oxford Knee Score (OKS), Western Ontario and McMaster Universities Osteoarthritis Index (WOMAC), Activity Rating Scale (ARS), and Tegner Activity Score (TAS). *Arthritis Care & Research* 63(S11):S208-S228. https://doi.org/10.1002/acr.20632.

Conners, K. C. 2014. *Conners' Continuous Performance Test*, 3rd ed. https://www.pearsonclinical.co.uk/store/ukassessments/en/Store/Professional-Assessments/Behavior/Attention-ADHD/Conners%27-Continuous-Performance-Test-3rd-Edition/p/P100009211.html (accessed January 4, 2022).

Cook, K. F., A. M. Bamer, D. Amtmann, I. R. Molton, and M. P. Jensen. 2012. Six Patient-Reported Outcome Measurement Information System short form measures have negligible age- or diagnosis-related differential item functioning in individuals with disabilities. *Archives of Physical Medicine and Rehabilitation* 93(7):1289-1291. https://doi.org/10.1016/j.apmr.2011.11.022.

Copetti, M., S. Morlino, M. Colombi, P. Grammatico, A. Fontana, and M. Castori. 2019. Severity classes in adults with hypermobile Ehlers–Danlos syndrome/hypermobility spectrum disorders: A pilot study of 105 Italian patients. *Rheumatology* 58(10):1722-1730. https://doi.org/10.1093/rheumatology/kez029.

Corbett, J. J., P. J. Savino, H. S. Thompson, T. Kansu, N. J. Schatz, L. S. Orr, and D. Hopson. 1982. Visual loss in pseudotumor cerebri. Follow-up of 57 patients from 5 to 41 years and a profile of 14 patients with permanent severe visual loss. *Archives of Neurology* 39(8):461-474. https://doi.org/10.1001/archneur.1982.00510200003001.

Culbertson, W. C., and E. A. Zillmer. 2005. *Tower of LondonDX™*, 2nd ed. https://storefront.mhs.com/collections/toldx-2nd-ed (accessed January 4, 2022).

Culver, B. H., B. L. Graham, A. L. Coates, J. Wanger, C. E. Berry, P. K. Clarke, T. S. Hallstrand, J. L. Hankinson, D. A. Kaminsky, N. R. MacIntyre, M. C. McCormack, M. Rosenfeld, S. Stanojevic, and D. J. Weiner. 2017. Recommendations for a standardized pulmonary function report. An official American Thoracic Society technical statement. *American Journal of Respiratory and Critical Care Medicine* 196(11):1463-1472. https://doi.org/10.1164/rccm.201710-1981ST.

D'Hondt, S., T. Van Damme, and F. Malfait. 2018. Vascular phenotypes in nonvascular subtypes of the Ehlers-Danlos syndrome: A systematic review. *Genetics in Medicine* 20(6):562-573. https://doi.org/10.1038/gim.2017.138.

Dabul, B. L. 2000. *Apraxia Battery for Adults*, 2nd ed. https://www.proedinc.com/Products/9100/aba2-apraxia-battery-for-adultssecond-edition.aspx (accessed January 3, 2022).

Daley, D., L. P. Payne, J. Galper, A. Cheung, L. Deal, M. Despres, J. D. Garcia, F. Kistner, N. Mackenzie, T. Perry, C. Richards, and R. Escorpizo. 2021. Clinical guidance to optimize work participation after injury or illness: The role of physical therapists. *Journal of Orthopaedic and Sports Physical Therapy* 51(8):CPG1-CPG102. https://doi.org/10.2519/jospt.2021.0303.

Dang, M. T., A. Ambort, and A. Arrey-Mensah. 2019. Recurrent swelling and pain in the abdomen and joints in a patient with hereditary angioedema and Ehlers-Danlos syndrome. *BMJ Case Reports* 12(11):e231484. https://doi.org/10.1136/bcr-2019-231484.

De Baets, S., P. Calders, L. Verhoost, M. Coussens, I. Dewandele, F. Malfait, G. Vanderstraeten, G. Van Hove, and D. Van de Velde. 2021. Patient perspectives on employment participation in the "hypermobile Ehlers-Danlos syndrome." *Disability and Rehabilitation* 43(5):668-677. https://doi.org/10.1080/09638288.2019.1636316.

de Leeuw, K., J. F. Goorhuis, I. F. Tielliu, S. Symoens, F. Malfait, A. de Paepe, J. P. van Tintelen, and J. B. Hulscher. 2012. Superior mesenteric artery aneurysm in a 9-year-old boy with classical Ehlers-Danlos syndrome. *American Journal of Medical Genetics Part A* 158(3):626-629. https://doi.org/10.1002/ajmg.a.34420.

De Martino, A., R. Morganti, G. Falcetta, G. Scioti, A. D. Milano, A. Pucci, and U. Bortolotti. 2019. Acute aortic dissection and pregnancy: Review and meta-analysis of incidence, presentation, and pathologic substrates. *Journal of Cardiac Surgery* 34(12):1591-1597. https://doi.org/10.1111/jocs.14305.

De Toma, G., M. Plocco, V. Nicolanti, G. Cavallaro, D. Amato, and C. Letizia. 2000. Arterial aneurysms associated with cystic hepato-renal disease. *Presse Medicale* 29(28):1559-1561.

De Wandele, I., L. Rombaut, T. De Backer, W. Peersman, H. Da Silva, S. De Mits, A. De Paepe, P. Calders, and F. Malfait. 2016. Orthostatic intolerance and fatigue in the hypermobility type of Ehlers-Danlos syndrome. *Rheumatology* 55(8):1412-1420. https://doi.org/10.1093/rheumatology/kew032.

Delis, D. C., E. Kaplan, and J. H. Kramer. 2001. *Delis-Kaplan Executive Function System™*. https://www.pearsonassessments.com/store/usassessments/en/Store/Professional-Assessments/Cognition-%26-Neuro/Delis-Kaplan-Executive-Function-System/p/100000618.html (accessed January 4, 2022).

Demirdas, S., E. Dulfer, L. Robert, M. Kempers, D. van Beek, D. Micha, B. G. van Engelen, B. Hamel, J. Schalkwijk, B. Loeys, A. Maugeri, and N. C. Voermans. 2017. Recognizing the tenascin-X deficient type of Ehlers-Danlos syndrome: A cross-sectional study in 17 patients. *Clinical Genetics* 91(3):411-425. https://doi.org/10.1111/cge.12853.

Di Stefano, G., C. Celletti, R. Baron, M. Castori, M. Di Franco, S. La Cesa, C. Leone, A. Pepe, G. Cruccu, A. Truini, and F. Camerota. 2016. Central sensitization as the mechanism underlying pain in joint hypermobility syndrome/Ehlers-Danlos syndrome, hypermobility type. *European Journal of Pain (London, England)* 20(8):1319-1325. https://doi.org/10.1002/ejp.856.

Dixon, D., M. Johnston, M. McQueen, and C. Court-Brown. 2008. The Disabilities of the Arm, Shoulder and Hand Questionnaire (DASH) can measure the impairment, activity limitations and participation restriction constructs from the International Classification of Functioning, Disability and Health (ICF). *BMC Musculoskeletal Disorders* 9(1):114. https://doi.org/10.1186/1471-2474-9-114.

Dobbs, B. M., A. R. Dobbs, and I. Kiss. 2001. Working memory deficits associated with chronic fatigue syndrome. *Journal of the International Neuropsychological Society* 7(3):285-293. https://doi.org/10.1017/S1355617701733024.

Doğan, Ş. K., Y. Taner, and D. Evcik. 2011. Benign joint hypermobility syndrome in patients with attention deficit/hyperactivity disorders. *Archives of Rheumatology* 26(3):187-192. https://dx.doi.org/10.5606/tjr.2011.029.

Domany, K. A., S. Hantragool, D. F. Smith, Y. Xu, M. Hossain, and N. Simakajornboon. 2018. Sleep disorders and their management in children with Ehlers-Danlos syndrome referred to sleep clinics. *Journal of Clinical Sleep Medicine* 14(4):623-629. https://doi.org/10.5664/jcsm.7058.

Donkervoort, S., C. G. Bonnemann, B. Loeys, H. Jungbluth, and N. C. Voermans. 2015. The neuromuscular differential diagnosis of joint hypermobility. *American Journal of Medical Genetics Part C: Seminars in Medical Genetics* 169(1):23-42. https://doi.org/10.1002/ajmg.c.31433.

Donnez, J. 2011. Menometrorrhagia during the premenopause: An overview. *Gynecological Endocrinology* 27(sup1):1114-1119. https://doi.org/10.3109/09513590.2012.637341.

Dordoni, C., M. Ritelli, M. Venturini, N. Chiarelli, L. Pezzani, A. Vascellaro, P. Calzavara-Pinton, and M. Colombi. 2013. Recurring and generalized visceroptosis in Ehlers-Danlos syndrome hypermobility type. *American Journal of Medical Genetics Part A* 161(5):1143-1147. https://doi.org/10.1002/ajmg.a.35825.

Drera, B., N. Zoppi, M. Ritelli, G. Tadini, M. Venturini, A. Wischmeijer, M. A. Nicolazzi, A. Musumeci, S. Penco, L. Buscemi, S. Crivelli, C. Danesino, M. Clementi, P. Calzavara-Pinton, S. Viglio, M. Valli, S. Barlati, and M. Colombi. 2011. Diagnosis of vascular Ehlers-Danlos syndrome in Italy: Clinical findings and novel *COL3A1* mutations. *Journal of Dermatological Science* 64(3):237-240. https://doi.org/10.1016/j.jdermsci.2011.09.002.

Dunn, D. M. 2018. *Peabody Picture Vocabulary Test*, 5th ed. https://www.pearsonassessments.com/store/usassessments/en/Store/Professional-Assessments/Academic-Learning/Brief/Peabody-Picture-Vocabulary-Test-%7C-Fifth-Edition/p/100001984.html (accessed January 12, 2022).

Dutil, É., A. Forget, M. Vanier, and C. Gaudreault. 1990. Development of the ADL profile: An evaluation for adults with severe head injury. In *Occupational therapy approaches to traumatic brain injury*, edited by L. H. Krefting and J. A. Johnson. New York: Routledge. Pp. 16-31. https://doi.org/10.4324/9780203057803-3.

Eccles, J., V. Iodice, N. Dowell, A. Owens, L. Hughes, S. Skipper, Y. Lycette, K. Humphries, N. Harrison, C. Mathias, and H. Critchley. 2014. Joint hypermobility and autonomic hyperactivity: Relevance to neurodevelopmental disorders. *Journal of Neurology, Neurosurgery and Psychiatry* 85(8):e3. https://doi.org/10.1136/jnnp-2014-308883.9.

Elliott, C. D. 2007. *Differential Ability Scales-II*. https://www.pearsonassessments.com/store/usassessments/en/Store/Professional-Assessments/Cognition-%26-Neuro/Comprehensive-Ability/Differential-Ability-Scales-II/p/100000468.html (accessed February 16, 2022).

Enderby, P., and R. Palmer. 2008. *Frenchay Dysarthria Assessment*, 2nd ed. https://www.proedinc.com/Products/12685/fda2-frenchay-dysarthria-assessmentsecond-edition.aspx (accessed January 3, 2022).

Enseki, K., M. Harris-Hayes, D. M. White, M. T. Cibulka, J. Woehrle, T. L. Fagerson, and J. C. Clohisy. 2014. Nonarthritic hip joint pain. *Journal of Orthopaedic and Sports Physical Therapy* 44(6):A1-A32. https://doi.org/10.2519/jospt.2014.0302.

Erickson, M., M. Lawrence, C. W. S. Jansen, D. Coker, P. Amadio, and C. Cleary. 2019. Hand pain and sensory deficits: Carpal tunnel syndrome. *Journal of Orthopaedic and Sports Physical Therapy* 49(5):CPG1-CPG85. https://doi.org/10.2519/jospt.2019.0301.

EuroQol Group. 1990. EuroQol—A new facility for the measurement of health-related quality of life. *Health Policy* 16(3):199-208. https://doi.org/10.1016/0168-8510(90)90421-9.

Exercise for knee injury prevention: A summary of clinical practice guideline recommendations—Using the evidence to guide physical therapist practice. 2018. *Journal of Orthopaedic and Sports Physical Therapy* 48(9):732-733.

Ezzeddine, H., P. Sabouraud, C. Eschard, O. El Tourjuman, N. Bednarek, and J. Motte. 2005. Bilateral frontal polymicrogyria and Ehlers-Danlos syndrome. *Archives de Pédiatrie* 12(2):173-175. https://doi.org/10.1016/j.arcped.2004.11.021.

Fikree, A., G. Chelimsky, H. Collins, K. Kovacic, and Q. Aziz. 2017. Gastrointestinal involvement in the Ehlers-Danlos syndromes. *American Journal of Medical Genetics Part C: Seminars in Medical Genetics* 175(1):181-187. https://doi.org/10.1002/ajmg.c.31546.

Finucane, L. M., A. Downie, C. Mercer, S. M. Greenhalgh, W. G. Boissonnault, A. L. Pool-Goudzwaard, J. M. Beneciuk, R. L. Leech, and J. Selfe. 2020. International framework for red flags for potential serious spinal pathologies. *Journal of Orthopaedic and Sports Physical Therapy* 50(7):350-372. https://doi.org/10.2519/jospt.2020.9971.

Fisher, A. G., and K. B. James. 2012. *Assessment of Motor and Process Skills*. 7th ed. Fort Collins, CO: Three Star Press.

Fore, L., Y. Perez, R. Neblett, S. Asih, T. G. Mayer, and R. J. Gatchel. 2015. Improved functional capacity evaluation performance predicts successful return to work one year after completing a functional restoration rehabilitation program. *PM&R* 7(4):365-375. https://doi.org/10.1016/j.pmrj.2014.09.013.

Frank, M., S. Adham, F. Zinzindohoué, and X. Jeunemaitre. 2019. Natural history of gastrointestinal manifestations in vascular Ehlers-Danlos syndrome: A 17-year retrospective review. *Journal of Gastroenterology and Hepatology* 34(5):857-863. https://doi.org/10.1111/jgh.14522.

Frattali, C. M., C. K. Thompson, A. L. Holland, C. B. Wohl, C. J. Wenck, S. C. Slater, and D. Paul. 2017. *American Speech-Language-Hearing Association Functional Assessment of Communication Skills for Adults (ASHA FACS)*. Rockville, MD: ASHA.

Freeman, R., W. Wieling, F. B. Axelrod, D. G. Benditt, E. Benarroch, I. Biaggioni, W. P. Cheshire, T. Chelimsky, P. Cortelli, C. H. Gibbons, D. S. Goldstein, R. Hainsworth, M. J. Hilz, G. Jacob, H. Kaufmann, J. Jordan, L. A. Lipsitz, B. D. Levine, P. A. Low, C. Mathias, S. R. Raj, D. Robertson, P. Sandroni, I. Schatz, R. Schondorff, J. M. Stewart, and J. G. van Dijk. 2011. Consensus statement on the definition of orthostatic hypotension, neurally mediated syncope and the postural tachycardia syndrome. *Clinical Autonomic Research* 21(2):69-72. https://doi.org/10.1007/s10286-011-0119-5.

Frieri, M. 2018. Mast cell activation syndrome. *Clinical Reviews in Allergy and Immunology* 54(3):353-365. https://doi.org/10.1007/s12016-015-8487-6.

Fu, Q., and B. D. Levine. 2015. Exercise in the postural orthostatic tachycardia syndrome. *Autonomic Neuroscience* 188:86-89. https://doi.org/10.1016/j.autneu.2014.11.008.

Fu, Q., and B. D. Levine. 2018. Exercise and non-pharmacological treatment of POTS. *Autonomic Neuroscience* 215:20-27. https://doi.org/10.1016/j.autneu.2018.07.001.

Galan, E., and B. G. Kousseff. 1995. Peripheral neuropathy in Ehlers-Danlos syndrome. *Pediatric Neurology* 12(3):242-245. https://doi.org/10.1016/0887-8994(95)00003-x.

Galli, M., V. Cimolin, L. Vismara, G. Grugni, F. Camerota, C. Celletti, G. Albertini, C. Rigoldi, and P. Capodaglio. 2011. The effects of muscle hypotonia and weakness on balance: A study on Prader-Willi and Ehlers-Danlos syndrome patients. *Research in Developmental Disabilities* 32(3):1117-1121. https://doi.org/10.1016/j.ridd.2011.01.015.

Gangadharan, V., and R. Kuner. 2013. Pain hypersensitivity mechanisms at a glance. *Disease Models & Mechanisms* 6(4):889-895. https://dx.doi.org/10.1242/dmm.011502.

Gao, F., J. Wang, J. Chen, X. Wang, Y. Chen, and X. Sun. 2021. Etiologies and clinical characteristics of young patients with angle-closure glaucoma: A 15-year single-center retrospective study. *Graefe's Archive for Clinical and Experimental Ophthalmology* 259(8):2379-2387. https://doi.org/10.1007/s00417-021-05172-6.

Gardarsdóttir, S., and S. Kaplan. 2002. Validity of the Arnadóttir OT-ADL Neurobehavioral Evaluation (A-ONE): Performance in activities of daily living and neurobehavioral impairments of persons with left and right hemisphere damage. *American Journal of Occupational Therapy* 56(5):499-508. https://doi.org/10.5014/ajot.56.5.499.

Gatehouse, S., and W. Noble. 2004. The Speech, Spatial and Qualities of Hearing Scale (SSQ). *International Journal of Audiology* 43(2):85-99. https://doi.org/10.1080/14992020400050014.

Genovese, E., and J. S. Galper. 2009. *Guide to the evaluation of functional ability: How to request, interpret, and apply functional capacity evaluations*. Chicago, IL: American Medical Association.

George, S. Z., T. A. Lentz, and C. M. Goertz. 2021. Back and neck pain: In support of routine delivery of non-pharmacologic treatments as a way to improve individual and population health. *Translational Research: The Journal of Laboratory and Clinical Medicine* 234(August):129-140. https://doi.org/10.1016/j.trsl.2021.04.006.

Giguère, C., C. Laroche, S. D. Soli, and V. Vaillancourt. 2008. Functionally-based screening criteria for hearing-critical jobs based on the Hearing in Noise Test. *International Journal of Audiology* 47(6):319-328. https://doi.org/10.1080/14992020801894824.

Gilliam, E., J. D. Hoffman, and G. Yeh. 2020. Urogenital and pelvic complications in the Ehlers-Danlos syndromes and associated hypermobility spectrum disorders: A scoping review. *Clinical Genetics* 97(1):168-178. https://doi.org/10.1111/cge.13624.

Glayzer, J. E., B. L. McFarlin, M. Castori, M. L. Suarez, M. C. Meinel, W. H. Kobak, A. D. Steffen, and J. M. Schlaeger. 2021. High rate of dyspareunia and probable vulvodynia in Ehlers-Danlos syndromes and hypermobility spectrum disorders: An online survey. *American Journal of Medical Genetics Part C: Seminars in Medical Genetics* 187(4):599-608. https://doi.org/10.1002/ajmg.c.31939.

Global Initiative for Asthma. 2021. *Global strategy for asthma management and prevention*. https://ginasthma.org/ (accessed March 2, 2022).

Goldstein, D., C. Holmes, S. Frank, R. Dendi, R. Cannon, Y. Sharabi, M. Esler, and G. Eisenhofer. 2002. Cardiac sympathetic dysautonomia in chronic orthostatic intolerance syndromes. *Circulation* 106(18):2358-2365. https://doi.org/10.1161/01.CIR.0000036015.54619.B6.

Goodman, B. P. 2018. Evaluation of postural tachycardia syndrome (POTS). *Autonomic Neuroscience* 215(December):12-19. https://doi.org/10.1016/j.autneu.2018.04.004.

Grabb, P. A., T. B. Mapstone, and W. J. Oakes. 1999. Ventral brain stem compression in pediatric and young adult patients with Chiari I malformations. *Neurosurgery* 44(3):520-527. https://doi.org/10.1097/00006123-199903000-00050.

Graf, C. 2008. The Lawton Instrumental Activities of Daily Living Scale. *American Journal of Nursing* 108(4):52-62. https://doi.org/10.1097/01.NAJ.0000314810.46029.74.

Graham, B. L., I. Steenbruggen, M. R. Miller, I. Z. Barjaktarevic, B. G. Cooper, G. L. Hall, T. S. Hallstrand, D. A. Kaminsky, K. McCarthy, M. C. McCormack, C. E. Oropez, M. Rosenfeld, S. Stanojevic, M. P. Swanney, and B. R. Thompson. 2019. Standardization of spirometry 2019 update. An official American Thoracic Society and European Respiratory Society technical statement. *American Journal of Respiratory and Critical Care Medicine* 200(8):e70-e88. https://doi.org/10.1164/rccm.201908-1590ST.

Granata, G., L. Padua, C. Celletti, M. Castori, V. M. Saraceni, and F. Camerota. 2013. Entrapment neuropathies and polyneuropathies in joint hypermobility syndrome/Ehlers-Danlos syndrome. *Clinical Neurophysiology* 124(8):1689-1694. https://doi.org/10.1016/j.clinph.2012.12.051.

Grant, D. A., and E. A. Berg. 1981. *Wisconsin Card Sorting Test.* https://www.wpspublish.com/wcst-wisconsin-card-sorting-test (accessed January 4, 2022).

Greally, M. T. 2020. Shprintzen-Goldberg syndrome. In *GeneReviews® [Internet]*, edited by M. P. Adam, H. H. Ardinger, R. A. Pagon, S. E. Wallace, L. J. Bean, K. W. Gripp, G. M. Mirzaa, and A. Amemiya. Seattle, WA: University of Washington; 1993-2022. https://www.ncbi.nlm.nih.gov/books/NBK1277/.

Greenberg, L., C. Holder, C. L. Kindschi, and T. R. Dupuy. 2017. *Test of Variables of Attention, version 9 (TOVA®9).* https://www.parinc.com/Products/Pkey/510 (accessed January 4, 2022).

Guerrerio, A. L., P. A. Frischmeyer-Guerrerio, C. Huang, Y. Wu, T. Haritunians, D. P. B. McGovern, G. L. MacCarrick, S. R. Brant, and H. C. Dietz. 2016. Increased prevalence of inflammatory bowel disease in patients with mutations in genes encoding the receptor subunits for TGFβ. *Inflammatory Bowel Diseases* 22(9):2058-2062. https://doi.org/10.1097/mib.0000000000000872.

Gupta, A., J. Gaikwad, A. Khaira, and D. S. Rana. 2010. Marfan syndrome and focal segmental glomerulosclerosis: A novel association. *Saudi Journal of Kidney Diseases and Transplantation* 21(4):754-755. https://www.sjkdt.org/text.asp?2010/21/4/754/64672.

Gupta, K., and I. T. Harvima. 2018. Mast cell-neural interactions contribute to pain and itch. *Immunological Reviews* 282(1):168-187. https://doi.org/10.1111/imr.12622.

Hakim, A., I. De Wandele, C. O'Callaghan, A. Pocinki, and P. Rowe. 2017a. Chronic fatigue in Ehlers-Danlos syndrome-hypermobile type. *American Journal of Medical Genetics Part C: Seminars in Medical Genetics* 175(1):175-180. https://doi.org/10.1002/ajmg.c.31542.

Hakim, A., C. O'Callaghan, I. De Wandele, L. Stiles, A. Pocinki, and P. Rowe. 2017b. Cardiovascular autonomic dysfunction in Ehlers-Danlos syndrome-hypermobile type. *American Journal of Medical Genetics Part C: Seminars in Medical Genetics* 175(1):168-174. https://doi.org/10.1002/ajmg.c.31543.

Hakim, A. J., B. T. Tinkle, and C. A. Francomano. 2021. Ehlers-Danlos syndromes, hypermobility spectrum disorders, and associated co-morbidities: Reports from EDS ECHO. *American Journal of Medical Genetics Part C: Seminars in Medical Genetics* 187(4):413-415. https://doi.org/10.1002/ajmg.c.31954.

Halko, G. J., R. Cobb, and M. Abeles. 1995. Patients with type IV Ehlers-Danlos syndrome may be predisposed to atlantoaxial subluxation. *Journal of Rheumatology* 22(11):2152-2155.

Halvorsen, T., E. S. Walsted, C. Bucca, A. Bush, G. Cantarella, G. Friedrich, F. J. F. Herth, J. H. Hull, H. Jung, R. Maat, L. Nordang, M. Remacle, N. Rasmussen, J. A. Wilson, and J. H. Heimdal. 2017. Inducible laryngeal obstruction: An official joint European Respiratory Society and European Laryngological Society statement. *European Respiratory Journal* 50(3):1602221. https://doi.org/10.1183/13993003.02221-2016.

Hamberis, A. O., C. H. Mehta, T. A. Valente, J. R. Dornhoffer, S. A. Nguyen, and T. A. Meyer. 2020. The pattern and progression of hearing loss in Marfan syndrome: A study of children and young adults. *International Journal of Pediatric Otorhinolaryngology* 138(November):110207. https://doi.org/10.1016/j.ijporl.2020.110207.

Hamilton, M. J. 2018. Nonclonal mast cell activation syndrome: A growing body of evidence. *Immunology and Allergy Clinics of North America* 38(3):469-481. https://doi.org/10.1016/j.iac.2018.04.002.

Hamilton, M. J., M. Zhao, M. P. Giannetti, E. Weller, R. Hufdhi, P. Novak, L. B. Mendoza-Alvarez, J. Hornick, J. J. Lyons, S. C. Glover, M. C. Castells, and O. Pozdnyakova. 2021. Distinct small intestine mast cell histologic changes in patients with hereditary alpha-tryptasemia and mast cell activation syndrome. *American Journal of Surgical Pathology* 45(7):997-1004. https://doi.org/10.1097/pas.0000000000001676.

Harrison, P., and T. Oakland. 2015. *Adaptive Behavior Assessment System*, 3rd ed. https://www.pearsonassessments.com/store/usassessments/en/Store/Professional-Assessments/Behavior/Brief/Adaptive-Behavior-Assessment-System-%7C-Third-Edition/p/100001262.html (accessed January 12, 2022).

Harvard Health Publishing. 2017. *Depression and pain.* https://www.health.harvard.edu/mind-and-mood/depression-and-pain (accessed March 7, 2022).

Hassan, I., T. Rasmussen, U. Schwarze, P. Rose, D. Whiteman, and P. Gloviczki. 2002. Ehlers-Danlos syndrome type IV and a novel mutation of the type III procollagen gene as a cause of abdominal apoplexy. *Mayo Clinic Proceedings* 77(8):861-863. https://doi.org/10.4065/77.8.861.

HealthMeasures. 2021. *Pain interference: A brief guide to the PROMIS© pain interference instruments.* http://www.healthmeasures.net/images/PROMIS/manuals/PROMIS_Pain_Interference_Scoring_Manual.pdf (accessed December 20, 2021).

Hear.com. n.d. *Conductive hearing loss.* https://www.hear.com/hearing-loss/conductive/ (accessed December 17, 2021).

Hegedus, E. J., S. M. McDonough, C. Bleakley, D. Baxter, and C. E. Cook. 2015. Clinician-friendly lower extremity physical performance tests in athletes: A systematic review of measurement properties and correlation with injury. Part 2—the tests for the hip, thigh, foot and ankle including the star excursion balance test. *British Journal of Sports Medicine* 49(10):649-656. https://doi.org/10.1136/bjsports-2014-094341.

Henderson, F. C., Sr., C. Austin, E. Benzel, P. Bolognese, R. Ellenbogen, C. A. Francomano, C. Ireton, P. Klinge, M. Koby, D. Long, S. Patel, E. L. Singman, and N. C. Voermans. 2017. Neurological and spinal manifestations of the Ehlers-Danlos syndromes. *American Journal of Medical Genetics. Part C: Seminars in Medical Genetics* 175(1):195-211. https://doi.org/10.1002/ajmg.c.31549.

Henderson, F. C., C. A. Francomano, M. Koby, K. Tuchman, J. Adcock, and S. Patel. 2019. Cervical medullary syndrome secondary to craniocervical instability and ventral brainstem compression in hereditary hypermobility connective tissue disorders: 5-year follow-up after craniocervical reduction, fusion, and stabilization. *Neurosurgical Review* 42(4):915-936. https://doi.org/10.1007/s10143-018-01070-4.

Henneberger, P. K., C. A. Redlich, D. B. Callahan, P. Harber, C. Lemière, J. Martin, S. M. Tarlo, O. Vandenplas, and K. Torén. 2011. An official American Thoracic Society statement: Work-exacerbated asthma. *American Journal of Respiratory and Critical Care Medicine* 184(3):368-378. https://doi.org/10.1164/rccm.812011ST.

Hentzen, C., N. Turmel, C. Chesnel, F. Le Breton, S. Sheikh Ismael, and G. Amarenco. 2018. Urinary disorders and Marfan syndrome: A series of 4 cases. *Urologia Internationalis* 101(3):369-371. https://doi.org/10.1159/000484696.

Herbowski, L. 2017. The major influence of the atmosphere on intracranial pressure: An observational study. *International Journal of Biometeorology* 61(1):181-188. https://doi.org/10.1007/s00484-016-1202-3.

Herbowski, L. 2019. From paradigm to paradox: Divergency between intracranial pressure and intracranial pulse pressure during atmospheric pressure fall: A case study. *Journal of Neurosurgical Sciences* 66(2):103-111. https://doi.org/10.23736/s0390-5616.19.04737-4.

Hernandez, A. M. C., and J. E. Dietrich. 2020. Gynecologic management of pediatric and adolescent patients with Ehlers-Danlos syndrome. *Journal of Pediatric and Adolescent Gynecology* 33(3):291-295. https://doi.org/10.1016/j.jpag.2019.12.011.

Hershenfeld, S. A., S. Wasim, V. McNiven, M. Parikh, P. Majewski, H. Faghfoury, and J. So. 2016. Psychiatric disorders in Ehlers-Danlos syndrome are frequent, diverse and strongly associated with pain. *Rheumatology International* 36(3):341-348. https://doi.org/10.1007/s00296-015-3375-1.

Higgins, D. M., A. M. Martin, D. G. Baker, J. J. Vasterling, and V. Risbrough. 2018. The relationship between chronic pain and neurocognitive function: A systematic review. *The Clinical Journal of Pain* 34(3). https://doi.org/10.1097/AJP.0000000000000536.

Hofman, K. J., B. A. Bernhardt, and R. E. Pyeritz. 1988. Marfan syndrome: Neuropsychological aspects. *American Journal of Medical Genetics* 31(2):331-338. https://doi.org/10.1002/ajmg.1320310210.

Holguin, F., J. C. Cardet, K. F. Chung, S. Diver, D. S. Ferreira, A. Fitzpatrick, M. Gaga, L. Kellermeyer, S. Khurana, S. Knight, V. M. McDonald, R. L. Morgan, V. E. Ortega, D. Rigau, P. Subbarao, T. Tonia, I. M. Adcock, E. R. Bleecker, C. Brightling, L. P. Boulet, M. Cabana, M. Castro, P. Chanez, A. Custovic, R. Djukanovic, U. Frey, B. Frankemölle, P. Gibson, D. Hamerlijnck, N. Jarjour, S. Konno, H. Shen, C. Vitary, and A. Bush. 2020. Management of severe asthma: A European Respiratory Society/American Thoracic Society guideline. *European Respiratory Journal* 55(1):1900588. https://doi.org/10.1183/13993003.00588-2019.

Holland, A. E., M. A. Spruit, T. Troosters, M. A. Puhan, V. Pepin, D. Saey, M. C. McCormack, B. W. Carlin, F. C. Sciurba, F. Pitta, J. Wanger, N. MacIntyre, D. A. Kaminsky, B. H. Culver, S. M. Revill, N. A. Hernandes, V. Andrianopoulos, C. A. Camillo, K. E. Mitchell, A. L. Lee, C. J. Hill, and S. J. Singh. 2014. An official European Respiratory Society/American Thoracic Society technical standard: Field walking tests in chronic respiratory disease. *European Respiratory Journal* 44(6):1428-1446. https://doi.org/10.1183/09031936.00150314.

Holland, A. E., N. S. Cox, L. Houchen-Wolloff, C. L. Rochester, C. Garvey, R. ZuWallack, L. Nici, T. Limberg, S. C. Lareau, B. P. Yawn, M. Galwicki, T. Troosters, M. Steiner, R. Casaburi, E. Clini, R. S. Goldstein, and S. J. Singh. 2021. Defining modern pulmonary rehabilitation. An official American Thoracic Society workshop report. *Annals of the American Thoracic Society* 18(5):e12-e29. https://doi.org/10.1513/AnnalsATS.202102-146ST.

Houston, D., S. L. Williams, J. Bloomer, and W. C. Mann. 1989. The Bay Area Functional Performance Evaluation: Development and standardization. 43:170-183. https://doi.org/10.5014/ajot.43.3.170.

Huang, J., C. Du, J. Liu, and G. Tan. 2020. Meta-analysis on intervention effects of physical activities on children and adolescents with autism. *International Journal of Environmental Research and Public Health* 17(6):1950. https://doi.org/10.3390/ijerph17061950.

Hugon-Rodin, J., G. Lebègue, S. Becourt, C. Hamonet, and A. Gompel. 2016. Gynecologic symptoms and the influence on reproductive life in 386 women with hypermobility type Ehlers-Danlos syndrome: A cohort study. *Orphanet Journal of Rare Diseases* 11(1):124. https://doi.org/10.1186/s13023-016-0511-2.

Hunter, A., A. W. Morgan, and H. A. Bird. 1998. A survey of Ehlers-Danlos syndrome: Hearing, voice, speech and swallowing difficulties. Is there an underlying relationship? *British Journal of Rheumatology* 37(7):803-804. https://doi.org/10.1093/rheumatology/37.7.803.

Hurst, B. S., S. S. Lange, S. M. Kullstam, R. S. Usadi, M. L. Matthews, P. B. Marshburn, M. A. Templin, and K. S. Merriam. 2014. Obstetric and gynecologic challenges in women with Ehlers-Danlos syndrome. *Obstetrics and Gynecology* 123(3):506-513. https://doi.org/10.1097/aog.0000000000000123.

Hurwitz, B. E., V. T. Coryell, M. Parker, P. Martin, A. Laperriere, N. G. Klimas, G. N. Sfakianakis, and M. S. Bilsker. 2009. Chronic fatigue syndrome: Illness severity, sedentary lifestyle, blood volume and evidence of diminished cardiac function. *Clinical Science (London, England: 1979)* 118(2):125-135. https://doi.org/10.1042/cs20090055.
Huynh, D. T. K., K. Shamash, M. Burch, E. Phillips, S. Cunneen, R. J. Van Allan, and D. Shouhed. 2019. Median arcuate ligament syndrome and its associated conditions. *American Surgeon* 85(10):1162-1165. https://doi.org/10.1177/000313481908501019.
IASP (International Association for the Study of Pain). 2021. Terminology: Nociplastic pain. https://www.iasp-pain.org/resources/terminology/ (accessed May 31, 2022).
Ilmarinen, J. 2007. The Work Ability Index (WAI). *Occupational Medicine* 57(2):160. https://doi.org/10.1093/occmed/kqm008.
Inayet, N., J. O. Hayat, A. Kaul, M. Tome, A. Child, and A. Poullis. 2018. Gastrointestinal symptoms in Marfan syndrome and hypermobile Ehlers-Danlos syndrome. *Gastroenterology Research and Practice* 2018:4854701-4854701. https://doi.org/10.1155/2018/4854701.
Islam, M., C. Chang, and M. E. Gershwin. 2020. Ehlers-Danlos syndrome: Immunologic contrasts and connective tissue comparisons. *Journal of Translational Autoimmunity* 4(December):100077. https://doi.org/10.1016/j.jtauto.2020.100077.
Iverson, G. L., and M. S. Koehle. 2013. Normative data for the Balance Error Scoring System in adults. *Rehabilitation Research and Practice* 2013:846418. https://doi.org/10.1155/2013/846418.
Iwama, T., H. Sato, T. Matsuzaki, S. Mitaka, K. Deguchi, and Y. Mishima. 1989. Ehlers-Danlos syndrome complicated by eventration of the diaphragm, colonic perforation and jejunal perforation—A case report. *Japanese Journal of Surgery* 19(3):376-380. https://doi.org/10.1007/bf02471417.
Jabs, C., and A. H. Child. 2016. Genitourinary tract in women with Marfan syndrome. In *Diagnosis and management of Marfan syndrome*, edited by A. H. Child. London: Springer. Pp. 219-225. https://doi.org/10.1007/978-1-4471-5442-6_20.
Jacobs, J. W., M. R. Bernhard, A. Delgado, and J. J. Strain. 1977. Screening for organic mental syndromes in the medically ill. *Annals of Internal Medicine* 86(1):40-46. https://doi.org/10.7326/0003-4819-86-1-40.
Jacome, D. E. 1999. Epilepsy in Ehlers-Danlos syndrome. *Epilepsia* 40(4):467-473. https://doi.org/10.1111/j.1528-1157.1999.tb00742.x.
Jahn, W. T., L. N. Cupon, and J. H. Steinbaugh. 2004. Functional and work capacity evaluation issues. *Journal of Chiropractic Medicine* 3(1):1-5. https://doi.org/10.1016/s0899-3467(07)60059-7.
Jayarajan, S. N., B. D. Downing, L. A. Sanchez, and J. Jim. 2020. Trends of vascular surgery procedures in Marfan syndrome and Ehlers-Danlos syndrome. *Vascular* 28(6):834-841. https://doi.org/10.1177/1708538120925597.
Jaycox, L. H., B. D. Stein, S. Paddock, J. N. Miles, A. Chandra, L. S. Meredith, T. Tanielian, S. Hickey, and M. A. Burnam. 2009. Impact of teen depression on academic, social, and physical functioning. *Pediatrics* 124(4):e596-e605. https://doi.org/10.1542/peds.2008-3348.
Jeon, J. W., J. Christensen, J. Chisholm, C. Zalewski, M. Rasooly, C. Dempsey, A. Magnani, P. Frischmeyer-Guerrerio, C. C. Brewer, and H. J. Kim. 2022. Audiologic and otologic clinical manifestations of Loeys-Dietz syndrome: A heritable connective tissue disorder. *Otolaryngology and Head and Neck Surgery* 166(2):357-362. https://doi.org/10.1177/01945998211008899.
Jester, A., A. Harth, G. Wind, G. Germann, and M. Sauerbier. 2005. Disabilities of the Arm, Shoulder and Hand (DASH) Questionnaire: Determining functional activity profiles in patients with upper extremity disorders. *Journal of Hand Surgery (Edinburgh, Scotland)* 30(1):23-28. https://doi.org/10.1016/j.jhsb.2004.08.008.

Jesudas, R., A. Chaudhury, and C. M. Laukaitis. 2019. An update on the new classification of Ehlers-Danlos syndrome and review of the causes of bleeding in this population. *Haemophilia* 25(4):558-566. https://doi.org/10.1111/hae.13800.

Ji, R. R., A. Nackley, Y. Huh, N. Terrando, and W. Maixner. 2018. Neuroinflammation and central sensitization in chronic and widespread pain. *Anesthesiology* 129(2):343-366. https://doi.org/10.1097/aln.0000000000002130.

Johannessen, E. C., H. S. Reiten, H. Løvaas, S. Maeland, and B. Juul-Kristensen. 2016. Shoulder function, pain and health related quality of life in adults with joint hypermobility syndrome/Ehlers–Danlos syndrome-hypermobility type. *Disability and Rehabilitation* 38(14):1382-1390. https://doi.org/10.3109/09638288.2015.1102336.

JOSPT infographic: Diagnosing and treating patellofemoral pain. 2021. *Journal of Orthopaedic and Sports Physical Therapy* 51(6):316-316. https://www.jospt.org/doi/abs/10.2519/jospt.2021.9001.

Joyce, E., S. Blumenthal, and S. Wessely. 1996. Memory, attention, and executive function in chronic fatigue syndrome. *Journal of Neurology, Neurosurgery and Psychiatry* 60(5):495-503. https://doi.org/10.1136/jnnp.60.5.495.

Kahn, T., M. Reiser, J. Gmeinwieser, and A. Heuck. 1988. The Ehlers-Danlos syndrome, type IV, with an unusual combination of organ malformations. *Cardiovascular and Interventional Radiology* 11(5):288-291. https://doi.org/10.1007/bf02577038.

Kalava, K., C. Roberts, J. D. Adair, and V. Raman. 2013. Response of primary erythromelalgia to pregabalin therapy. *Journal of Clinical Rheumatology* 19(5):284-285. https://doi.org/10.1097/RHU.0b013e31829cf8a2.

Kandola, A., and B. Stubbs. 2020. Exercise and anxiety. *Advances in Experimental Medicine and Biology* 1228:345-352. https://doi.org/10.1007/978-981-15-1792-1_23.

Kandola, A., D. Vancampfort, M. Herring, A. Rebar, M. Hallgren, J. Firth, and B. Stubbs. 2018. Moving to beat anxiety: Epidemiology and therapeutic issues with physical activity for anxiety. *Current Psychiatry Reports* 20(8):63. https://doi.org/10.1007/s11920-018-0923-x.

Kanigowska, K., M. Grałek, and D. Klimczak-Slaczka. 2006. The estimation of functional results after surgical treatment for ectopia lentis in children. *Klinika Oczna* 107(7-9):460-463. https://www.unboundmedicine.com/medline/citation/16416997/.

Kareha, S. M., P. W. McClure, and A. Fernandez-Fernandez. 2021. Reliability and concurrent validity of shoulder tissue irritability classification. *Physical Therapy* 101(3):pzab022. https://doi.org/10.1093/ptj/pzab022.

Katz, S. 1983. Assessing self-maintenance: Activities of daily living, mobility, and instrumental activities of daily living. *Journal of the American Geriatrics Society* 31(12):721-727. https://doi.org/10.1111/j.1532-5415.1983.tb03391.x.

Katz, S., and C. A. Akpom. 1976. Index of ADL. *Medical Care* 14(5 Suppl):116-118. https://doi.org/10.1097/00005650-197605001-00018.

Katzman, R., T. Brown, P. Fuld, A. Peck, R. Schechter, and H. Schimmel. 1983. Validation of a short Orientation-Memory-Concentration Test of cognitive impairment. *American Journal of Psychiatry* 140(6):734-739. https://doi.org/10.1176/ajp.140.6.734.

Kaufman, A. S., and N. L. Kaufman. 2004. *Kaufman Brief Intelligence Test*, 2nd ed. https://www.wpspublish.com/kbit-2-kaufman-brief-intelligence-test-second-edition (accessed January 4, 2022).

Kaufman, A. S., and N. L. Kaufman. 2018. *Kaufman Assessment Battery for Children Normative Update*, 2nd ed. https://www.pearsonassessments.com/store/usassessments/en/Store/Professional-Assessments/Cognition-%26-Neuro/Gifted-%26-Talented/Kaufman-Assessment-Battery-for-Children-%7C-Second-Edition-Normative-Update/p/100000088.html (accessed February 16, 2022).

Keefe, R. S. E., T. E. Goldberg, P. D. Harvey, J. M. Gold, M. P. Poe, and L. Coughenour. 2004. The Brief Assessment of Cognition in Schizophrenia: Reliability, sensitivity, and comparison with a standard neurocognitive battery. *Schizophrenia Research* 68(2):283-297. https://doi.org/10.1016/j.schres.2003.09.011.

Keefe, R. S. E., P. D. Harvey, T. E. Goldberg, J. M. Gold, T. M. Walker, C. Kennel, and K. Hawkins. 2008. Norms and standardization of the Brief Assessment of Cognition in Schizophrenia (BACS). *Schizophrenia Research* 102(1):108-115. https://doi.org/10.1016/j.schres.2008.03.024.

Kennedy, C. A., D. E. Beaton, P. Smith, D. Van Eerd, K. Tang, T. Inrig, S. Hogg-Johnson, D. Linton, and R. Couban. 2013. Measurement properties of the QuickDASH (disabilities of the arm, shoulder and hand) outcome measure and cross-cultural adaptations of the QuickDASH: A systematic review. *Quality of Life Research* 22(9):2509-2547. https://doi.org/10.1007/s11136-013-0362-4.

Kennedy, M., K. Loomba, H. Ghani, and B. Riley. 2022. The psychological burden associated with Ehlers-Danlos syndromes: A systematic review. *Journal of Osteopathic Medicine* 122(8):381-392. https://doi.org/10.1515/jom-2021-0267.

Khan, D. A. 2013. Alternative agents in refractory chronic urticaria: Evidence and considerations on their selection and use. *Journal of Allergy and Clinical Immunology: In Practice* 1(5):433-440. https://doi.org/10.1016/j.jaip.2013.06.003.

Khatri, S. B., J. M. Iaccarino, A. Barochia, I. Soghier, P. Akuthota, A. Brady, R. A. Covar, J. S. Debley, Z. Diamant, A. M. Fitzpatrick, D. A. Kaminsky, N. J. Kenyon, S. Khurana, B. J. Lipworth, K. McCarthy, M. Peters, L. G. Que, K. R. Ross, E. K. Schneider-Futschik, C. A. Sorkness, and T. S. Hallstrand. 2021. Use of fractional exhaled nitric oxide to guide the treatment of asthma: An official American Thoracic Society clinical practice guideline. *American Journal of Respiratory and Critical Care Medicine* 204(10):e97-e109. https://doi.org/10.1164/rccm.202109-2093ST.

Khera, T., and V. Rangasamy. 2021. Cognition and pain: A review. *Frontiers in Psychology* 12 (May):673962. https://doi.org/10.3389/fpsyg.2021.673962.

Kho, K. A., and J. K. Shields. 2020. Diagnosis and management of primary dysmenorrhea. *JAMA* 323(3):268-269. https://doi.org/10.1001/jama.2019.16921.

Kliethermes, C. J., M. Shah, S. Hoffstetter, J. A. Gavard, and A. Steele. 2016. Effect of vestibulectomy for intractable vulvodynia. *Journal of Minimally Invasive Gynecology* 23(7):1152-1157. https://doi.org/10.1016/j.jmig.2016.08.822.

Klinge, P. M. 2015. Histopathological evidence of clinically relevant filum pathology in tethered cord syndromes with little radiographic evidence including hypermobility syndromes. In *CSF Research Colloquium, September 26, 2015*. New Orleans, Louisiana. https://s3.amazonaws.com/csf.production/apps/uploads/2019/08/27202553/2015_Colloquium_Booklet_5.pdf.

Knee ligament sprain guidelines: Revision 2017: Using the evidence to guide physical therapist practice. 2017. *Journal of Orthopaedic and Sports Physical Therapy* 47(11):822-823. https://doi.org/10.2519/jospt.2017.0510.

Kohlman-Thomson, L. 1992. *Kohlman evaluation of living skills*. Rockville, MD: American Occupational Therapy Association.

Kornhuber, K. T. I., H. Seidel, C. Pujol, C. Meierhofer, F. Röschenthaler, A. Pressler, A. Stöckl, N. Nagdyman, R. C. Neidenbach, P. von Hundelshausen, M. Halle, S. Holdenrieder, P. Ewert, H. Kaemmerer, and M. Hauser. 2019. Hemostatic abnormalities in adult patients with Marfan syndrome. *Cardiovascular Diagnosis and Therapy* 9 (Suppl 2):S209-S220. https://cdt.amegroups.com/article/view/29689.

Krupp, L. B., N. G. LaRocca, J. Muir-Nash, and A. D. Steinberg. 1989. The fatigue severity scale: Application to patients with multiple sclerosis and systemic lupus erythematosus. *Archives of Neurology* 46(10):1121-1123. https://doi.org/10.1001/archneur.1989.00520460115022.

Kucera, S., and S. N. Sullivan. 2017. Visceroptosis and the Ehlers-Danlos syndrome. *Cureus* 9(11):e1828. https://doi.org/10.7759/cureus.1828.

Kuijer, P. P. F. M., V. Gouttebarge, S. Brouwer, M. F. Reneman, and M. H. W. Frings-Dresen. 2012. Are performance-based measures predictive of work participation in patients with musculoskeletal disorders? A systematic review. *International Archives of Occupational and Environmental Health* 85(2):109-123. https://doi.org/10.1007/s00420-011-0659-y.

Lambez, B., A. Harwood-Gross, E. Z. Golumbic, and Y. Rassovsky. 2020. Non-pharmacological interventions for cognitive difficulties in ADHD: A systematic review and meta-analysis. *Journal of Psychiatric Research* 120(January):40-55. https://doi.org/10.1016/j.jpsychires.2019.10.007.

Langhinrichsen-Rohling, J., C. L. Lewis, S. McCabe, E. C. Lathan, G. A. Agnew, C. N. Selwyn, and M. E. Gigler. 2021. They've been BITTEN: Reports of institutional and provider betrayal and links with Ehlers-Danlos syndrome patients' current symptoms, unmet needs and healthcare expectations. *Therapeutic Advances in Rare Disease* 2:263300402110220. https://dx.doi.org/10.1177/26330040211022033.

Lannoo, E., A. De Paepe, B. Leroy, and E. Thiery. 1996. Neuropsychological aspects of Marfan syndrome. *Clinical Genetics* 49(2):65-69. https://doi.org/10.1111/j.1399-0004.1996.tb04329.x.

Laroche, C., S. Soli, C. Giguère, J. Lagacé, V. Vaillancourt, and M. Fortin. 2003. An approach to the development of hearing standards for hearing-critical jobs. *Noise and Health* 6(21):17-37. https://www.noiseandhealth.org/text.asp?2003/6/21/17/31684.

Laszkowska, M., A. Roy, B. Lebwohl, P. H. R. Green, H. E. K. Sundelin, and J. F. Ludvigsson. 2016. Nationwide population-based cohort study of celiac disease and risk of Ehlers-Danlos syndrome and joint hypermobility syndrome. *Digestive and Liver Disease* 48(9):1030-1034. https://doi.org/10.1016/j.dld.2016.05.019.

Lee, D. M., N. Pendleton, A. Tajar, T. W. O'Neill, D. B. O'Connor, G. Bartfai, S. Boonen, F. F. Casanueva, J. D. Finn, G. Forti, A. Giwercman, T. S. Han, I. T. Huhtaniemi, K. Kula, M. E. J. Lean, M. Punab, A. J. Silman, D. Vanderschueren, C. M. Moseley, F. C. W. Wu, and J. McBeth. 2010. Chronic widespread pain is associated with slower cognitive processing speed in middle-aged and older European men. *Pain* 151(1):30-36. https://doi.org/10.1016/j.pain.2010.04.024.

Leganger, J., M.-L. Kulas Søborg, L. Q. Mortensen, R. Gregersen, J. Rosenberg, and J. Burcharth. 2016. Association between diverticular disease and Ehlers-Danlos syndrome: A 13-year nationwide population-based cohort study. *International Journal of Colorectal Disease* 31(12):1863-1867. https://doi.org/10.1007/s00384-016-2650-2.

Leganger, J., S. Fonnes, M.-L. Kulas Søborg, J. Rosenberg, and J. Burcharth. 2022. The most common comorbidities in patients with Ehlers-Danlos syndrome: A 15-year nationwide population-based cohort study. *Disability and Rehabilitation* 44(2):189-193. https://doi.org/10.1080/09638288.2020.1761890.

Levine, D., B. Work, S. McDonald, N. Harty, C. Mabe, A. Powell, and G. Sanford. 2021. Occupational therapy interventions for clients with Ehlers-Danlos syndrome (EDS) in the presence of postural orthostatic tachycardia syndrome (POTS). *Occupational Therapy in Health Care*: 36(3):253-270. https://doi.org/10.1080/07380577.2021.1975200.

Levine, N. A., and B. R. Rigby. 2018. Thoracic outlet syndrome: Biomechanical and exercise considerations. *Healthcare (Basel)* 6(2):68. https://doi.org/10.3390/healthcare6020068.

Liguori, G., and American College of Sports Medicine. 2021. *ACSM's guidelines for exercise testing and prescription*. 11th ed. Philadelphia, PA: Lippincott Williams & Wilkins.

Lin, I., L. Wiles, R. Waller, R. Goucke, Y. Nagree, M. Gibberd, L. Straker, C. G. Maher, and P. P. B. O'Sullivan. 2020. What does best practice care for musculoskeletal pain look like? Eleven consistent recommendations from high-quality clinical practice guidelines: Systematic review. *British Journal of Sports Medicine* 54(2):79-86. https://doi.org/10.1136/bjsports-2018-099878.

Lind, J., and H. C. Wallenburg. 2002. Pregnancy and the Ehlers-Danlos syndrome: A retrospective study in a Dutch population. *Acta Obstetricia et Gynecologica Scandinavica* 81(4):293-300. https://doi.org/10.1034/j.1600-0412.2002.810403.x.

Liu, D., A. Ahmet, L. Ward, P. Krishnamoorthy, E. D. Mandelcorn, R. Leigh, J. P. Brown, A. Cohen, and H. Kim. 2013. A practical guide to the monitoring and management of the complications of systemic corticosteroid therapy. *Allergy, Asthma, and Clinical Immunology: Official Journal of the Canadian Society of Allergy and Clinical Immunology* 9:30. https://doi.org/10.1186/1710-1492-9-30.

Logerstedt, D. S., D. Scalzitti, M. A. Risberg, L. Engebretsen, K. E. Webster, J. Feller, L. Snyder-Mackler, M. J. Axe, and C. M. McDonough. 2017. Knee stability and movement coordination impairments: Knee ligament sprain revision 2017. *Journal of Orthopaedic and Sports Physical Therapy* 47(11):a1-a47. https://doi.org/10.2519/jospt.2017.0303.

Logerstedt, D. S., D. A. Scalzitti, K. L. Bennell, R. S. Hinman, H. Silvers-Granelli, J. Ebert, K. Hambly, J. L. Carey, L. Snyder-Mackler, M. J. Axe, and C. M. McDonough. 2018. Knee pain and mobility impairments: Meniscal and articular cartilage lesions revision 2018. *Journal of Orthopaedic and Sports Physical Therapy* 48(2):A1-A50. https://doi.org/10.2519/jospt.2018.0301.

Louisias, M., S. Silverman, and A. Maitland. 2013. Prevalence of allergic disorders and mast cell activation syndrome in patients with Ehlers Danlos syndrome. *Annals of Allergy, Asthma & Immunology* 111 (1):A12-A13. https://doi.org/10.1002/ajmg.c.31555.

Low, P. A., P. Sandroni, M. Joyner, and W. K. Shen. 2009. Postural tachycardia syndrome (POTS). *Journal of Cardiovascular Electrophysiology* 20(3):352-358. https://doi.org/10.1111/j.1540-8167.2008.01407.x.

Luskin, K. T., A. A. White, and J. J. Lyons. 2021. The genetic basis and clinical impact of hereditary alpha-tryptasemia. *Journal of Allergy and Clinical Immunology: In Practice* 9(6):2235-2242. https://doi.org/10.1016/j.jaip.2021.03.005.

Lybil, M. A., and B. Genie. 2019. Loeys-Dietz syndrome presenting with inflammatory bowel disease symptoms. *The American Journal of Gastroenterology* 114:S17. https://doi.org/10.14309/01.ajg.0000578324.00040.06.

Lyons, J. J., X. Yu, J. D. Hughes, Q. T. Le, A. Jamil, Y. Bai, N. Ho, M. Zhao, Y. Liu, M. P. O'Connell, N. N. Trivedi, C. Nelson, T. DiMaggio, N. Jones, H. Matthews, K. L. Lewis, A. J. Oler, R. J. Carlson, P. D. Arkwright, C. Hong, S. Agama, T. M. Wilson, S. Tucker, Y. Zhang, J. J. McElwee, M. Pao, S. C. Glover, M. E. Rothenberg, R. J. Hohman, K. D. Stone, G. H. Caughey, T. Heller, D. D. Metcalfe, L. G. Biesecker, L. B. Schwartz, and J. D. Milner. 2016. Elevated basal serum tryptase identifies a multisystem disorder associated with increased *TPSAB1* copy number. *Nature Genetics* 48(12):1564-1569. https://doi.org/10.1038/ng.3696.

MacCarrick, G., J. H. Black, 3rd, S. Bowdin, I. El-Hamamsy, P. A. Frischmeyer-Guerrerio, A. L. Guerrerio, P. D. Sponseller, B. Loeys, and H. C. Dietz, 3rd. 2014. Loeys-Dietz syndrome: A primer for diagnosis and management. *Genetics in Medicine* 16(8):576-587. https://doi.org/10.1038/gim.2014.11.

MacDermid, J. C., T. Turgeon, R. S. Richards, M. Beadle, and J. H. Roth. 1998. Patient rating of wrist pain and disability: A reliable and valid measurement tool. *Journal of Orthopaedic Trauma* 12(8):577-586. https://doi.org/10.1097/00005131-199811000-00009.

Mackay, M. 2015. Lupus brain fog: A biologic perspective on cognitive impairment, depression, and fatigue in systemic lupus erythematosus. *Immunologic Research* 63(1-3):26-37. https://doi.org/10.1007/s12026-015-8716-3.

Madonna Rehabilitation Hospitals. n.d. *Speech Intelligibility Test.* https://www.madonna.org/institute/software (accessed March 7, 2022).

Makatsariya, A., L. Radetskaya, V. Bitsadze, J. Khizroeva, N. Khamani, and N. Makatsariya. 2020. Prenatal care and labor in patients with mesenchimal dysplasias (Marfan syndrome, Ehlers-Danlos syndrome, hereditary hemorrhagic telangiectasia). *Journal of Maternal-Fetal & Neonatal Medicine* 33(3):373-379. https://doi.org/10.1080/14767058.2018.1493102.

Malfait, F., C. Francomano, P. Byers, J. Belmont, B. Berglund, J. Black, L. Bloom, J. M. Bowen, A. F. Brady, N. P. Burrows, M. Castori, H. Cohen, M. Colombi, S. Demirdas, J. De Backer, A. De Paepe, S. Fournel-Gigleux, M. Frank, N. Ghali, C. Giunta, R. Grahame, A. Hakim, X. Jeunemaitre, D. Johnson, B. Juul-Kristensen, I. Kapferer-Seebacher, H. Kazkaz, T. Kosho, M. E. Lavallee, H. Levy, R. Mendoza-Londono, M. Pepin, F. M. Pope, E. Reinstein, L. Robert, M. Rohrbach, L. Sanders, G. J. Sobey, T. Van Damme, A. Vandersteen, C. van Mourik, N. Voermans, N. Wheeldon, J. Zschocke, and B. Tinkle. 2017. The 2017 international classification of the Ehlers-Danlos syndromes. *American Journal of Medical Genetics Part C: Seminars in Medical Genetics* 175(1):8-26. https://doi.org/10.1002/ajmg.c.31552.

Malyuk, D. F., N. Campeau, and J. C. Benson. 2022. Loeys-Dietz syndrome: Case report and review of the literature. *Radiology Case Reports* 17(3):767-770. https://doi.org/10.1016/j.radcr.2021.12.024.

Marfan Foundationm, The. 2017. *Physical activity guidelines*. https://info.marfan.org/hubfs/FINAL%20Physical%20Activity%20Guidelines%2011_17.pdf (accessed January 18, 2022).

Marfeo, E. E., P. Ni, S. M. Haley, A. M. Jette, K. Bogusz, M. Meterko, C. M. McDonough, L. Chan, D. E. Brandt, and E. K. Rasch. 2013. Development of an instrument to measure behavioral health function for work disability: Item pool construction and factor analysis. *Archives of Physical Medicine and Rehabilitation* 94(9):1670-1678. https://doi.org/10.1016/j.apmr.2013.03.013.

Marfeo, E. E., C. McDonough, P. Ni, K. Peterik, J. Porcino, M. Meterko, E. Rasch, L. Kazis, and L. Chan. 2019. Measuring work related physical and mental health function: Updating the Work Disability Functional Assessment Battery (WD-FAB) using item response theory. *Journal of Occupational and Environmental Medicine* 61(3):219-224. https://doi.org/10.1097/jom.0000000000001521.

Marmura, M. J. 2018. Triggers, protectors, and predictors in episodic migraine. *Current Pain and Headache Reports* 22(12):81. https://doi.org/10.1007/s11916-018-0734-0.

Martin, R. L., T. E. Davenport, J. J. Fraser, J. Sawdon-Bea, C. R. Carcia, L. A. Carroll, B. R. Kivlan, and D. Carreira. 2021. Ankle stability and movement coordination impairments: Lateral ankle ligament sprains revision 2021. *Journal of Orthopaedic and Sports Physical Therapy* 51(4):CPG1-CPG80. https://doi.org/10.2519/jospt.2021.0302.

Martin, V. T., and D. Neilson. 2014. Joint hypermobility and headache: The glue that binds the two together—Part 2. *Headache* 54(8):1403-1411. https://doi.org/10.1111/head.12417.

Matsuda, M., Y. Huh, and R. R. Ji. 2019. Roles of inflammation, neurogenic inflammation, and neuroinflammation in pain. *Journal of Anesthesia* 33(1):131-139. https://doi.org/10.1007/s00540-018-2579-4.

Mayo Clinic. 2022a. *Anxiety disorders*. https://www.mayoclinic.org/diseases-conditions/anxiety/symptoms-causes/syc-20350961 (accessed May 20, 2022).

Mayo Clinic. 2022b. *Depression*. https://www.mayoclinic.org/diseases-conditions/depression/symptoms-causes/syc-20356007 (accessed May 20, 2022).

Mazzone, L., F. Ducci, M. C. Scoto, E. Passaniti, V. G. D'Arrigo, and B. Vitiello. 2007. The role of anxiety symptoms in school performance in a community sample of children and adolescents. *BMC Public Health* 7(December):347. https://doi.org/10.1186/1471-2458-7-347.

McBride, W. S., C. D. Mulrow, C. Aguilar, and M. R. Tuley. 1994. Methods for screening for hearing loss in older adults. *American Journal of the Medical Sciences* 307(1):40-42. https://doi.org/10.1097/00000441-199401000-00007.

Meterko, M., E. E. Marfeo, C. M. McDonough, A. M. Jette, P. Ni, K. Bogusz, E. K. Rasch, D. E. Brandt, and L. Chan. 2015. Work Disability Functional Assessment Battery: Feasibility and psychometric properties. *Archives of Physical Medicine and Rehabilitation* 96(6):1028-1035. https://doi.org/10.1016/j.apmr.2014.11.025.

Meterko, M., M. Marino, P. Ni, E. Marfeo, C. M. McDonough, A. Jette, K. Peterik, E. Rasch, D. E. Brandt, and L. Chan. 2019. Psychometric evaluation of the improved Work-Disability Functional Assessment Battery. *Archives of Physical Medicine and Rehabilitation* 100(8):1442-1449. https://doi.org/10.1016/j.apmr.2018.09.125.

Milhorat, T. H., P. A. Bolognese, M. Nishikawa, N. B. McDonnell, and C. A. Francomano. 2007. Syndrome of occipitoatlantoaxial hypermobility, cranial settling, and Chiari malformation type I in patients with hereditary disorders of connective tissue. *Journal of Neurosurgery: Spine* 7(6):601-609. https://doi.org/10.3171/spi-07/12/601.

Minhas, D. 2021. Practical management strategies for benign hypermobility syndromes. *Current Opinion in Rheumatology* 33(3):249-254. https://doi.org/10.1097/bor.0000000000000798.

Mitakides, J., and B. T. Tinkle. 2017. Oral and mandibular manifestations in the Ehlers–Danlos syndromes. *American Journal of Medical Genetics Part C: Seminars in Medical Genetics* 175(1):220-225. https://doi.org/10.1002/ajmg.c.31541.

Molderings, G. J., B. Haenisch, S. Brettner, J. Homann, M. Menzen, F. L. Dumoulin, J. Panse, J. Butterfield, and L. B. Afrin. 2016. Pharmacological treatment options for mast cell activation disease. *Naunyn-Schmiedeberg's Archives of Pharmacology* 389(7):671-694. https://doi.org/10.1007/s00210-016-1247-1.

Møller, A. R. 2007. Tinnitus: Presence and future. In *Progress in Brain Research*. Vol. 166, edited by B. Langguth, G. Hajak, T. Kleinjung, A. Cacace and A. R. Møller. Amsterdam: Elsevier. Pp. 3-16. https://doi.org/10.1016/S0079-6123(07)66001-4.

Morey, L. 1991. *The Personality Assessment Inventory professional manual*. Odessa, FL: Psychological Assessment Resources.

Morgan, A. W., S. B. Pearson, S. Davies, H. C. Gooi, and H. A. Bird. 2007. Asthma and airways collapse in two heritable disorders of connective tissue. *Annals of the Rheumatic Diseases* 66(10):1369-1373. https://doi.org/10.1136/ard.2006.062224.

Moriarty, O., B. E. McGuire, and D. P. Finn. 2011. The effect of pain on cognitive function: A review of clinical and preclinical research. *Progress in Neurobiology* 93(3):385-404. https://doi.org/10.1016/j.pneurobio.2011.01.002.

Morosini, P. L., L. Magliano, L. Brambilla, S. Ugolini, and R. Pioli. 2000. Development, reliability and acceptability of a new version of the DSM-IV Social and Occupational Functioning Assessment Scale (SOFAS) to assess routine social functioning. *Acta Psychiatrica Scandinavica* 101(4):323-329. https://doi.org/10.1034/j.1600-0447.2000.101004323.x.

Morrison, M. T., G. M. Giles, J. D. Ryan, C. M. Baum, A. W. Dromerick, H. J. Polatajko, and D. F. Edwards. 2013. Multiple Errands Test–Revised (MET–R): A performance-based measure of executive function in people with mild cerebrovascular accident. *American Journal of Occupational Therapy* 67(4):460-468. https://doi.org/10.5014/ajot.2013.007880.

Moss, C., J. Fernandez-Mendoza, J. Schubart, T. Sheehan, A. Schilling, C. Francomano, and R. Bascom. 2018. Nighttime sleep and daytime functioning in Ehlers-Danlos syndrome: A cohort study of syndrome subtypes. *Sleep* 41(suppl 1):A343. https://doi.org/10.1093/sleep/zsy061.923.

Mott, T., G. Jones, and K. Roman. 2021. Costochondritis: Rapid evidence review. *American Family Physician* 104(1):73-78. https://www.aafp.org/afp/2021/0700/p73.

Murray, M. L., M. Pepin, S. Peterson, and P. H. Byers. 2014. Pregnancy-related deaths and complications in women with vascular Ehlers–Danlos syndrome. *Genetics in Medicine* 16(12):874-880. https://doi.org/10.1038/gim.2014.53.

NASEM (National Academies of Sciences, Engineering, and Medicine). 2016. *Hearing health care for adults: Priorities for improving access and affordability.* Edited by D. G. Blazer, S. Domnitz, and C. T. Liverman. Washington, DC: The National Academies Press. doi: 10.17226/23446.

NASEM. 2017. *The promise of assistive technology to enhance activity and work participation.* Edited by A. M. Jette, C. M. Spicer and J. L. Flaubert. Washington, DC: The National Academies Press. https://doi.org/10.17226/24740.

NASEM. 2019. *Functional assessment for adults with disabilities.* Edited by P. A. Volberding, C. M. Spicer and J. L. Flaubert. Washington, DC: The National Academies Press. https://doi.org/10.17226/25376.

Nasreddine, Z. S., N. A. Phillips, V. Bédirian, S. Charbonneau, V. Whitehead, I. Collin, J. L. Cummings, and H. Chertkow. 2005. The Montreal Cognitive Assessment, MoCA: A brief screening tool for mild cognitive impairment. *Journal of the American Geriatrics Society* 53(4):695-699. https://doi.org/10.1111/j.1532-5415.2005.53221.x.

Nelson, A. D., M. A. Mouchli, N. Valentin, D. Deyle, P. Pichurin, A. Acosta, and M. Camilleri. 2015a. Ehlers Danlos syndrome and gastrointestinal manifestations: A 20-year experience at Mayo Clinic. *Neurogastroenterology and Motility* 27(11):1657-1666. https://doi.org/10.1111/nmo.12665.

Nelson, A. M., D. R. Walega, and R. J. McCarthy. 2015b. The incidence and severity of physical pain symptoms in Marfan syndrome: A survey of 993 patients. *Clinical Journal of Pain* 31(12):1080-1086. https://doi.org/10.1097/ajp.0000000000000202.

Newcastle upon Tyne Hospitals: NHS Foundation Trust. 2020. *CRESTA Fatigue Clinic: Managing your energy.* Edited by K. Ratcliffe, V. Ewan, V. Strassheim, K. Hackett, V. Deary and J. Newton. London, United Kingdom: NHS Foundation Trust. https://www.newcastle-hospitals.nhs.uk/content/uploads/2021/02/CRESTA-booklet-060720-contents-revised_sr.pdf (accessed January 13, 2022).

Newman, C. W., B. E. Weinstein, G. P. Jacobson, and G. A. Hug. 1990. The Hearing Handicap Inventory for Adults: Psychometric adequacy and audiometric correlates. *Ear and Hearing* 11(6):430-433. https://doi.org/10.1097/00003446-199012000-00004.

Nijs, J., O. Mairesse, D. Neu, L. Leysen, L. Danneels, B. Cagnie, M. Meeus, M. Moens, K. Ickmans, and D. Goubert. 2018. Sleep disturbances in chronic pain: Neurobiology, assessment, and treatment in physical therapist practice. *Physical Therapy* 98(5):325-335. https://doi.org/10.1093/ptj/pzy020.

Niv, N., A. N. Cohen, G. Sullivan, and A. S. Young. 2007. The MIRECC version of the Global Assessment of Functioning scale: Reliability and validity. *Psychiatric Services (Washington, D.C.)* 58(4):529-535. https://doi.org/10.1176/ps.2007.58.4.529.

NLM (National Library of Medicine). 2022. *Anxiety.* https://medlineplus.gov/anxiety.html (accessed May 20, 2022).

NORD (National Organization for Rare Disorders). 2017a. *Rare disease database: Ehlers Danlos syndromes.* https://rarediseases.org/rare-diseases/ehlers-danlos-syndrome/ (accessed February 16, 2022).

NORD. 2017b. *Rare disease database: Shprintzen goldberg syndrome.* https://rarediseases.org/rare-diseases/shprintzen-goldberg-syndrome/ (accessed March 3, 2022).

Oaklander, A. L., and M. M. Klein. 2013. Evidence of small-fiber polyneuropathy in unexplained, juvenile-onset, widespread pain syndromes. *Pediatrics* 131(4):e1091-e1100. https://doi.org/10.1542/peds.2012-2597.

Ocon, A. 2013. Caught in the thickness of brain fog: Exploring the cognitive symptoms of chronic fatigue syndrome. *Frontiers in Physiology* 4(April):63. https://doi.org/10.3389/fphys.2013.00063.

Okamoto, L. E., S. R. Raj, A. Peltier, A. Gamboa, C. Shibao, A. Diedrich, B. K. Black, D. Robertson, and I. Biaggioni. 2012. Neurohumoral and haemodynamic profile in postural tachycardia and chronic fatigue syndromes. *Clinical Science (London, England: 1979)* 122(4):183-192. https://doi.org/10.1042/cs20110200.

Oliveira, C. B., C. G. Maher, R. Z. Pinto, A. C. Traeger, C. C. Lin, J. F. Chenot, M. van Tulder, and B. W. Koes. 2018a. Clinical practice guidelines for the management of non-specific low back pain in primary care: An updated overview. *European Spine Journal* 27(11):2791-2803. https://doi.org/10.1007/s00586-018-5673-2.

Oliveira, M. J. P., F. Rodrigues, J. Firmino-Machado, I. T. Ladeira, R. Lima, S. D. Conde, and M. Guimarães. 2018b. Assessment of respiratory muscle weakness in subjects with neuromuscular disease. *Respiratory Care* 63(10):1223-1230. https://doi.org/10.4187/respcare.06136.

Oppizzi, L. M., and R. Umberger. 2018. The effect of physical activity on PTSD. *Issues in Mental Health Nursing* 39(2):179-187. https://doi.org/10.1080/01612840.2017.1391903.

Ottenbacher, K. J., Y. Hsu, C. V. Granger, and R. C. Fiedler. 1996. The reliability of the functional independence measure: A quantitative review. *Archives of Physical Medicine and Rehabilitation* 77(12):1226-1232. https://doi.org/10.1016/s0003-9993(96)90184-7.

Overbeek, C. L., S. P. Nota, P. Jayakumar, M. G. Hageman, and D. Ring. 2015. The PROMIS physical function correlates with the QuickDASH in patients with upper extremity illness. *Clinical Orthopaedics and Related Research* 473(1):311-317. https://doi.org/10.1007/s11999-014-3840-2.

Packham, T., and J. C. MacDermid. 2013. Measurement properties of the Patient-Rated Wrist and Hand Evaluation: Rasch analysis of responses from a traumatic hand injury population. *Journal of Hand Therapy* 26(3):216-223; quiz 224. https://doi.org/10.1016/j.jht.2012.12.006.

Palmer, S., I. Davey, L. Oliver, A. Preece, L. Sowerby, and S. House. 2021. The effectiveness of conservative interventions for the management of syndromic hypermobility: A systematic literature review. *Clinical Rheumatology* 40(3):1113-1129. https://doi.org/10.1007/s10067-020-05284-0.

Palomo-Toucedo, I. C., F. Leon-Larios, M. Reina-Bueno, M. D. C. Vázquez-Bautista, P. V. Munuera-Martínez, and G. Domínguez-Maldonado. 2020. Psychosocial influence of Ehlers-Danlos syndrome in daily life of patients: A qualitative study. *International Journal of Environmental Research and Public Health* 17(17):6425. https://doi.org/10.3390/ijerph17176425.

Papapetropoulos, T., C. Tsankanikas, and M. Spengos. 1981. Brachial neuropathy and Ehlers-Danlos syndrome. *Neurology* 31(5):642-643. https://doi.org/10.1212/WNL.31.5.642-a

Paris, M.-J., and Brigham and Women's Hospital. 2008. *Standard of care: Marfan syndrome*. https://www.brighamandwomens.org/assets/bwh/patients-and-families/rehabilitation-services/pdfs/general-marfan-syndrome-bwh.pdf (accessed March 8, 2022).

Pasquini, M., C. Celletti, I. Berardelli, V. Roselli, S. Mastroeni, M. Castori, M. Biondi, and F. Camerota. 2014. Unexpected association between joint hypermobility syndrome/Ehlers-Danlos syndrome hypermobility type and obsessive-compulsive personality disorder. *Rheumatology International* 34(5):631-636. https://doi.org/10.1007/s00296-013-2901-2.

Patterson, M. B., and J. L. Mack. 2001. The Cleveland Scale for Activities of Daily Living (CSADL): Its reliability and validity. *Journal of Clinical Geropsychology* 7(1):15-28. https://doi.org/10.1023/A:1026408600751.

Paul, D. R., C. Frattali, A. L. Holland, C. K. Thompson, C. J. Caperton, S. C. Slater, and American Speech-Language-Hearing Association. 2004. *Quality of communication life scale: Manual*. Rockville, MD: American Speech-Language-Hearing Association.

Perez-Roustit, S., D. T. Nguyen, O. Xerri, M. P. Robert, N. De Vergnes, Z. Mincheva, K. Benistan, and D. Bremond-Gignac. 2019. Ocular manifestations in Ehlers-Danlos syndromes: Clinical study of 21 patients. *Journal Français d'Ophtalmologie* 42(7):722-729. https://doi.org/10.1016/j.jfo.2019.01.005.

Pescatello, L. S., R. Arena, D. Riebe, P. D. Thompson, and American College of Sports Medicine. 2014. *American College of Sport Medicine's guidelines for exercise testing and prescription*. 9th ed. Philadelphia: Wolters Kluwer Health/Lippincott Williams & Wilkins.

Peters, K., F. Kong, R. Horne, C. Francomano, and B. Biesecker. 2001. Living with Marfan syndrome I. Perceptions of the condition. *Clinical Genetics* 60(4):273-282. https://doi.org/10.1034/j.1399-0004.2001.600405.x.

Physical therapy after an ankle sprain: Using the evidence to guide physical therapist practice. 2021. *Journal of Orthopaedic and Sports Physical Therapy* 51(4):159-160.

Physiopedia. n.d. *10 metre walk test*. https://www.physio-pedia.com/10_Metre_Walk_Test (accessed December 20, 2021).

Plaisier I., A. T. Beekman, R. de Graaf, J. H. Smit, R. van Dyck, and B.W. Penninx. 2010. Work functioning in persons with depressive and anxiety disorders: The role of specific psychopathological characteristics. *Journal of Affective Disorders* 125(1-3):198-206. doi: 10.1016/j.jad.2010.01.072.

Powell, L. E., and A. M. Myers. 1995. The Activities-specific Balance Confidence (ABC) Scale. *Journals of Gerontology. Series A: Biological Sciences and Medical Sciences* 50A(1):M28-M34. https://doi.org/10.1093/gerona/50a.1.m28.

Practice Bulletin No. 176: Pelvic organ prolapse. 2017. *Obstetrics and Gynecology* 129(4):e56-e72.

Pretorius, M. E., and I. J. Butler. 1983. Neurologic manifestations of Ehlers-Danlos syndrome. *Neurology* 33(8):1087-1089. https://doi.org/10.1212/wnl.33.8.1087.

Price, J., A. Rushton, I. Tyros, V. Tyros, and N. R. Heneghan. 2020. Effectiveness and optimal dosage of exercise training for chronic non-specific neck pain: A systematic review with a narrative synthesis. *PloS One* 15(6):e0234511. https://doi.org/10.1371/journal.pone.0234511.

Puledda, F., A. Viganò, C. Celletti, B. Petolicchio, M. Toscano, E. Vicenzini, M. Castori, G. Laudani, D. Valente, F. Camerota, and V. Di Piero. 2015. A study of migraine characteristics in joint hypermobility syndrome a.k.a. Ehlers-Danlos syndrome, hypermobility type. *Neurological Sciences* 36(8):1417-1424. https://doi.org/10.1007/s10072-015-2173-6.

Qiu, J., Y. Lou, Y. Zhu, M. Wang, H. Peng, Y. Hao, H. Jiang, and Y. Mao. 2021. Clinical characteristics and genetic analysis of a family with Birt-Hogg-Dubé syndrome and congenital contractural arachnodactyly. *Frontiers in Genetics* 12(January):768342. https://doi.org/10.3389/fgene.2021.768342.

Quinn, T. J., P. Langhorne, and D. J. Stott. 2011. Barthel index for stroke trials: Development, properties, and application. *Stroke* 42(4):1146-1151. https://doi.org/10.1161/strokeaha.110.598540.

Rabin, J., M. Brown, and S. Alexander. 2017. Update in the treatment of chronic pain within pediatric patients. *Current Problems in Pediatric and Adolescent Health Care* 47(7):167-172. https://doi.org/10.1016/j.cppeds.2017.06.006.

Raj, V., M. Opie, and A. C. Arnold. 2018. Cognitive and psychological issues in postural tachycardia syndrome. *Autonomic Neuroscience* 215(December):46-55. https://doi.org/10.1016/j.autneu.2018.03.004.

Randolph, C. 2012. *Repeatable Battery for the Assessment of Neuropsychological Status update (RBANS update)*. https://www.pearsonassessments.com/store/usassessments/en/Store/Professional-Assessments/Cognition-%26-Neuro/Repeatable-Battery-for-the-Assessment-of-Neuropsychological-Status-Update/p/100000726.html (accessed January 3, 2022).

Ratiu, I., T. B. Virden, H. Baylow, M. Flint, and M. Esfandiarei. 2018. Executive function and quality of life in individuals with Marfan syndrome. *Quality of Life Research* 27(8):2057-2065. https://doi.org/10.1007/s11136-018-1859-7.

Reinstein, E., M. Pimentel, M. Pariani, S. Nemec, T. Sokol, and D. L. Rimoin. 2012. Visceroptosis of the bowel in the hypermobility type of Ehlers-Danlos syndrome: Presentation of a rare manifestation and review of the literature. *European Journal of Medical Genetics* 55(10):548-551. https://doi.org/10.1016/j.ejmg.2012.06.012.

Reisberg, B., S. H. Ferris, M. J. De Leon, and T. Crook. 1982. The Global Deterioration Scale for assessment of primary degenerative dementia. *American Journal of Psychiatry* 139(9):1136-1139. https://doi.org/10.1176/ajp.139.9.1136.

Reischl, S., A. Dabbagh, and J. C. MacDermid. 2020. Appraisal of clinical practice guideline: OPTIMa revised recommendations for non-pharmacological management of persistent headaches associated with neck pain. *Journal of Physiotherapy* 66(3):201. https://doi.org/10.1016/j.jphys.2020.05.009.

Reychler, G., G. Liistro, G. E. Piérard, T. Hermanns-Lê, and D. Manicourt. 2019. Inspiratory muscle strength training improves lung function in patients with the hypermobile Ehlers–Danlos syndrome: A randomized controlled trial. *American Journal of Medical Genetics Part A* 179(3):356-364. https://doi.org/10.1002/ajmg.a.61016.

Reychler, G., M. M. De Backer, E. Piraux, W. Poncin, and G. Caty. 2021. Physical therapy treatment of hypermobile Ehlers-Danlos syndrome: A systematic review. *American Journal of Medical Genetics Part A* 185(10):2986-2994. https://doi.org/10.1002/ajmg.a.62393.

Reynolds, C. R., and R. W. Kamphaus. 2015. *Reynolds Intellectual Assessment Scales*, 2nd ed. https://www.wpspublish.com/rias-2-reynolds-intellectual-assessment-scales-second-edition (accessed January 4, 2022).

Rezar-Dreindl, S., E. Stifter, T. Neumayer, A. Papp, A. Gschliesser, and U. Schmidt-Erfurth. 2019. Visual outcome and surgical results in children with Marfan syndrome. *Clinical & Experimental Ophthalmology* 47(9):1138-1145. https://doi.org/10.1111/ceo.13596.

Rich, E. M., A. Vas, V. Boyette, and C. Hollingsworth. 2020. Daily life experiences: Challenges, strategies, and implications for therapy in postural tachycardia syndrome (POTS). *Occupational Therapy in Health Care*: 36(3):306-323. https://doi.org/10.1080/07380577.2020.1824303.

Ritelli, M., C. Dordoni, M. Venturini, N. Chiarelli, S. Quinzani, M. Traversa, N. Zoppi, A. Vascellaro, A. Wischmeijer, E. Manfredini, L. Garavelli, P. Calzavara-Pinton, and M. Colombi. 2013. Clinical and molecular characterization of 40 patients with classic Ehlers-Danlos syndrome: Identification of 18 *COL5A1* and 2 *COL5A2* novel mutations. *Orphanet Journal of Rare Diseases* 8(April):58. https://doi.org/10.1186/1750-1172-8-58.

Ritelli, M., M. Venturini, V. Cinquina, N. Chiarelli, and M. Colombi. 2020. Multisystemic manifestations in a cohort of 75 classical Ehlers-Danlos syndrome patients: Natural history and nosological perspectives. *Orphanet Journal of Rare Diseases* 15(July):197. https://doi.org/10.1186/s13023-020-01470-0.

Røe, Y. 2014. *Shoulder pain within the ICF framework; patient experiences of functioning and assessment methods*. Doctoral thesis, Department of Physical Medicine and Rehabilitation: University of Oslo, Norway.

Roeser, R. J., K. A. Buckley, and G. S. Stickney. 2000. Pure tone tests. In *Audiology diagnosis*, edited by R. J. Roeser, M. Valente, and H. Hosford-Dunn. New York: Thieme. Pp. 227-251.

Roid, G. H. 2003. *Stanford-Binet Intelligence Scales*, 5th ed. https://www.wpspublish.com/sb-5-stanford-binet-intelligence-scales-fifth-edition (accessed January 5, 2022).

Roid, G. H., L. J. Miller, M. Pomplun, and C. Koch. 2013. *Leiter International Performance Scale*, 3rd ed. https://www.wpspublish.com/leiter-3-leiter-international-performance-scale-third-edition (accessed January 5, 2022).

Roma, M., C. L. Marden, I. De Wandele, C. A. Francomano, and P. C. Rowe. 2018. Postural tachycardia syndrome and other forms of orthostatic intolerance in Ehlers-Danlos syndrome. *Autonomic Neuroscience* 215(December):89-96. https://doi.org/10.1016/j.autneu.2018.02.006.

Romano, P. E., N. C. Kerr, and G. M. Hope. 2002. Bilateral ametropic functional amblyopia in genetic ectopia lentis: Its relation to the amount of subluxation, an indicator for early surgical management. *Binocular Vision and Strabismus Quarterly* 17(3):235-241.

Rombaut, L., F. Malfait, A. Cools, A. De Paepe, and P. Calders. 2010. Musculoskeletal complaints, physical activity and health-related quality of life among patients with the Ehlers-Danlos syndrome hypermobility type. *Disability and Rehabilitation* 32(16):1339-1345. https://doi.org/10.3109/09638280903514739.

Rombaut, L., F. Malfait, I. De Wandele, A. Cools, Y. Thijs, A. De Paepe, and P. Calders. 2011. Medication, surgery, and physiotherapy among patients with the hypermobility type of Ehlers-Danlos syndrome. *Archives of Physical Medicine and Rehabilitation* 92(7):1106-1112. https://doi.org/10.1016/j.apmr.2011.01.016.

Rombaut, L., M. Scheper, I. De Wandele, J. De Vries, M. Meeus, F. Malfait, R. Engelbert, and P. Calders. 2015. Chronic pain in patients with the hypermobility type of Ehlers-Danlos syndrome: Evidence for generalized hyperalgesia. *Clinical Rheumatology* 34(6):1121-1129. https://doi.org/10.1007/s10067-014-2499-0.

Rosa, A. C., and R. Fantozzi. 2013. The role of histamine in neurogenic inflammation. *British Journal of Pharmacology* 170(1):38-45. https://doi.org/10.1111/bph.12266.

Rosen, S. G., and P. E. Creyer. 1982. Postural tachycardia syndrome. Reversal of sympathetic hyper-responsiveness and clinical improvement during sodium loading. *American Journal of Medicine* 72(5):847-850. https://doi.org/10.1016/00002-9343(82)90559-9.

Rosen, R., Y. Vandenplas, M. Singendonk, M. Cabana, C. DiLorenzo, F. Gottrand, S. Gupta, M. Langendam, A. Staiano, N. Thapar, N. Tipnis, and M. Tabbers. 2018. Pediatric gastroesophageal reflux clinical practice guidelines: Joint recommendations of the North American Society for Pediatric Gastroenterology, Hepatology, and Nutrition and the European Society for Pediatric Gastroenterology, Hepatology, and Nutrition. *Journal of Pediatric Gastroenterology and Nutrition* 66(3):516-554. https://doi.org/10.1097/mpg.0000000000001889.

Rosen, N. O., S. J. Dawson, M. Brooks, and S. Kellogg-Spadt. 2019. Treatment of vulvodynia: Pharmacological and non-pharmacological approaches. *Drugs* 79(5):483-493. https://doi.org/10.1007/s40265-019-01085-1.

Ross, A. J., M. S. Medow, P. C. Rowe, and J. M. Stewart. 2013. What is brain fog? An evaluation of the symptom in postural tachycardia syndrome. *Clinical Autonomic Research* 23(6):305-311. https://doi.org/10.1007/s10286-013-0212-z.

Rowe, P. C. 2016. Fatigue and the chronic fatigue syndrome. In *Neinstein's adolescent and young adult health care*. 6th ed., edited by L. S. Neinstein. Philadelphia, PA: Wolters Kluwer.

Rowe, P. C. 2022. *The functional impact of orthostatic intolerance in Ehlers-Danlos syndrome*. Paper commissioned by the Committee on Selected Heritable Disorders of Connective Tissue and Disability, National Academies of Sciences, Engineering, and Medicine, Washington, DC.

Rowe, P. C., R. Underhill, K. Friedman, A. Gurwitt, M. Medow, M. Schwartz, N. Speight, J. Stewart, R. Vallings, and K. Rowe. 2017. Myalgic encephalomyelitis/chronic fatigue syndrome diagnosis and management in young people: A primer. *Frontiers in Pediatrics*, 5(June):121. https://doi.org/10.3389/fped.2017.00121.

Rozen, T. D., J. M. Roth, and N. Denenberg. 2006. Cervical spine joint hypermobility: A possible predisposing factor for new daily persistent headache. *Cephalalgia* 26(10):1182-1185. https://doi.org/10.1111/j.1468-2982.2006.01187.x.

Rubinstein, M. K., and N. H. Cohen. 1964. Ehlers-Danlos syndrome associated with multiple intracranial aneurysms. *Neurology* 14(2):125-125. https://doi.org/10.1212/wnl.14.2.125.

Rueda, J. R., I. Mugueta-Aguinaga, J. Vilaró, and M. Rueda-Etxebarria. 2020. Myofunctional therapy (oropharyngeal exercises) for obstructive sleep apnoea. *Cochrane Database of Systematic Reviews* 11(11):CD013449. https://doi.org/10.1002/14651858.CD013449.pub2.

Russo, M. L., N. Sukhavasi, V. Mathur, and S. A. Morris. 2018. Obstetric management of Loeys-Dietz syndrome. *Obstetrics and Gynecology* 131(6):1080-1084. https://doi.org/10.1097/AOG.0000000000002615.

Rybarczyk, B. 2011. Social and Occupational Functioning Assessment Scale (SOFAS). In *Encyclopedia of clinical neuropsychology*, edited by J. S. Kreutzer, J. DeLuca, and B. Caplan. New York: Springer. P. 171. https://doi.org/10.1007/978-0-387-79948-3_428.

Sacheti, A., J. Szemere, B. Bernstein, T. Tafas, N. Schechter, and P. Tsipouras. 1997. Chronic pain is a manifestation of the Ehlers-Danlos syndrome. *Journal of Pain and Symptom Management* 14(2):88-93. https://doi.org/10.1016/s0885-3924(97)00007-9.

Sadler, B., T. Kuensting, J. Strahle, T. S. Park, M. Smyth, D. D. Limbrick, M. B. Dobbs, G. Haller, and C. A. Gurnett. 2020. Prevalence and impact of underlying diagnosis and comorbidities on Chiari 1 malformation. *Pediatric Neurology* 106(May):32-37. https://doi.org/10.1016/j.pediatrneurol.2019.12.005.

Samuel Merritt University. n.d. *Function in Sitting Test (FIST)*. https://www.samuelmerritt.edu/fist (accessed December 20, 2021).

Savasta, S., P. Merli, M. Ruggieri, L. Bianchi, and M. V. Spartà. 2011. Ehlers-Danlos syndrome and neurological features: A review. *Child's Nervous System* 27(3):365-371. https://doi.org/10.1007/s00381-010-1256-1.

Schievink, W. I., M. Limburg, J. W. Oorthuys, P. Fleury, and F. M. Pope. 1990. Cerebrovascular disease in Ehlers-Danlos syndrome type IV. *Stroke* 21(4):626-632. https://doi.org/10.1161/01.str.21.4.626.

Schievink, W. I., F. B. Meyer, J. L. Atkinson, and B. Mokri. 1996. Spontaneous spinal cerebrospinal fluid leaks and intracranial hypotension. *Journal of Neurosurgery* 84(4):598-605. https://doi.org/10.3171/jns.1996.84.4.0598.

Schondorf, R., and P. Low. 1993. Idiopathic postural orthostatic tachycardia syndrome: An attenuated form of acute pandysautonomia? *Neurology* 43(1):132-137. https://doi.org/10.1212/wnl.43.1_part_1.132.

Schoolman, A., and J. J. Kepes. 1967. Bilateral spontaneous carotid-cavernous fistulae in Ehlers-Danlos syndrome. Case report. *Journal of Neurosurgery* 26(1):82-86. https://doi.org/10.3171/jns.1967.26.1part1.0082.

SchoolToolkit (SchoolToolkit for EDS and JHS). 2022. *Resonable adjustments in school.* https://theschooltoolkit.org/reasonable-adjustments/ (accessed May 31, 2022).

Schoser, B., E. Fong, T. Geberhiwot, D. Hughes, J. T. Kissel, S. C. Madathil, D. Orlikowski, M. I. Polkey, M. Roberts, H. A. Tiddens, and P. Young. 2017. Maximum inspiratory pressure as a clinically meaningful trial endpoint for neuromuscular diseases: A comprehensive review of the literature. *Orphanet Journal of Rare Diseases* 12(1):52. https://doi.org/10.1186/s13023-017-0598-0.

Schubert-Hjalmarsson, E., A. Öhman, M. Kyllerman, and E. Beckung. 2012. Pain, balance, activity, and participation in children with hypermobility syndrome. *Pediatric Physical Therapy* 24(4):339-344. https://doi.org/10.1097/PEP.0b013e318268e0ef.

Schuling, J., R. de Haan, M. Limburg, and K. H. Groenier. 1993. The Frenchay Activities Index. Assessment of functional status in stroke patients. *Stroke* 24(8):1173-1177. https://doi.org/10.1161/01.str.24.8.1173.

Seaton, L., and T. Brown. 2018. The relationship between body function and structure factors and the activity-participation of healthy community-dwelling older adults. *Physical & Occupational Therapy in Geriatrics* 36(2-3):121-135. https://doi.org/10.1080/02703181.2018.1443193.

Segev, F., E. Héon, W. G. Cole, R. J. Wenstrup, F. Young, A. R. Slomovic, D. S. Rootman, D. Whitaker-Menezes, I. Chervoneva, and D. E. Birk. 2006. Structural abnormalities of the cornea and lid resulting from collagen V mutations. *Investigative Ophthalmology and Visual Science* 47(2):565-573. https://doi.org/10.1167/iovs.05-0771.

Seneviratne, S. L., A. Maitland, and L. Afrin. 2017. Mast cell disorders in Ehlers-Danlos syndrome. *American Journal of Medical Genetics Part C: Seminars in Medical Genetics* 175(1):226-236. https://doi.org/10.1002/ajmg.c.31555.

Shauver, M. J., and K. C. Chung. 2013. The Michigan Hand Outcomes Questionnaire after 15 years of field trial. *Plastic and Reconstructive Surgery* 131(5):779e-787e. https://doi.org/10.1097/PRS.0b013e3182865d83.

Sheehan, D. V. 1983. The Sheehan Disability Scale. In *The anxiety disease*. New York: Charles Scribner and Sons. p. 151.

Sheehan, K. H., and D. V. Sheehan. 2008. Assessing treatment effects in clinical trials with the Discan metric of the Sheehan Disability Scale. *International Clinical Psychopharmacology* 23(2):70-83. https://doi.org/10.1097/YIC.0b013e3282f2b4d6.

Sheldon, R. S., B. P. Grubb, 2nd, B. Olshansky, W. K. Shen, H. Calkins, M. Brignole, S. R. Raj, A. D. Krahn, C. A. Morillo, J. M. Stewart, R. Sutton, P. Sandroni, K. J. Friday, D. T. Hachul, M. I. Cohen, D. H. Lau, K. A. Mayuga, J. P. Moak, R. K. Sandhu, and K. Kanjwal. 2015. 2015 Heart Rhythm Society expert consensus statement on the diagnosis and treatment of postural tachycardia syndrome, inappropriate sinus tachycardia, and vasovagal syncope. *Heart Rhythm* 12(6):e41-e63. https://doi.org/10.1016/j.hrthm.2015.03.029.

Sheslow, D., and W. Adams. 2003. *Wide Range Assessment of Memory and Learning*, 2nd ed. https://www.wpspublish.com/wraml2-wide-range-assessment-of-memory-and-learning-second-edition (accessed January 4, 2022).

Shiari, R., F. Saeidifard, and G. Zahed. 2013. Evaluation of the prevalence of joint laxity in children with attention deficit/hyperactivity disorder. *Annals of Paediatric Rheumatology* 2:78-80. https://doi.org/10.5455/apr.032420131219.

Shin, B., S. L. Cole, S. J. Park, D. K. Ledford, and R. F. Lockey. 2010. A new symptom-based questionnaire for predicting the presence of asthma. *Journal of Investigational Allergology and Clinical Immunology* 20(1):27-34. http://www.jiaci.org/issues/vol20issue1/vol20issue01-5.htm.

Shirley Ryan AbilityLab. 2013a. *30 Second Sit to Stand Test*. https://www.sralab.org/rehabilitation-measures/30-second-sit-stand-test (accessed December 20, 2021).

Shirley Ryan AbilityLab. 2013b. *Lower Extremity Functional Scale*. https://www.sralab.org/rehabilitation-measures/lower-extremity-functional-scale (May 26, 2022).

Shirley Ryan AbilityLab. 2013c. *Numeric Pain Rating Scale*. https://www.sralab.org/rehabilitation-measures/numeric-pain-rating-scale (accessed February 16, 2022).

Shirley Ryan AbilityLab. 2013d. *Oswestry Disability Index*. https://www.sralab.org/rehabilitation-measures/oswestry-disability-index (accessed May 26, 2022).

Shirley Ryan AbilityLab. 2013e. *Romberg Test*. https://www.sralab.org/rehabilitation-measures/romberg-test (accessed May 26, 2022).

Shirley Ryan AbilityLab. 2013f. *Sensory Organization Test*. https://www.sralab.org/rehabilitation-measures/sensory-organization-test (accessed December 20, 2021).

Shirley Ryan AbilityLab. 2015a. *Foot and Ankle Mobility Measures*. https://www.sralab.org/rehabilitation-measures/foot-and-ankle-ability-measures (May 26, 2022).

Shirley Ryan AbilityLab. 2015b. *Neck Disability Index*. https://www.sralab.org/rehabilitation-measures/neck-disability-index (accessed May 26, 2022).

Shirley Ryan AbilityLab. 2016. *Fatigue Severity Scale*. https://www.sralab.org/rehabilitation-measures/fatigue-severity-scale (accessed May 26, 2022).

Shirley Ryan AbilityLab. 2017. *Functional Dexterity Test*. https://www.sralab.org/rehabilitation-measures/functional-dexterity-test (accessed December 20, 2021).

Shirley Ryan AbilityLab. 2019. *Assessment of Motor and Process Skills.* https://www.sralab.org/rehabilitation-measures/assessment-motor-and-process-skills (accessed February 16, 2022).
Shirley Ryan AbilityLab. 2020a. *Berg Balance Scale.* https://www.sralab.org/rehabilitation-measures/berg-balance-scale (accessed May 26, 2022).
Shirley Ryan AbilityLab. 2020b. *Multidimensional Assessment of Fatigue.* https://www.sralab.org/rehabilitation-measures/multidimensional-assessment-fatigue (accessed May 26, 2022).
Shusterman, D., F. M. Baroody, T. Craig, S. Friedlander, T. Nsouli, and B. Silverman. 2017. Role of the allergist-immunologist and upper airway allergy in sleep-disordered breathing. *The Journal of Allergy and Clinical Immunology: In Practice* 5(3):628-639. https://doi.org/10.1016/j.jaip.2016.10.007.
Sletten, D. M., G. A. Suarez, P. A. Low, J. Mandrekar, and W. Singer. 2012. COMPASS 31: A refined and abbreviated Composite Autonomic Symptom Score. *Mayo Clinic Proceedings* 87(12):1196-1201. https://doi.org/10.1016/j.mayocp.2012.10.013.
Smith, A. 1973. *Symbol Digit Modalities Test.* https://www.wpspublish.com/sdmt-symbol-digit-modalities-test (accessed January 4, 2022).
Smith, T. O., V. Easton, H. Bacon, E. Jerman, K. Armon, F. Poland, and A. J. Macgregor. 2013. The relationship between benign joint hypermobility syndrome and psychological distress: A systematic review and meta-analysis. *Rheumatology* 53(1):114-122. https://doi.org/10.1093/rheumatology/ket317.
Smits, C., T. S. Kapteyn, and T. Houtgast. 2004. Development and validation of an automatic speech-in-noise screening test by telephone. *International Journal of Audiology* 43(1):15-28. https://doi.org/10.1080/14992020400050004.
Soer, R., C. P. van der Schans, J. W. Groothoff, J. H. Geertzen, and M. F. Reneman. 2008. Towards consensus in operational definitions in functional capacity evaluation: A Delphi survey. *Journal of Occupational Rehabilitation* 18(4):389-400. https://doi.org/10.1007/s10926-008-9155-y.
Song, B., P. Yeh, D. Nguyen, U. Ikpeama, M. Epstein, and J. Harrell. 2020. Ehlers-Danlos syndrome: An analysis of the current treatment options. *Pain Physician* 23(4):429-438. https://doi.org/10.36076/ppj.2020/23/429.
Sorokin, Y., M. P. Johnson, N. Rogowski, D. A. Richardson, and M. I. Evans. 1994. Obstetric and gynecologic dysfunction in the Ehlers-Danlos syndrome. *Journal of Reproductive Medicine* 39(4):281-284. https://doi.org/10.1097/AOG.0000000000000123.
Sparrow, S. S., D. V. Cicchetti, and C. A. Saulnier. 2016. *Vineland Adaptive Behavior Scales,* 3rd ed. https://www.pearsonassessments.com/store/usassessments/en/Store/Professional-Assessments/Behavior/Adaptive/Vineland-Adaptive-Behavior-Scales-%7C-Third-Edition/p/100001622.html (accessed January 12, 2022).
Speed, T. J., V. A. Mathur, M. Hand, B. Christensen, P. D. Sponseller, K. A. Williams, and C. M. Campbell. 2017. Characterization of pain, disability, and psychological burden in Marfan syndrome. *American Journal of Medical Genetics Part A* 173(2):315-323. https://doi.org/10.1002/ajmg.a.38051.
SSA (U.S. Social Security Administration). 2009. *SSR 09-1p: Title XVI: Determining childhood disability under the functional equivalence rule—The "whole child" approach.* https://www.ssa.gov/OP_Home/rulings/ssi/02/SSR2009-01-ssi-02.html#fn4 (accessed May 26, 2022).
SSA. 2020. *Disability report—adult. Form SSA-3368-BK.* https://www.ssa.gov/forms/ssa-3368-bk.pdf (accessed February 27, 2022).
SSA. 2021. *DI 24510.057 sustainability and the residual functional capacity (RFC) assessment* http://policy.ssa.gov/poms.nsf/lnx/0424510057 (accessed January 26, 2022).

SSA. 2022. *Occupational information system project.* https://www.ssa.gov/disabilityresearch/occupational_info_systems.html (accessed February 27, 2022).

SSA. n.d.-a. *Benefit offset national demonstration.* https://www.ssa.gov/disabilityresearch/ois_project_faqs.html (accessed February 27, 2022).

SSA. n.d.-b. *Disability evaluation under Social Security: Listing of impairments—Adult listings (Part A).* https://www.ssa.gov/disability/professionals/bluebook/AdultListings.htm (accessed May 17, 2022).

SSA. n.d.-c. *Disability evaluation under Social Security: 12.00 mental disorders—Adult.* https://www.ssa.gov/disability/professionals/bluebook/12.00-MentalDisorders-Adult.htm (accessed March 7, 2022).

SSA. n.d.-d. *Disability evaluation under Social Security: 112.00 mental disorders—Childhood.* https://www.ssa.gov/disability/professionals/bluebook/112.00-MentalDisorders-Childhood.htm (accessed March 7, 2022).

SSA. n.d.-e. *SSR 83-10. Titles II and XVI: Determining capability to do other work—The medical-vocational rules of Appendix 2.* https://www.ssa.gov/OP_Home/rulings/di/02/SSR83-10-di-02.html (accessed March 7, 2022).

SSA. n.d.-f. *SSR 85-15. Titles II and XVI: Capability to do other work—The medical-vocational rules as a framework for evaluating solely nonexertional impairments.* https://www.ssa.gov/OP_Home/rulings/di/02/SSR85-15-di-02.html (accessed March 29, 2022).

Stachler, R. J., D. O. Francis, S. R. Schwartz, C. C. Damask, G. P. Digoy, H. J. Krouse, S. J. McCoy, D. R. Ouellette, R. R. Patel, C. C. W. Reavis, L. J. Smith, M. Smith, S. W. Strode, P. Woo, and L. C. Nnacheta. 2018. Clinical practice guideline: Hoarseness (dysphonia) (update). *Otolaryngology and Head and Neck Surgery* 158(1 Suppl):S1-S42. https://doi.org/10.1177/0194599817751030.

Stand. n.d. Stand. *The Britannica dictionary.* https://www.britannica.com/dictionary/stand (accessed May 26, 2022).

Stasi, C., C. Nisita, S. Cortopassi, G. Corretti, D. Gambaccini, N. De Bortoli, B. Fani, N. Simonetti, A. Ricchiuti, L. Dell'Osso, S. Marchi, and M. Bellini. 2017. Subthreshold psychiatric psychopathology in functional gastrointestinal disorders: Can it be the bridge between gastroenterology and psychiatry? *Gastroenterology Research and Practice* 2017:1953435. https://doi.org/10.1155/2017/1953435.

Steinberg, N., S. Tenenbaum, A. Zeev, M. Pantanowitz, G. Waddington, G. Dar, and I. Siev-Ner. 2021. Generalized joint hypermobility, scoliosis, patellofemoral pain, and physical abilities in young dancers. *BMC Musculoskeletal Disorders* 22(1):161. https://doi.org/10.1186/s12891-021-04023-z.

Stevens, M. L., C. C. Lin, and C. G. Maher. 2016. The Roland Morris Disability Questionnaire. *Journal of Physiotherapy* 62(2):116. https://doi.org/10.1016/j.jphys.2015.10.003.

Stewart, J. M., J. R. Boris, G. Chelimsky, P. R. Fischer, J. E. Fortunato, B. P. Grubb, G. L. Heyer, I. T. Jarjour, M. S. Medow, M. T. Numan, P. T. Pianosi, W. Singer, S. Tarbell, T. C. Chelimsky, and Pediatric Writing Group of the American Autonomic Society. 2018. Pediatric disorders of orthostatic intolerance. *Pediatrics* 141(1):e20171673. https://doi.org/10.1542/peds.2017-1673.

Strand, E. A., J. R. Duffy, H. M. Clark, and K. Josephs. 2014. The Apraxia of Speech Rating Scale: A tool for diagnosis and description of apraxia of speech. *Journal of Communication Disorders* 51:43-50. https://doi.org/10.1016/j.jcomdis.2014.06.008.

Streeten, D. H. P., and D. S. Bell. 1998. Circulating blood volume in chronic fatigue syndrome. *Journal of Chronic Fatigue Syndrome* 4(1):3-11. https://doi.org/10.1300/J092v04n01_02.

Suster, S. M., M. Ronnen, and J. J. Bubis. 1984. Diverticulosis coli in association with Marfan's syndrome. *Archives of Internal Medicine* 144(1):203.

Syx, D., I. De Wandele, L. Rombaut, and F. Malfait. 2017. Hypermobility, the Ehlers-Danlos syndromes and chronic pain. *Clinical and Experimental Rheumatology* 35 Suppl 107(5):116-122.

Tang, Z., Z. Chen, B. Tang, and H. Jiang. 2015. Primary erythromelalgia: A review. *Orphanet Journal of Rare Diseases* 10(September):127. https://doi.org/10.1186/s13023-015-0347-1.

Theoharides, T. C., P. Valent, and C. Akin. 2015. Mast cells, mastocytosis, and related disorders. *New England Journal of Medicine* 373(2):163-172. https://doi.org/10.1056/NEJMra1409760.

Toprak Celenay, S., and D. Ozer Kaya. 2017. Effects of spinal stabilization exercises in women with benign joint hypermobility syndrome: A randomized controlled trial. *Rheumatology International* 37(9):1461-1468. https://doi.org/10.1007/s00296-017-3713-6.

Treede, R.-D., W. Rief, A. Barke, Q. Aziz, M. I. Bennett, R. Benoliel, M. Cohen, S. Evers, N. B. Finnerup, M. B. First, M. A. Giamberardino, S. Kaasa, E. Kosek, P. Lavand'homme, M. Nicholas, S. Perrot, J. Scholz, S. Schug, B. H. Smith, P. Svensson, J. W. S. Vlaeyen, and S.-J. Wang. 2015. A classification of chronic pain for ICD-11. *Pain* 156(6):1003-1007. https://doi.org/10.1097/j.pain.0000000000000160.

Tsui, P., A. Deptula, and D. Y. Yuan. 2017. Conversion disorder, functional neurological symptom disorder, and chronic pain: Comorbidity, assessment, and treatment. *Current Pain and Headache Reports* 21(6):29. https://doi.org/10.1007/s11916-017-0627-7.

Tun, M. H., B. Borg, M. Godfrey, N. Hadley-Miller, and E. D. Chan. 2021. Respiratory manifestations of Marfan syndrome: A narrative review. *Journal of Thoracic Disease* 13(10):6012-6025. https://doi.org/10.21037/jtd-21-1064.

Tuomi, K., J. Ilmarinen, A. Jahkola, L. Katajarinne, and A. Tulkki. 1998. *Work Ability Index*. 2nd revised ed. Helsinki: Finnish Institute of Occupational Health.

University of California San Fransico Health. n.d. *Hearing loss & diagnosis*. https://www.ucsfhealth.org/conditions/hearing-loss/diagnosis (accessed December 14, 2021).

Vadivelu, N., A. M. Kai, G. Kodumudi, K. Babayan, M. Fontes, and M. M. Burg. 2017. Pain and psychology—A reciprocal relationship. *Ochsner Journal* 17(2):173-180. https://www.ncbi.nlm.nih.gov/pmc/articles/PMC5472077/.

van Campen, C. M. C., P. C. Rowe, F. W. A. Verheugt, and F. C. Visser. 2020. Physical activity measures in patients with myalgic encephalomyelitis/chronic fatigue syndrome: Correlations between peak oxygen consumption, the physical functioning scale of the SF-36 questionnaire, and the number of steps from an activity meter. *Journal of Translational Medicine* 18(1):228. https://doi.org/10.1186/s12967-020-02397-7.

van de Laar, I. M. B. H., R. A. Oldenburg, G. Pals, J. W. Roos-Hesselink, B. M. de Graaf, J. M. A. Verhagen, Y. M. Hoedemaekers, R. Willemsen, L.-A. Severijnen, H. Venselaar, G. Vriend, P. M. Pattynama, M. Collée, D. Majoor-Krakauer, D. Poldermans, I. M. E. Frohn-Mulder, D. Micha, J. Timmermans, Y. Hilhorst-Hofstee, S. M. Bierma-Zeinstra, P. J. Willems, J. M. Kros, E. H. G. Oei, B. A. Oostra, M. W. Wessels, and A. M. Bertoli-Avella. 2011. Mutations in *SMAD3* cause a syndromic form of aortic aneurysms and dissections with early-onset osteoarthritis. *Nature Genetics* 43(2):121-126. https://doi.org/10.1038/ng.744.

van de Laar, I. M. B. H., D. van der Linde, E. H. G. Oei, P. K. Bos, J. H. Bessems, S. M. Bierma-Zeinstra, B. L. van Meer, G. Pals, R. A. Oldenburg, J. A. Bekkers, A. Moelker, B. M. de Graaf, G. Matyas, I. M. E. Frohn-Mulder, J. Timmermans, Y. Hilhorst-Hofstee, J. M. Cobben, H. T. Bruggenwirth, L. van Laer, B. Loeys, J. De Backer, P. J. Coucke, H. C. Dietz, P. J. Willems, B. A. Oostra, A. De Paepe, J. W. Roos-Hesselink, A. M. Bertoli-Avella, and M. W. Wessels. 2012. Phenotypic spectrum of the *SMAD3*-related aneurysms–osteoarthritis syndrome. *Journal of Medical Genetics* 49(1):47. https://doi.org/10.1136/jmedgenet-2011-100382.

van der Linde, D., I. M. B. H. van de Laar, A. M. Bertoli-Avella, R. A. Oldenburg, J. A. Bekkers, F. U. S. Mattace-Raso, A. H. van den Meiracker, A. Moelker, F. van Kooten, I. M. E. Frohn-Mulder, J. Timmermans, E. Moltzer, J. M. Cobben, L. van Laer, B. Loeys, J. De Backer, P. J. Coucke, A. De Paepe, Y. Hilhorst-Hofstee, M. W. Wessels, and J. W. Roos-Hesselink. 2012. Aggressive cardiovascular phenotype of aneurysms-osteoarthritis syndrome caused by pathogenic *SMAD3* variants. *Journal of the American College of Cardiology* 60(5):397-403. https://doi.org/10.1016/j.jacc.2011.12.052.

van Dijk, N., M. C. Boer, B. J. M. Mulder, G. A. van Montfrans, and W. Wieling. 2008. Is fatigue in Marfan syndrome related to orthostatic intolerance? *Clinical Autonomic Research* 18(4):187. https://doi.org/10.1007/s10286-008-0475-y.

van Lankveld, W., P. van't Pad Bosch, J. Bakker, S. Terwindt, M. Franssen, and P. van Kiel. 1996. Sequential occupational dexterity assessment (SODA): A new test to measure hand disability. *Journal of Hand Therapy* 9(1):27-32. https://doi.org/10.1016/S0894-1130(96)80008-1.

van Rossom, S., C. R. Smith, D. G. Thelen, B. Vanwanseele, D. Van Assche, and I. Jonkers. 2018. Knee joint loading in healthy adults during functional exercises: Implications for rehabilitation guidelines. *Journal of Orthopaedic and Sports Physical Therapy* 48(3):162-173. https://doi.org/10.2519/jospt.2018.7459.

Varni, J. W., M. Seid, and P. S. Kurtin. 2001. PedsQL 4.0: Reliability and validity of the Pediatric Quality of Life Inventory version 4.0 generic core scales in healthy and patient populations. *Medical Care* 39(8):800-812. https://doi.org/10.1097/00005650-200108000-00006.

Velvin, G., T. Bathen, S. Rand-Hendriksen, and A. Ø. Geirdal. 2015. Work participation in adults with Marfan syndrome: Demographic characteristics, MFS related health symptoms, chronic pain, and fatigue. *American Journal of Medical Genetics Part A* 167(12):3082-3090. https://doi.org/10.1002/ajmg.a.37370.

Vitaliti, G., P. Pavone, N. Matin, O. Tabatabaie, S. Cocuzza, M. Vecchio, L. Maiolino, P. Di Mauro, A. Conti, R. Lubrano, A. Serra, and R. Falsaperla. 2017. Therapeutic approaches to pediatric pseudotumor cerebri: New insights from literature data. *International Journal of Immunopathology and Pharmacology* 30(1):94-97. https://doi.org/10.1177/0394632016681578.

Voermans, N. C., H. Knoop, G. Bleijenberg, and B. G. van Engelen. 2010a. Pain in Ehlers-Danlos syndrome is common, severe, and associated with functional impairment. *Journal of Pain and Symptom Management* 40(3):370-378. https://doi.org/10.1016/j.jpainsymman.2009.12.026.

Voermans, N. C., H. Knoop, N. van de Kamp, B. C. Hamel, G. Bleijenberg, and B. G. van Engelen. 2010b. Fatigue is a frequent and clinically relevant problem in Ehlers-Danlos syndrome. *Seminars in Arthritis and Rheumatism* 40(3):267-274. https://doi.org/10.1016/j.semarthrit.2009.08.003.

von Kodolitsch, Y., A. Demolder, E. Girdauskas, H. Kaemmerer, K. Kornhuber, L. Muino Mosquera, S. Morris, E. Neptune, R. Pyeritz, S. Rand-Hendriksen, A. Rahman, N. Riise, L. Robert, I. Staufenbiel, K. Szöcs, T. T. Vanem, S. J. Linke, M. Vogler, A. Yetman, and J. De Backer. 2019. Features of Marfan syndrome not listed in the Ghent nosology—The dark side of the disease. *Expert Review of Cardiovascular Therapy* 17(12):883-915. https://doi.org/10.1080/14779072.2019.1704625.

Walker, L. S., and J. W. Greene. 1991. The Functional Disability Inventory: Measuring a neglected dimension of child health status. *Journal of Pediatric Psychology* 16(1):39-58. https://doi.org/10.1093/jpepsy/16.1.39.

Wallace, S. L., L. D. Miller, and K. Mishra. 2019. Pelvic floor physical therapy in the treatment of pelvic floor dysfunction in women. *Current Opinion in Obstetrics and Gynecology* 31(6):485-493. https://doi.org/10.1097/gco.0000000000000584.

Wallis, J. A., L. Roddy, J. Bottrell, S. Parslow, and N. F. Taylor. 2021. A systematic review of clinical practice guidelines for physical therapist management of patellofemoral pain. *Physical Therapy* 101(3):pzab021. https://doi.org/10.1093/ptj/pzab021.

Ware, J. E., Jr., and C. D. Sherbourne. 1992. The MOS 36-item short-form health survey (SF-36). I. Conceptual framework and item selection. *Medical Care* 30(6):473-483.

Warnink-Kavelaars, J., A. Beelen, S. Dekker, F. Nollet, L. A. Menke, and R. H. H. Engelbert. 2019. Marfan syndrome in childhood: Parents' perspectives of the impact on daily functioning of children, parents and family; a qualitative study. *BMC Pediatrics* 19(1):262. https://doi.org/10.1186/s12887-019-1612-6.

Wasim, S., J. S. Suddaby, M. Parikh, S. Leylachian, B. Ho, A. Guerin, and J. So. 2019. Pain and gastrointestinal dysfunction are significant associations with psychiatric disorders in patients with Ehlers–Danlos syndrome and hypermobility spectrum disorders: A retrospective study. *Rheumatology International* 39(7):1241-1248. https://doi.org/10.1007/s00296-019-04293-w.

Watson, C. S., G. R. Kidd, J. D. Miller, C. Smits, and L. E. Humes. 2012. Telephone screening tests for functionally impaired hearing: Current use in seven countries and development of a US version. *Journal of the American Academy of Audiology* 23(10):757-767. https://doi.org/10.3766/jaaa.23.10.2.

Wechsler, D. 2008. *Wechsler Adult Intelligence Scale*, 4th ed. https://www.pearsonassessments.com/store/usassessments/en/Store/Professional-Assessments/Cognition-%26-Neuro/Wechsler-Adult-Intelligence-Scale-%7C-Fourth-Edition/p/100000392.html (accessed January 4, 2022).

Wechsler, D. 2011. *Wechsler Abbreviated Scale of Intelligence*, 2nd ed. https://www.pearsonassessments.com/store/usassessments/en/Store/Professional-Assessments/Cognition-%26-Neuro/Wechsler-Abbreviated-Scale-of-Intelligence-%7C-Second-Edition/p/100000593.html (accessed January 4, 2022).

Wechsler, D. 2012. *Wechsler Preschool and Primary Scale of Intelligence*, 4th ed. https://www.pearsonassessments.com/store/usassessments/en/Store/Professional-Assessments/Cognition-%26-Neuro/Gifted-%26-Talented/Wechsler-Preschool-and-Primary-Scale-of-Intelligence-%7C-Fourth-Edition/p/100000102.html (accessed January 5, 2022).

Wechsler, D. 2014. *Wechsler Intelligence Scale for Children*, 5th ed. https://www.pearsonassessments.com/store/usassessments/en/Store/Professional-Assessments/Cognition-%26-Neuro/Gifted-%26-Talented/Wechsler-Intelligence-Scale-for-Children-%7C-Fifth-Edition-/p/100000771.html (accessed January 5, 2022).

Weiler, C. R., K. F. Austen, C. Akin, M. S. Barkoff, J. A. Bernstein, P. Bonadonna, J. H. Butterfield, M. Carter, C. C. Fox, A. Maitland, T. Pongdee, S. S. Mustafa, A. Ravi, M. C. Tobin, H. Vliagoftis, and L. B. Schwartz. 2019. AAAAI Mast Cell Disorders Committee Work Group report: Mast cell activation syndrome (MCAS) diagnosis and management. *Journal of Allergy and Clinical Immunology* 144(4):883-896. https://doi.org/10.1016/j.jaci.2019.08.023.

Wells, K. F., and E. K. Dillon. 1952. The sit and reach—A test of back and leg flexibility. *Research Quarterly. American Association for Health, Physical Education and Recreation* 23(1):115-118. https://doi.org/10.1080/10671188.1952.10761965.

Wells, R., F. Paterson, S. Bacchi, A. Page, M. Baumert, and D. H. Lau. 2020. Brain fog in postural tachycardia syndrome: An objective cerebral blood flow and neurocognitive analysis. *Journal of Arrhythmia* 36(3):549-552. https://doi.org/10.1002/joa3.12325.

Whitmore, K. E., and T. C. Theoharides. 2011. When to suspect interstitial cystitis. *Journal of Family Practice* 60(6):340-348. https://www.mdedge.com/familymedicine/article/64347/womens-health/when-suspect-interstitial-cystitis.

WHO (World Health Organization). 2001. *International classification of functioning, disability and health*. Geneva, Switzerland: WHO. https://apps.who.int/iris/bitstream/handle/10665/42407/9241545429.pdf;jsessionid=5136600A7DDE039504C0BDD0D57 4CEB9?sequence=1.

WHO. 2021. *ICD-11 for mortality and morbidity statistics: MG30 chronic pain*. https://icd.who.int/browse11/l-m/en#/http%3a%2f%2fid.who.int%2ficd%2fentity%2f1581976053 (accessed October 14, 2021).

WHO. 2022. *Depression*. https://www.who.int/news-room/fact-sheets/detail/depression (accessed May 20, 2022).

Williams, K. T. 2018. *Expressive Vocabulary Test*, 3rd ed. https://www.pearsonassessments.com/store/usassessments/en/Store/Professional-Assessments/Academic-Learning/Brief/Expressive-Vocabulary-Test-%7C-Third-Edition/p/100001982.html (accessed January 12, 2022).

Willy, R. W., L. T. Hoglund, C. J. Barton, L. A. Bolgla, D. A. Scalzitti, D. S. Logerstedt, A. D. Lynch, L. Snyder-Mackler, and C. M. McDonough. 2019. Patellofemoral pain. *Journal of Orthopaedic and Sports Physical Therapy* 49(9):CPG1-CPG95. https://doi.org/10.2519/jospt.2019.0302.

Wyller, V. B., J. A. Evang, K. Godang, K. K. Solhjell, and J. Bollerslev. 2010. Hormonal alterations in adolescent chronic fatigue syndrome. *Acta Paediatrica* 99(5):770-773. https://doi.org/10.1111/j.1651-2227.2010.01701.x.

Yasuda, S., K. Imoto, K. Uchida, D. Machida, H. Yanagi, T. Sugiura, K. Kurosawa, and M. Masuda. 2013. Successful endovascular treatment of a ruptured superior mesenteric artery in a patient with Ehlers-Danlos syndrome. *Annals of Vascular Surgery* 27(7):e971-e975. https://doi.org/10.1016/j.avsg.2013.01.004.

Yorkston, K. M., and D. R. Beukelman. 1984. *Assessment of intelligibility of dysarthric speech*. Austin, TX: PRO-ED.

Yueh, B., N. Shapiro, C. H. MacLean, and P. G. Shekelle. 2003. Screening and management of adult hearing loss in primary care: Scientific review. *JAMA* 289(15):1976-1985. https://doi.org/10.1001/jama.289.15.1976.

Zhang, L., and T. F. Yuan. 2019. Exercise and substance abuse. *International Review of Neurobiology* 147:269-280. https://doi.org/10.1016/bs.irn.2019.07.007.

ANNEX TABLE 5-1
Levels of Work Based on Physical Exertion Requirements

Level of Work	Definition
Sedentary	Sedentary work involves "lifting no more than 10 pounds at a time and occasionally lifting or carrying articles like docket files, ledgers, and small tools" (SSA, n.d.-e). Although a sedentary job is defined as one that involves sitting,
	a certain amount of walking and standing is often necessary in carrying out job duties. Jobs are sedentary if walking and standing are required occasionally and other sedentary criteria are met. By its very nature, work performed primarily in a seated position entails no significant stooping. Most unskilled sedentary jobs require good use of the hands and fingers for repetitive hand-finger actions.
	"Occasionally" means occurring from very little up to one-third of the time. Since being on one's feet is required "occasionally" at the sedentary level of exertion, periods of standing or walking should generally total no more than about 2 hours of an 8-hour workday, and sitting should generally total approximately 6 hours of an 8-hour workday. Work processes in specific jobs will dictate how often and how long a person will need to be on his or her feet to obtain or return small articles. (SSA, n.d.-e; see also CFR § 416.967)
Light	Light work involves
	lifting no more than 20 pounds at a time with frequent lifting or carrying of objects weighing up to 10 pounds. Even though the weight lifted in a particular light job may be very little, a job is in this category when it requires a good deal of walking or standing—the primary difference between sedentary and most light jobs. A job is also in this category when it involves sitting most of the time but with some pushing and pulling of arm-hand or leg-foot controls, which require greater exertion than in sedentary work; e.g., mattress sewing machine operator, motor-grader operator, and road-roller operator (skilled and semiskilled jobs in these particular instances). Relatively few unskilled light jobs are performed in a seated position.
	"Frequent" means occurring from one-third to two-thirds of the time. Since frequent lifting or carrying requires being on one's feet up to two-thirds of a workday, the full range of light work requires standing or walking, off and on, for a total of approximately 6 hours of an 8-hour workday. Sitting may occur intermittently during the remaining time. The lifting requirement for the majority of light jobs can be accomplished with occasional, rather than frequent, stooping. Many unskilled light jobs are performed primarily in one location, with the ability to stand being more critical than the ability to walk. They require use of arms and hands to grasp and to hold and turn objects, and they generally do not require use of the fingers for fine activities to the extent required in much sedentary work. (SSA, n.d.-e; see also CFR § 416.967)

continued

ANNEX TABLE 5-1
Continued

Level of Work	Definition
Medium	Medium work involves
	lifting no more than 50 pounds at a time with frequent lifting or carrying of objects weighing up to 25 pounds. A full range of medium work requires standing or walking, off and on, for a total of approximately 6 hours in an 8-hour workday in order to meet the requirements of frequent lifting or carrying objects weighing up to 25 pounds. As in light work, sitting may occur intermittently during the remaining time. Use of the arms and hands is necessary to grasp, hold, and turn objects, as opposed to the finer activities in much sedentary work, which require precision use of the fingers as well as use of the hands and arms.
	The considerable lifting required for the full range of medium work usually requires frequent bending-stooping. (Stooping is a type of bending in which a person bends his or her body downward and forward by bending the spine at the waist.) Flexibility of the knees as well as the torso is important for this activity. (Crouching is bending both the legs and spine in order to bend the body downward and forward.) However, there are relatively few occupations in the national economy which require exertion in terms of weights that must be lifted at time (or involve equivalent exertion in pushing and pulling), but are performed primarily in a sitting position, e.g., taxi driver, bus driver, and tank-truck driver (semi-skilled jobs). In most medium jobs, being on one's feet for most of the workday is critical. Being able to do frequent lifting or carrying of objects weighing up to 25 pounds is often more critical than being able to lift up to 50 pounds at a time. (SSA, n.d.-e; see also CFR § 416.967)
Heavy	"Heavy work involves lifting no more than 100 pounds at a time with frequent lifting or carrying of objects weighing up to 50 pounds" (CFR § 416.967).
Very heavy	"Very heavy work involves lifting objects weighing more than 100 pounds at a time with frequent lifting or carrying of objects weighing 50 pounds or more" (CFR § 416.967).

SOURCES: SSA, n.d.-e; CFR § 416.967.

ANNEX TABLE 5-2
Physical Activities; Vision, Hearing, and Speech; and Mental Activities

Activity	Definition
Physical Activities	
Sitting	For the purpose of collecting occupational data, the U.S. Bureau of Labor Statistics considers sitting to be present when any of the following conditions exists: • Workers remain in a seated position. This includes active sitting. For example, bicyclists sit but push/pull with their feet/legs. • Workers are lying down. This includes active lying down. For example, a mechanic lying on a dolly working underneath a vehicle is sitting. • Workers may choose between sitting and standing for a given task. For example, office workers can choose a standing desk. (BLS, 2020, p. 112) From a functional perspective, however, sitting as a physical activity involves resting one's lower body (buttocks) on a seat or the ground, while maintaining one's upper body (torso, neck, head) in an upright position. In addition to strong neck, shoulder, and core muscles, sitting requires balance and good proprioception. Although lying on a raised surface (e.g., a bed) may be grouped with sitting, sitting is distinct from lying down on the ground (e.g., lying on a dolly underneath a vehicle), which this report groups under low work.
Standing	For the purpose of collecting occupational data, the Occupational Requirements Survey distinguishes only between sitting (as defined previously) and standing/walking defined as "whenever workers are not sitting or lying down," including "time spent stooping, crawling, kneeling, crouching, or climbing" (BLS, 2020, p. 112). In other words, "a worker is always either sitting or standing/walking" (BLS, 2020, p. 112). From a functional perspective, standing is distinct from walking, which in turn is distinct from low work (stooping, crawling, kneeling, crouching), or climbing. For the purpose of this report, standing is defined as being "in an upright position with all of [one's] weight on [one's] feet" (*Stand,* n.d.).
Walking	Moving along on foot or advancing by steps, with one foot always on the ground. Distance (long or short) and surface type (uneven, rough) can affect an individual's ability to walk.
Strenuous physical activity	Strenuous physical activity captures activities that require exertion and stamina—for example, running, jumping, swimming, throwing, catching, and the like. It potentially includes all other physical activities, in addition to running and other impact activities.
Lifting (floor to waist and overhead)	Use of upper and/or lower extremities to raise or lower an object from one level to another, including upward pulling (BLS, 2020, p. 118).
Carrying	"Transporting an object, usually by holding it in the hands or arms, or wearing it on the body, usually around the waist or upper torso" (BLS, 2020, p. 118). Carrying usually also requires the ability to stand, lift, and walk.

continued

ANNEX TABLE 5-2
Continued

Activity	Definition
Pushing/pulling	Use of upper and/or lower extremities to exert force upon an object so that the object moves away from or toward the origin of the force (BLS, 2020, p. 125).
Reaching	"Extending the hand(s) and arm(s) in any direction, requiring the straightening and extending of the arm(s) and elbow(s) and the engagement of the shoulder(s)" (BLS, 2020, p. 130). Reaching may require standing.
Overhead reaching	Extending the arm(s) with the hand(s) higher than the head and (1) the elbow is bent and the angle at the shoulders is about 90 degrees or more or (2) the elbow is extended and the angle at the shoulder is about 120 degrees or more (BLS, 2020, p. 130). Overhead reaching requires neck extension and may require standing.
At/below the shoulder reaching	Reaching that does not meet the threshold for overhead reaching described above (BLS, 2020, p. 130). At/below the shoulder reaching may require standing.
Gross manipulation	Gross manipulation involves "seizing, holding, grasping, turning, or otherwise working with the hand(s). Fingers are involved only to the extent that they are an extension of the hand to hold or operate an object or tool, such as hammer" (BLS, 2020, p. 187). It includes handling of large objects.
Fine manipulation	Fine manipulation involves "touching, picking, pinching, or otherwise working primarily with fingers rather than with the whole hand or arm" (BLS, 2020, p. 133). It includes writing, typing, or handling small objects (fingering).
Foot/leg controls	Refers to the "use of one or both feet or legs to move controls on machinery or equipment. Controls include, but are not limited to, pedals, buttons, levers, and cranks" (BLS, 2020, p. 133).
Climbing	"The act of ascending or descending stairs, ramps, ladders, ropes or scaffolding and similar structures using feet, legs, hands, and/or arms" (BLS, 2020, p. 142).

ANNEX TABLE 5-2
Continued

Activity	Definition
Low work	Low work is a group of activities that includes stooping, crouching, kneeling, crawling, and lying on the ground.
	Stooping is the act of "bending the body forward and down while bending the spine at the waist 45 degrees or more either over something below waist level or down towards an object on or near the ground" (BLS, 2020, p. 193). Must be performed standing.
	Crouching is "bending the body downward and forward by bending the legs and spine" (BLS, 2020, p. 138).
	Kneeling is "bending the legs at the knees to come to rest on the knee or knees" (BLS, 2020, p. 139).
	Crawling is "moving about on hands and knees or hands and feet" (BLS, 2020, p. 139).
	Lying on the ground includes the need to get down and up from the ground (e.g., lying down on a trolley on the ground).
	Clustering the low work activities is appropriate because one generally has to be able to stoop, crouch, and kneel to be able to crawl. There might be an occasion when someone only has to kneel momentarily (e.g., to lift a child) that might be less difficult for some people, but most of the difficulties are shared among these activities.
	From a functional perspective, lying on the ground has more in common with other low work activities in that it includes the need to get up and down from the ground and potentially squirming around to do work while on the ground. These are difficult tasks that are equivalent to the other low work activities.
Vision, Hearing, and Speaking Activities	
Near visual acuity	"Clarity of vision at approximately 20 inches or less, as when working with small objects or reading small print" (BLS, 2020, p. 154), including the use of a computer in support of a critical job function, regardless of distance.
Far visual acuity	"Clarity of vision at a distance of 20 feet or more, involving the ability to distinguish features of a person or objects at a distance" (BLS, 2020, p. 154).
Peripheral vision	"What is seen above, below, to the left or right by the eye while staring straight ahead" (BLS, 2020, p. 154).
Hearing	"Ability to hear, understand, and distinguish speech and/or other sounds" (BLS, 2020, p. 149). Includes hearing in-person one-on-one and group or conference communication; telephones and similar devices, such as radios, walkie-talkies, intercoms, and public address systems; and other such sounds as machinery alarms and equipment sounds. Passing a hearing test may be required for certain jobs.

continued

ANNEX TABLE 5-2
Continued

Activity	Definition
Speaking	"Expressing or exchanging ideas by means of the spoken word to impart oral information to clients or the public and to convey detailed spoken instructions to other workers accurately, loudly, or quickly" (BLS, 2020, p. 149).
Mental Activities	
Understand, remember, and apply information	The abilities to learn, recall, and use (apply) information (SSA, n.d.-c, n.d.-d).
Concentrate, persist, or maintain pace	The abilities to focus attention on work/school activities and stay on task at a sustained rate (SSA, n.d.-c, n.d.-d).
Problem solve	"Analyze issues and make decisions that have a moderate to significant level of difficulty (e.g., the full extent of issues may not be readily apparent and requires independent judgment and research or investigation). The defining characteristics of problem solving are that there is no obvious, immediate solution to a problem or issue, and the worker must identify and weigh alternatives to arrive at a solution" (BLS, 2020, p. 99).
Interact with others	The abilities to relate to and work with supervisors, coworkers, the public, teachers, peers, and others—for example, cooperating with others; asking for help when needed; handling conflicts with others; stating [one's] point of view; initiating or sustaining conversation; understanding and responding to social cues (physical, verbal, emotional); responding to requests, suggestions, criticism, correction, and challenges; and keeping social interactions free of excessive irritability, sensitivity, argumentativeness, or suspiciousness. (SSA, n.d.-c; see also SSA, n.d.-d)
Adapt or manage oneself	The abilities to "regulate emotions, control behavior, and maintain well-being" in a work or school setting—for example, responding to demands; adapting to changes; managing [one's] psychologically based symptoms; distinguishing between acceptable and unacceptable work performance; setting realistic goals; making plans for [oneself] independently of others; maintaining personal hygiene and [appropriate attire]; and being aware of normal hazards and taking appropriate precautions. (SSA, n.d.-c; see also SSA, n.d.-d)

SOURCES: BLS, 2020; SSA, n.d.-c, n.d.-d.

ANNEX TABLE 5-3
Selected Musculoskeletal Manifestations Associated with Heritable Disorders of Connective Tissue

Manifestations		HDCTs (Selected)	Common Diagnostic Techniques	Potential Treatments
Subluxations and dislocations	Patella	• Hypermobile EDS (hEDS)/HSD • EDS (many other subtypes) • MFS	• Physical exam • X-ray for dislocation and risk factors; imaging might not detect subluxation • Advanced imaging (e.g., MRI, CT)	• Physical therapy[a] • Self-administered interventions[b] • Medications (oral and topical) • Surgical intervention • Orthoses (e.g., braces, splints), assistive devices (e.g., crutches, wheelchair); custom orthoses may be important • Environmental modifications
	Shoulder	• hEDS/HSD • Classical EDS (cEDS) • MFS	• Physical exam • X-ray for dislocation; imaging might not detect subluxation • Advanced imaging	• Physical therapy[a] • Self-administered interventions[b] • Occupational therapy[c] • Medications (oral and topical) • Surgical intervention • Orthoses, compression clothing • Environmental modifications
	Hip	• hEDS/HSD • MFS	• Physical exam • X-ray for dislocation; imaging might not detect subluxation • Advanced imaging	• Physical therapy[a] • Self-administered interventions[b] • Medications (oral and topical) • Compression clothing, assistive devices (e.g., crutches, wheelchair); less often orthoses • Surgical intervention • Environmental modifications

continued

ANNEX TABLE 5-3
Continued

Manifestations	HDCTs (Selected)	Common Diagnostic Techniques	Potential Treatments
Ankle/subtalar joint	• HSD • EDS (all types) • MFS	• Physical exam • X-ray • Advanced imaging	• Medications (oral) • Physical therapy[a] • Self-administered interventions[b] • Orthoses, assistive devices • Surgical intervention • Environmental modifications
Temporomandibular joint (TMJ)	• hEDS/HSD • EDS (many other subtypes)	• Physical exam • Advanced imaging	• Liquid diet • Physical therapy[a] • Self-administered interventions[b] • Speech therapy • Surgical intervention • Medications (oral, topical, injected) • Dental appliance • Psychological support for pain or stress management; cognitive behavioral therapy (CBT) training for patients • Botox injections (muscles of mastication; use extreme caution if injecting cervical muscles due to likelihood of cervical instability)

Rib	• hEDS/HSD • EDS (other subtypes)	• Physical exam (Imaging often cannot pick up subtle malalignments.)	• Physical therapy[a] • Self-administered interventions[b] • Medications (oral and topical) • Orthoses, straps, compression garments, etc. • Breathing arts, such as yoga, tai chi, Pilates • Environmental modifications
Other common joints	• hEDS/HSD • EDS (other subtypes)	• Physical exam	• Physical therapy[a] • Self-administered interventions[b] • Occupational therapy[c] • Orthoses, compression clothing, assistive devices • Environmental modifications

continued

ANNEX TABLE 5-3 Continued

Manifestations		HDCTs (Selected)	Common Diagnostic Techniques	Potential Treatments
Instability	Cervical	• HSD • EDS (all types) • LDS	• *Gentle* cervical traction for diagnostic purposes only • Physical exam for ligamentous laxity (e.g., Sharp-Purser, alar ligament, Aspinall, etc.) • Physical exam for cervical myelopathy (e.g., Hoffmann, Babinski, grip-release tests) • Testing should also address contributing factors, such as weakness or poor motor control of deep neck flexors (craniocervical flexion test with pressure biofeedback) and proprioceptive deficits (joint position error with laser).	• Physical therapy[a] (Mechanical cervical traction may be used for diagnostic purposes, but there is a precaution/contraindication in its use for treatment.) • Self-administered interventions[b] • Medications (oral and topical); topicals for trigger points • Pilates • Speech therapy (for swallowing disorders) • Rigid cervical stabilization braces • Surgical intervention • Environmental modifications • Occupational therapy[c]
	Lumbar and sacroiliac	• HSD • EDS (all types)	• Physical exam • Testing should also address contributing factors, such as weakness or poor motor control of stabilizing muscles.	• Mechanical lumbar traction is a precaution/contraindication, even if radicular signs are present. • Self-administered interventions[b] • Pilates, tai chi, some forms of yoga • Orthoses, compression clothing, etc. • Surgical intervention • Medications (oral and topical) • Environmental modifications • Occupational therapy[c]

Costochondritis	hEDS/HSD EDS (other subtypes)	• Physical exam • Other tests to rule out other conditions	• Physical therapy[a] • Self-administered interventions[b] • Medications (oral, topical, injectable) • Orthoses, compression clothing, etc. • Environmental modifications • Occupational therapy[c]
Hand/finger instability	hEDS/HSD EDS (other subtypes)	• Physical exam	• Physical therapy[a] • Self-administered interventions[b] • Occupational therapy[c] • Environmental modifications • Orthoses, splints, compression clothing, etc. • Medications (oral and topical)
Joint pain Pain	hEDS/HSD EDS (other subtypes) MFS	• Physical exam • Advanced imaging • Evaluation for presence of immune-mediated arthropathy (see Annex Table 5-7 [immunologic table])	• Medications (oral, topical, injectable) • Physical therapy[a] • Self-administered interventions[b] • Occupational therapy[c] • Orthoses, splints, compression clothing, assistive devices, etc. • Environmental modifications

continued

ANNEX TABLE 5-3 Continued

Manifestations	HDCTs (Selected)	Common Diagnostic Techniques	Potential Treatments
Chronic pain syndrome	• All	• Physical exam	• Physical therapy[a] • Self-administered interventions[b] • Occupational therapy[c] • Mind-body arts, such as yoga, Pilates, tai chi • Psychological support for pain management; CBT training for patients • Mast cell activation disease (MCAD) management • Postural orthostatic tachycardia syndrome (POTS) management • Orthoses, compression clothing, etc.
Spinal pain (including, but not limited to, instability, muscle spasm, nerve compression, facet joint syndromes)	• hEDS/HSD • EDS (other subtypes) • MFS	• Physical exam • Advanced imaging • Evaluation for neurological complications	• Medications (oral, topical, injectable) • Physical therapy[a] • Self-administered interventions[b] • Occupational therapy[c] • Orthoses, braces, compression clothing, assistive devices, etc. • Environmental modifications

Headache	• hEDS/HSD • EDS (other subtypes)	• Physical exam (looking for contributing factors, as well as pain generators) • Advanced imaging only if suspicion of serious spinal pathology is present	• Physical therapy[a], precaution with mechanical traction, especially when cervical instability present, though traction may be used for diagnostic purposes • Self-administered interventions[b] • Medications (oral, topical, injectable) • Neck braces if neck is unstable • Botox injections (Use caution when injecting muscles providing stability, especially in the neck. Those who are not knowledgeable about EDS should avoid doing Botox injections into cervical muscles in EDS.)
Tendon and ligament disorders			
Tendon abnormalities	• hEDS/HSD • EDS (other subtypes)	• Physical exam • Advanced imaging	• Physical therapy[a] • Self-administered interventions[b] • Orthoses, compression clothing, etc. • Occupational therapy[c] • Medications (oral and topical)
Plantar fasciitis	• All	• Physical exam • Advanced imaging	• Physical therapy[a] • Self-administered interventions[b] • Orthoses, compression clothing, etc; custom orthoses may be important

continued

ANNEX TABLE 5-3 Continued

Manifestations		HDCTs (Selected)	Common Diagnostic Techniques	Potential Treatments
Cartilage disorders	Meniscus tears	All	- Advanced imaging - CT arthrogram - Physical exam	- Physical therapy[a] - Self-administered interventions[b] - Orthoses, compression clothing, etc. - Surgical intervention
	Hip labrum tears, "snapping hip syndrome," hip impingement	All	- Advanced imaging - CT arthrogram - Physical exam	- Physical therapy[a] - Self-administered interventions[b] - Surgical intervention - Orthoses, compression clothing, assistive devices, mobility devices
	Shoulder labrum tears	hEDS/HSD EDS (other subtypes)	- Advanced imaging - CT arthrogram - Physical exam	- Physical therapy[a] - Self-administered interventions[b] - Surgical intervention - Orthoses, compression clothing, etc.
	Triangular fibrocartilage complex	hEDS/HSD EDS (other subtypes)	- Physical exam - Advanced imaging	- Physical therapy[a] - Self-administered interventions[b] - Occupational therapy[c] - Orthoses

Myofascial disorders	Muscle spasms/trigger points	hEDS/HSD EDS (other subtypes)	Physical exam	Physical therapy[a] Self-administered interventions[b] Occupational therapy[c] Massage therapy Movement art, such as Pilates, yoga, tai chi Orthoses, splints, compression clothing, etc. Botox injections (Use caution when injecting muscles providing stability, especially in the neck. Those who are not knowledgeable about EDS should avoid doing Botox injections into cervical muscles in EDS.)
	Myofascial restriction	hEDS/HSD EDS (other subtypes)	Physical exam	Physical therapy[a] Self-administered interventions[b] Massage therapy Orthoses, compression clothing, etc. Movement art, such as yoga, tai chi, qigong
	TMJ myofascial pain	hEDS/HSD EDS (other subtypes)	Physical exam	Physical therapy[a] Self-administered interventions[b] Dental appliance Speech therapy Psychological support for pain management
	Chronic pelvic pain	hEDS/HSD EDS (other subtypes)	Physical exam Internal EMG Advanced imaging Advanced diagnostic testing	Physical therapy[a] Self-administered interventions[b] Orthoses, compression clothing, etc. Psychological support

continued

ANNEX TABLE 5-3 Continued

Manifestations		HDCTs (Selected)	Common Diagnostic Techniques	Potential Treatments
Nerve compression disorders	Thoracic outlet syndrome	• hEDS/HSD • EDS (other subtypes)	• Physical exam • X-ray (1st rib) • Arteriogram • Electrodiagnostic testing	• Physical therapy[a] • Self-administered interventions[b] • Medications (oral and topical) • Movement arts that involve diaphragmatic breathing: yoga, tai chi, qigong • Surgical intervention
	Carpal tunnel	• hEDS/HSD • EDS (other subtypes)	• Physical exam • Electrodiagnostic testing	• Physical therapy[a] • Self-administered interventions[b] • Occupational therapy[c] • Medications (oral and topical) • Orthoses, compression clothing, etc. • Surgical intervention
	Cubital tunnel	• hEDS/HSD • EDS (other subtypes)	• Physical exam • Electrodiagnostic testing	• Physical therapy[a] • Self-administered interventions[b] • Occupational therapy[c] • Orthoses, compression clothing, etc. • Medications (oral and topical) • Surgical intervention
	Sciatica	• hEDS/HSD • EDS (other subtypes)	• Physical exam • Electrodiagnostic testing • Advanced imaging to rule out spinal source	• Physical therapy[a] • Self-administered interventions[b] • Medications (oral) • Orthoses, compression clothing, etc.

Morton's neuroma	MFS hEDS/HSD LDS	Physical exam Advanced imaging	Orthoses; custom orthoses may be important Physical therapy[a] Self-administered interventions[b] Medications (oral) Injections Surgical intervention
Scoliosis	MFS LDS CCA	Physical exam Advanced imaging	Physical therapy[a] Bracing Surgical intervention
Joint contractures	MFS CCA	Physical exam	Physical therapy[a] Occupational therapy[c] Botox injections Bracing Surgical release

NOTES: CCA = congenital contractural arachnodactyly; CT = computed tomography; EDS = Ehlers-Danlos syndromes; EMG = electromyogram; HDCT = heritable disorder of connective tissue; HSD = hypermobility spectrum disorders; LDS = Loeys-Dietz syndrome; MFS = Marfan syndrome.

[a]Physical therapy includes, but is not limited to, the following interventions:

- Education about posture, body mechanics, ergonomics, joint protection, trigger point management, pain neuroscience, physiological quieting, biofeedback, self-care), POTS self-care, MCAS self-care
- Neuromuscular reeducation: proprioception, motor control, stabilization, balance; may include forms of movement biofeedback; also includes breathing retraining
- Exercise, including range of motion, strengthening, muscle/fascia stretching, cardiovascular exercise; includes named exercise approaches, such as Pilates, tai chi, and yoga, if instructed by someone knowledgeable about EDS; also includes POTS-specific prescribed exercise
- Recommending, training, and/or fitting for braces, splints, orthotics, assistive devices, taping, compression clothing
- Gait training with or without assistive devices, particularly for lumbar and lower extremity conditions
- Physical modalities should not be the core of clinic management but may be helpful to permit active interventions. Modalities include heat/ice, transcutaneous electric nerve stimulation, with less evidence for ultrasound, laser, infrared, and shock wave. Cervical and lumbar traction are a precaution in hypermobility, so should only be used with caution.

ANNEX TABLE 5-3
Continued

- In addition to physical therapy, manual therapy approaches may be performed by a variety of professionals and include, but are not limited to, massage, soft-tissue mobilization, myofascial release, joint mobilizations (mobilizations are a precaution, and manipulations are contraindicated except by experts in manual therapy for EDS), acupuncture, dry needling, and other named manual therapy approaches (e.g., "Mobilization with Movement," "Visceral Mobilization," or "Strain Counter-strain"; many other terms are used).

[b]Self-administered interventions with guidance from a health care provider include, but are not limited to, the following interventions:

- Posture, joint protection principles, ergonomic modifications
- Exercise (including all types that could be recommended/instructed by a physical therapist, occupational therapist, or other qualified health care provider, including Pilates, tai chi, qigong, some forms of yoga, and breathing exercises)
- Physical modalities, such as ice, heat, transcutaneous electric nerve stimulation (TENS).
- Over-the-counter topicals (e.g., diclofenac cream, lidocaine spray, menthol spray/cream, salicylate, CBD, capsaicin) and oral analgesics (e.g., acetaminophen, ibuprofen).
- Using splints, braces, orthoses, compression clothing, assistive devices, taping, etc.
- Self-management of trigger points through exercise, self-manual therapy, topicals, etc.
- Pain self-management using principles of pain neuroscience, physiological quieting, biofeedback, pacing

[c]Occupational therapy includes, but is not limited to, the following interventions:

- Adapting of person, tasks, and environment to increase function and decrease pain
- Education about posture, body mechanics, ergonomics, joint protection, trigger point management, pain self-management (pain neuroscience, physiological quieting, biofeedback, self-care)
- Neuromuscular reeducation: proprioception, motor control, stabilization, including breathing retraining and, possibly, forms of movement biofeedback
- Exercise: including range of motion, strengthening, muscle/fascia stretching, cardiovascular exercise
- Recommending, training, fabrication, and/or fitting for braces, splints, assistive devices, taping, compression clothing
- Manual therapy: massage, soft-tissue mobilization, myofascial release, joint mobilizations/manipulations (manipulations and, to a lesser degree, mobilizations are a precaution), dry needling (where allowed), and other named manual therapy approaches (e.g., "Mobilization with Movement," or "Strain Counterstrain"; many terms are used)
- Physical modalities should not be the core of clinical management, but may be helpful to permit active interventions. These modalities include heat/ice and transcutaneous electroneural stimulation, with less evidence for ultrasound, laser, infrared, and shock wave.
- Cognitive retraining
- Work retraining

SOURCES: Barrett et al., 2021; Bier et al., 2018; Blanpied et al., 2017; Butts et al., 2017; Carpal tunnel syndrome, 2019; Celletti et al., 2021; Clinical guidance to optimize work participation after injury or illness, 2021; Daley et al., 2021; De Baets et al., 2021; Enseki et al., 2014; Erickson et al., 2019; Exercise for knee injury prevention, 2018; Finucane et al., 2020; George et al., 2021; JOSPT infographic, 2018; Kareha et al., 2021; Knee ligament sprain guidelines, 2017; Lin et al., 2020; Logerstedt et al., 2017; Logerstedt et al., 2018; Martin et al., 2021; Minhas, 2021; Oliveira et al., 2018a; Palmer et al., 2021; Physical therapy after an ankle sprain, 2021; Price et al., 2020; Reischl et al., 2020; Reychler et al., 2021; Røe, 2014; Steinberg et al., 2021; van Rossom et al., 2018; Wallis et al., 2021; Willy et al., 2019.

ANNEX TABLE 5-4
Selected Neurologic Manifestations Associated with Heritable Disorders of Connective Tissue

Manifestations		HDCTs (Selected)	Common Diagnostic Techniques	Potential Treatments
Cranial disorders	Migraines	• hEDS/HSD • EDS (other subtypes, unspecified) • MFS • LDS	• Clinical • Evaluation for postural orthostatic tachycardia syndrome (POTS) and mast cell activation disease	• Medications • Environmental modifications (e.g., avoid known triggers, such as foods, smoke, smells, stress) • Physical therapy • Occupational therapy • Psychological support for pain management; cognitive behavioral therapy training
	Empty sella turcica syndrome	• EDS (subtypes unspecified)	• Advanced imaging	• Medications
	Delayed cognitive development	• EDS (subtypes unspecified)	• Clinical	• Occupational therapy
	Craniosynostosis	• EDS (subtypes unspecified)	• Advanced imaging	• Surgical intervention
	Intracranial venous stenosis	• EDS (subtypes unspecified)	• Advanced imaging	• Surgical intervention
	Eagle syndrome	• hEDS/HSD • EDS (other subtypes unspecified	• Advanced imaging • Clinical	• Surgical intervention

continued

ANNEX TABLE 5-4 Continued

Manifestations		HDCTs (Selected)	Common Diagnostic Techniques	Potential Treatments
Intracranial pressure changes	Intracranial hypertension	• hEDS/HSD • EDS (other subtypes unspecified) • MFS • LDS	• Advanced imaging • Intracranial pressure monitoring	• Medications • Physical therapy • Occupational therapy • Environmental modifications • Surgical intervention
	Intracranial hypotension	• hEDS/HSD • EDS (other subtypes unspecified) • MFS • LDS	• Advanced imaging • Intracranial pressure monitoring	• Medications • Physical therapy • Occupational therapy • Environmental modifications • Autologous blood patch • Surgical intervention
Chiari malformation		• hEDS/HSD • EDS (other subtypes unspecified) • MFS • LDS	• MRI (brain, upright cervical, thoracic spine)	• Medications • Physical therapy • Surgical decompression
Spinal disorders	Atlanto-occipital instability	• hEDS/HSD • EDS (other subtypes unspecified) • MFS • LDS	• Advanced imaging	• Medications • Physical therapy • Occupational therapy • Environmental modifications • Surgical intervention

Atlanto-axial instability	• hEDS/HSD • EDS (other subtypes unspecified) • MFS • LDS	• Advanced imaging	• Medications • Physical therapy • Occupational therapy • Environmental modifications • Surgical intervention
Basilar invagination	• EDS (subtypes unspecified) • MFS • LDS	• Advanced imaging	• Medications • Physical therapy • Occupational therapy • Environmental modifications • Surgical intervention
Spontaneous CSF leak	• hEDS/HSD • EDS (other subtypes unspecified)	• Advanced imaging	• Medications • Physical therapy • Occupational therapy • Environmental modifications • Surgical intervention
Vertebral artery torsion	• EDS (subtypes unspecified)	• Advanced imaging	• Medications • Physical therapy • Occupational therapy • Environmental modifications • Surgical intervention
Myodural bridges	• hEDS/HSD • EDS (other subtypes unspecified)	• Advanced imaging	• Medications • Physical therapy • Occupational therapy • Environmental modifications • Surgical intervention
Tethered cord syndrome	• hEDS/HSD • EDS (other subtypes unspecified)	• Advanced imaging	• Physical therapy • Surgical intervention

continued

ANNEX TABLE 5-4 Continued

Manifestations	HDCTs (Selected)	Common Diagnostic Techniques	Potential Treatments
Segmental instability	• hEDS/HSD • EDS (other subtypes unspecified)	• Advanced imaging	• Medications • Physical therapy • Occupational therapy • Environmental modifications • Surgical intervention
Segmental kyphosis	• EDS (subtypes unspecified)	• Advanced imaging	• Medications • Physical therapy • Occupational therapy • Environmental modifications • Surgical intervention
Scoliosis	• hEDS/HSD • EDS (other subtypes unspecified) • MFS	• Advanced imaging	• Medications • Physical therapy • Occupational therapy • Environmental modifications • Surgical intervention
Tarlov cysts	• hEDS/HSD • EDS (other subtypes unspecified)	• Advanced imaging	• Surgical intervention
Dural ectasia	• EDS (subtypes unspecified)	• Advanced imaging	• Medications • Physical therapy • Occupational therapy • Environmental modifications • Surgical intervention

	Instability or malformation of the cervical and thoracic spine	• EDS (subtypes unspecified) • MFS • LDS	• Advanced imaging	• Medications • Physical therapy • Occupational therapy • Environmental modifications • Surgical intervention
Movement disorders	Dystonia	• hEDS/HSD • EDS (other subtypes unspecified) • MFS • LDS	• Advanced imaging • Clinical	• Medications • Physical therapy • Occupational therapy • Environmental modifications
	Tremor	• EDS (subtypes unspecified) • MFS • LDS	• Advanced imaging • Clinical	• Medications • Physical therapy • Occupational therapy • Environmental modifications
	Chorea	• EDS (subtypes unspecified) • MFS • LDS	• Advanced imaging • Clinical	• Medications • Physical therapy • Occupational therapy • Environmental modifications
	Myoclonus	• EDS (subtypes unspecified) • MFS • LDS	• Advanced imaging • Clinical	• Medications • Physical therapy • Occupational therapy • Environmental modifications
	Tic disorders	• EDS (subtypes unspecified) • MFS • LDS	• Advanced imaging • Clinical	• Medications • Physical therapy • Occupational therapy • Environmental modifications

continued

ANNEX TABLE 5-4 Continued

Manifestations		HDCTs (Selected)	Common Diagnostic Techniques	Potential Treatments
Neuropathies	Compression neuropathy	• hEDS/HSD • EDS (other subtypes unspecified)	• Advanced imaging • Clinical	• Medications • Physical therapy • Occupational therapy • Environmental modifications • Surgical intervention
	Overstretch neuropathy	• hEDS/HSD • EDS (other subtypes unspecified)	• Advanced imaging • Clinical	• Medications • Physical therapy • Occupational therapy • Environmental modifications • Surgical intervention
	Brachial plexopathy	• hEDS/HSD • EDS (other subtypes unspecified)	• Advanced imaging • Clinical	• Medications • Physical therapy • Occupational therapy • Environmental modifications • Surgical intervention
	Common peroneal neuralgia	• hEDS/HSD • EDS (other subtypes unspecified)	• Clinical	• Surgical intervention • Physical therapy
	Complex regional pain syndrome	• hEDS/HSD • EDS (other subtypes unspecified)	• Clinical	• Medications • Physical therapy • Occupational therapy • Environmental modifications
	Axonal polyneuropathy	• EDS (subtypes unspecified)	• Clinical • Laboratory testing	• Medications • Physical therapy • Occupational therapy • Environmental modifications

Condition		Subtype	Diagnosis	Treatment
Small fiber neuropathy		• hEDS/HSD • EDS (other subtypes unspecified)	• Clinical • Laboratory testing • Skin biopsy	• Medications • Physical therapy • Occupational therapy • Environmental modifications
Dysautonomia	POTS	• hEDS/HSD • EDS (other subtypes unspecified) • MFS • LDS	• Clinical • Laboratory testing	• Medications • Physical therapy • Occupational therapy • Environmental modifications • Self-care: diet, compression garments
	Hyperadrenergic POTS	• hEDS/HSD • EDS (other subtypes unspecified) • MFS • LDS	• Clinical • Laboratory testing	• Medications • Physical therapy • Occupational therapy • Environmental modifications
	Neurocardiogenic syncope	• hEDS/HSD • EDS (other subtypes unspecified) • MFS • LDS	• Clinical • Laboratory testing	• Medications • Physical therapy • Occupational therapy • Environmental modifications
	Multiple system atrophy	• hEDS/HSD • EDS (other subtypes unspecified) • MFS • LDS	• Clinical • Laboratory testing	• Medications • Physical therapy • Occupational therapy • Environmental modifications

continued

ANNEX TABLE 5-4 Continued

Manifestations	HDCTs (Selected)	Common Diagnostic Techniques	Potential Treatments
Pure autonomic failure	• EDS (subtypes unspecified) • MFS • LDS	• Clinical • Laboratory testing	• Medications • Physical therapy • Occupational therapy • Environmental modifications
Autoimmune autonomic ganglionopathy	• EDS (subtypes unspecified) • MFS • LDS	• Clinical • Laboratory testing	• Medications • Physical therapy • Occupational therapy • Environmental modifications
Thoracic outlet syndrome (TOS) Neurogenic TOS	• hEDS/HSD • EDS (other subtypes unspecified)	• Clinical • Advanced imaging	• Medications • Physical therapy • Occupational therapy • Environmental modifications • Surgical intervention
Venous TOS	• hEDS/HSD • EDS (other subtypes unspecified)	• Clinical • Advanced imaging	• Medications • Physical therapy • Occupational therapy • Environmental modifications • Surgical intervention
Arterial TOS	• hEDS/HSD • EDS (other subtypes unspecified)	• Clinical • Advanced imaging	• Medications • Physical therapy • Occupational therapy • Environmental modifications • Surgical intervention
Anterior cutaneous nerve entrapment syndrome	• hEDS/HSD • EDS (other subtypes unspecified)	• Clinical • Diagnostic nerve blocks	• Surgical intervention • Physical therapy

- Mitochondrial dysfunction, secondary
- EDS (subtypes unspecified)
- Clinical
- Laboratory testing
- Medications
- Physical therapy
- Occupational therapy
- Environmental modifications

NOTE: CSF = cerebrospinal fluid; EDS = Ehlers-Danlos syndrome; HDCT = heritable disorder of connective tissue; hEDS = hypermobile Ehlers-Danlos syndrome; HSD = hypermobility spectrum disorders; LDS = Loeys-Dietz syndrome; MFS = Marfan syndrome.

SOURCES: Bozkurt et al., 2018; Bragée et al., 2020; Carvalho et al., 2020; Castori et al., 2015a; Castori and Voermans, 2014; Cazzato et al., 2016; Collins and Orpin, 2021; Corbett et al., 1982; Donkervoort et al., 2015; Ezzeddine et al., 2005; Fu and Levine, 2015, 2018; Galan and Kousseff, 1995; Grabb et al., 1999; Granata et al., 2013; Halko et al., 1995; Henderson et al., 2017; 2019; Jacome, 1999; Klinge, 2015; Levine et al., 2021; Levine and Rigby, 2018; Martin and Neilson, 2014; Milhorat et al., 2007; Papapetropoulos et al., 1981; Pretorius and Butler, 1983; Puledda et al., 2015; Rozen et al., 2006; Rubinstein and Cohen, 1964; Sadler et al., 2020; Savasta et al., 2011; Schievink et al., 1990; 1996; Schoolman and Kepes, 1967; Song et al., 2020; Toprak Celenay and Ozer Kaya, 2017; Vitaliti et al., 2017; Voermans et al., 2010a.

ANNEX TABLE 5-5
Selected Cardiovascular and Hematologic Manifestations Associated with Heritable Disorders of Connective Tissue

Manifestations	HDCTs (Selected)	Common Diagnostic Techniques	Potential Treatments
Ascending aortic aneurysm	• MFS • LDS • CCA • SGS (rare) • Vascular EDS (vEDS) • Familial aortopathies	• Echocardiogram • Advanced imaging (e.g., CT, magnetic resonance axial imaging with image reconstruction)	• Limitations and restrictions • Beta-adrenergic blockade • Angiotension receptor blockade • Aortic replacement depending on diameter and gene mutation
Descending aortic dissection	• MFS • LDS • vEDS	• Advanced imaging	• Emergency evaluation in acute situation • Chest and abdominal imaging at 1 and 3 months following dissection, and every 6 months thereafter • Surgery to replace descending aorta when progression of aortic diameter or extent of dissection occurs
Ascending aortic dissection	• MFS • LDS • vEDS • Familial aortopathies	• Advanced imaging	• Emergency aortic surgery
Aortic regurgitation	• MFS • LDS • Familial aortopathies	• Echocardiogram	• Aortic valve replacement based on severity of regurgitation and left ventricular function
Bicuspid aortic valve	• ~1–1.5% in general population, higher in LDS	• Echocardiogram	• Aortic valve replacement • Surgery to replace a moderately or severely dilated ascending aorta • Surgery to repair aortic coarctation

Mitral valve prolapse	• MFS • LDS • CCA • EDS (most types)	• Echocardiogram	• Mitral valve repair or replacement • Treatment for atrial fibrillation
Arterial tortuosity	• MFS • LDS	• Advanced imaging	• Regular imaging; frequency depends of severity of tortuosity and association with arterial dilatation • Arterial surgery in cases of severity and rapid progression of dilatation • Beta-adrenergic blockade, angiotensin receptor blockade, or both
Arterial rupture	• vEDS		• Emergency surgery
Varicose veins	• MFS • LDS • EDS (most types)		• Compression sleeve if varicosities are superficial • Vein stripping of superficial varicosities • Anticoagulation if deep veins involved and clots formed
Anemia	• EDS (many types)	• CBC	• Iron, B12, and/or folate supplementation • Red cell transfusion

continued

ANNEX TABLE 5-5
Continued

Manifestations	HDCTs (Selected)	Common Diagnostic Techniques	Potential Treatments
Excessive bleeding associated with minor trauma, dental procedures, surgical interventions, menstruation, postpartum bleeding, etc.	• EDS (many types) • MFS (very rare)	• ISTH Bleeding Assessment Tool • CBC • Platelet function and coagulation tests • Factor VIII activity, vWF antigen, and activity assays	• Iron, B12, and/or folate supplementation • Red cell or platelet transfusion • Tranexamic acid

NOTE: CBC = complete blood count; CCA = congenital contractural arachnodactyly; CT = computed tomography; EDS = Ehlers-Danlos syndromes; HDCT = heritable disorder of connective tissue; ISTH = International Society on Thrombosis and Haemostasis; LDS = Loeys-Dietz syndrome; MFS = Marfan syndrome; SGS = Shprintzen Goldberg syndrome; vWF = von Willebrand Factor.

SOURCES: Beighton, 1969; Castori et al., 2012; D'Hondt et al., 2018; Drera et al., 2011; Gilliam et al., 2020; Jesudas et al., 2019; Kornhuber et al., 2019; Lind and Wallenburg, 2002; Makatsariya et al., 2020; Murray et al., 2014.

ANNEX TABLE 5-6
Selected Respiratory Manifestations Associated with Heritable Disorders of Connective Tissue

Manifestations		HDCTs (Selected)	Common Diagnostic Techniques	Potential Treatments

Inflammatory	Asthma	• EDS
		• Classical EDS (cEDS)
		• Hypermobile EDS (hEDS)/HSD
		• Kyphoscoliotic EDS (kEDS)
		• MFS
		• LDS
			Objective confirmation of diagnosis
			• Spirometry with flow-volume loops
			• Bronchodilator response with spirometry using flow-volume loops
			• Challenge testing (methacholine, cold air, exercise)
			• Exhaled nitric oxide
			Assessment of control
			• Spirometry
			• Patient Reported Outcome Measures
			Asthma phenotype screening
			• Eosinophilia
			• Atopic disease/allergy testing
			• Primary immunodeficiency disease (PIDD) Screen
			• Immunodeficiency evaluation
			Environmental screening
			• Tobacco product use/exposure
			• Uncontrolled moisture
			• Environmental allergens
			Exclusionary testing
			• Chest X-ray
			• Chest CT scan (if severe-persistent to bronchiectasis)
			• Rhinolaryngoscopy (if cough or extrathoracic airflow obstruction on flow-volume loops)
			• Evaluation for laryngopharyngeal reflux
				• Inhaled medications (corticosteroids, anticholinergic, beta-agonists) (Note: adverse effects of beta-agonists in MFS are possible; use caution)
				• Environmental restrictions
				• Treatment of comorbid disorders:
				  ○ Mast cell dysfunction (Annex Table 5-7, immunologic table)
				  ○ Atopy (see immunologic table)
				  ○ Eosinophilia (see immunologic table)
				  ○ Immunodeficiency (see immunologic table)
				  ○ GERD, LPR, (Annex Table 5-8, GI table)
				  ○ Rhinitis
				  ○ Sleep disorder
				  ○ Obesity
				  ○ Tobacco use disorder
				• Respiratory rehabilitation for moderate-severe asthma
				• Breathing arts, such as yoga, tai chi, Pilates

continued

ANNEX TABLE 5-6 Continued

Manifestations	HDCTs (Selected)	Common Diagnostic Techniques	Potential Treatments
Chronic or recurrent sinusitis	• EDS (subtypes unspecified) • MFS	• CT of sinuses—evaluation for structural abnormalities, chronic mucosal disease • Rhinoscopy • Complete blood count (CBC) and differential If chronic sinusitis: • Immune dysfunction evaluation (allergy testing, immunodeficiency evaluation) • Evaluation for cystic fibrosis and ciliary dykinesias	• Treatment of the underlying process (e.g., vaccination, immunoglobulin replacement, allergen immunotherapy, topical therapies [corticosteroids, biologics], sinus surgery) • Breathing arts, such as yoga, tai chi, qigong • See immunologic table
Recurrent bronchitis or pneumonia	• EDS (subtypes unspecified)	• CT sinuses • Rhinoscopy • CT chest (obstructing lesion—foreign body, neoplasm), bronchiectasis • Evaluation for GERD/aspiration • Immune dysfunction evaluation (allergy testing, immunodeficiency evaluation)	• Treatment of predisposing condition (aspiration, immunodeficiency, obstruction) • See Annex Table 5-7 (immunologic table)
Bronchiectasis	• EDS (subtypes unspecified) • MFS • Cutis laxa	• CT of chest • Culture for acid-fast and other bacteria, and fungi • Immunoglobin E test • CBC and differential • Evaluation for cystic fibrosis • Alpha-1-antitrypsin • Immunodeficiency evaluation • Evaluation for GERD/aspiration	• Mucous mobilization measures • Treat predisposing condition

	Condition	Subtype	Diagnostic	Management
	Costochondritis	• hEDS/HSD • EDS (other subtypes)	• Physical examination • Rib X-rays	• Physical therapy (see Annex Table 5-3, musculoskeletal table) • Self-administered interventions (see musculoskeletal table) • Medications (oral, topical, injectable) • Orthoses, compression clothing, etc. • Environmental modifications • Occupational therapy (see musculoskeletal table)
Functional	Obstructive sleep apnea	• Arthrochalasia EDS (aEDS) • cEDS • hEDS/HSD • Vascular EDS (vEDS) • MFS	• Polysomnography	• Nocturnal continuous positive airway pressure (CPAP) • Myofunctional therapy (may be provided by speech therapy)
	Central sleep apnea	• MFS	• Polysomnography	• Nocturnal bilevel positive airway pressure (BiPAP)
	Tracheomalacia	• vEDS	• Spirometry • Chest CT scan with inspiratory and expiratory maneuvers • Bronchoscopy	• CPAP/BiPAP • Surgical repair
	Reduced inspiratory muscle strength	• hEDS	• Negative inspiratory force • 6-minute walk distance (6MWD)	• Inspiratory muscle training • Breathing arts: yoga, tai chi, qigong
	Obstructive physiology	• MFS	• Spirometry, plethysmographic lung volumes, diffusion capacity • 6MWD	• Observation • Inhaler therapy
	Thoracic Insufficiency Syndrome	• MFS	• Spirometry • Arterial blood gases	• Aggressive conservative and/or surgical intervention

ANNEX TABLE 5-6 Continued

Manifestations		HDCTs (Selected)	Common Diagnostic Techniques	Potential Treatments
Structural, lung	Spontaneous pneumothorax	- vEDS - cEDS - Classical-like (clEDS) - MFS - LDS - Cutis Laxa - BHDS	- Chest X-ray - Chest CT scan	- Oxygen - Tube thoracostomy - Pleurodesis - Pleurectomy - Avoidance of extremes of barometric pressure, contact sports, high intensity exercise
	Pulmonary cysts, blebs, and/or bullae	- vEDS - MFS	- Chest CT scan	- Observation, bullectomy (rarely)
	Hemopneumothorax, lung hemorrhage	- vEDS	- Chest CT scan	- Tube thoracostomy - Surgical repair - Bronchial artery embolization
	Early onset emphysema	- MFS - Cutis laxa	- Spirometry and plethysmographic lung volumes - Diffusion capacity - 6MWD - Chest CT scan - Alpha-1-antitrypsin level	- Inhaled medications (corticosteroids, anticholinergic, beta agonists) - Intravenous replacement therapy (e.g., alpha-proteinase inhibitor) - Environmental restrictions - Treatment of comorbid disorders (e.g., GERD, LPR, rhinitis, sleep disorder, obesity) - Pulmonary rehabilitation
	Fibrous nodules	- vEDS	- Chest CT scan	- Monitoring to assure stability

Structural, musculoskeletal	Diaphragm rupture	• EDS (subtypes unspecified)	• Chest CT scan	• Surgical correction
	Cervical spine instability	• vEDS • EDS (other subtypes)	• Physical Exam • Spirometry • Negative inspiratory force	• See Annex Tables 5-3 and 5-4 (musculoskeletal and neurological tables)
	Kyphosis or scoliosis	• kEDS • MFS	• Spine films • Chest CT scan • Spirometry and plethysmographic lung volumes to assess degree of restriction • If advanced, arterial blood gas	• Observation • Physical therapy • Surgical correction
	Pectus excavatum or carinatum	• cEDS • hEDS • vEDS • EDS (other subtypes) • MFS	• Spirometry, plethysmographic lung volumes to assess for restrictive physiology • Comparison of seated and supine forced vital capacity • Negative inspiratory force (to evaluate diaphragmatic weakness) • 6MWD • Pulse oximetry • Arterial blood gas	• Observation • Surgical correction • Noninvasive ventilation • Mechanical ventilation
	Rib subluxation	• HSD • EDS (subtypes unspecified)	• Physical exam (imaging often cannot pick up subtle malalignments)	• Physical therapy (see Annex Table 5-3, musculoskeletal table) • Self-administered interventions (see musculoskeletal table)

continued

ANNEX TABLE 5-6 Continued

Manifestations	HDCTs (Selected)	Common Diagnostic Techniques	Potential Treatments
Procedural or postprocedural complications	Increased rates of respiratory failure post-vascular surgery	MFS	• Continuous pulse oximetry	• Noninvasive ventilation (e.g., BiPAP) • Mechanical ventilation
	Hemorrhage	EDS (subtypes unspecified)	• Radiographic imaging	• Emergency control of bleeding (surgical and nonsurgical management)

NOTE: BHDS = Birt-Hogg-Dubé syndrome; CT = computed tomography; EDS = Ehlers-Danlos syndrome; GERD = gastroesophageal reflux disease; GI = gastrointestinal; HDCT = heritable disorder of connective tissue; HSD = hypermobility spectrum disorder; LDS = Loeys-Dietz syndrome; LPR = laryngopharyngeal reflux; MFS = Marfan syndrome.

SOURCES: Abishek et al., 2019; American Thoracic Society and European Respiratory Society, 2002; Bascom et al., 2021; Bezerra et al., 2014; Birchall et al., 2021; Boone et al., 2019; Camacho et al., 2015; Chohan et al., 2021; Cloutier et al., 2020; Culver et al., 2017; Global Initiative for Asthma, 2021; Graham et al., 2019; Hakim et al., 2021; Halvorsen et al., 2017; Henderson et al., 2017; Henneberger et al., 2011; Holguin et al., 2020; Holland et al., 2014, 2021; Jayarajan et al., 2020; Khatri et al., 2021; Mott et al., 2021; Oliveira et al., 2018b; Qiu et al., 2021; Reychler et al., 2019; Rosen et al., 2018; Rueda et al., 2020; Schoser et al., 2017; Shusterman et al., 2017; Stachler et al., 2018; Tun et al., 2021.

ANNEX TABLE 5-7
Selected Immunologic Manifestations Associated with Heritable Disorders of Connective Tissue

Manifestations	HDCTs (Selected)	Common Diagnostic Techniques	Potential Treatments
Mast cell activation disease (MCAD)—single organ	<ul><li>Hypermobile EDS (hEDS)/HSD</li><li>EDS (unspecified subtypes)</li></ul>Skin<ul><li>Atopic dermatitis</li><li>Urticaria</li><li>Angioedema</li></ul>Airway<ul><li>Rhinitis</li><li>Asthma</li></ul>Gastrointestinal disorders<ul><li>Hypersensitivity/gastroenteritis</li><li>Eosinophilic esophagitis/gastroenteritis</li></ul>Neuropsychiatric<ul><li>Neurocognitive disorders</li><li>Some headache disorders</li><li>Mood disorders in the context of general medical condition</li></ul>	<ul><li>Allergen specific IgE testing</li><li>Complete blood count (CBC) with differential</li><li>Serum IgE total</li><li>Target organ biopsy</li><li>End organ challenge</li><li>Tryptase</li><li>Urine methylhistamine, prostaglandin metabolites</li></ul><ul><li>Allergen-specific IgE testing</li><li>Esophagogastroduodenoscopy (EGD)/colonoscopy</li><li>Tryptase levels</li><li>Urine methylhistamine, prostaglandin metabolites</li><li>Empirical trial of 6- or 8-food elimination diet</li><li>Fecal leukocyte stain</li><li>Calprotectin</li></ul><ul><li>Allergen specific IgE testing</li><li>CBC with differential</li><li>Serum IgE total</li><li>Tryptase</li><li>Urine methylhistamine, prostaglandin metabolites</li><li>Imaging (head, spinal cord)</li></ul>	<ul><li>Avoidance measures for suspected foods, medications, airborne allergens)</li><li>Oral medications: antihistamines, leukotriene antagonists, mast cell stabilizers</li><li>For asthmatics: bronchodilators</li><li>Topical medications</li><li>Biologics therapy</li><li>Immunotherapy</li><li>Anaphylaxis: epinephrine</li></ul><ul><li>Allergen avoidance (foods, medications)</li><li>Oral medications: antihistamines, leukotriene antagonists), mast cell stabilizers</li><li>Biologics therapies</li><li>Acute episodes: epinephrine</li></ul>

continued

ANNEX TABLE 5-7 Continued

Manifestations	HDCTs (Selected)	Common Diagnostic Techniques	Potential Treatments
Mast cell activation disease (MCAD)—single organ	Genitourinary • Interstitial cystitis		• Tryptase • Urine methylhistamine, prostaglandin metabolites • Digital and manometric pelvic floor muscle examination • Cystoscopy	• Oral medications (antihistamines) • Intravesical therapies
MCAD—multiorgan disease Mast cell activation syndrome (MCAS)	• Systemic mastocytosis • Monoclonal mast cell activation syndrome • Hereditary alpha tryptasemia • Anaphylaxis	• hEDS/HSD • EDS (unspecified subtypes)	• Tryptase • Allergen specific IgE testing • Urine methylhistamine prostaglandin metabolites • Positive KIT D816V mutation • Atypical mast cells in bone marrow or another extracutaneous biopsy • Cervical spine instability	• Oral medications: antihistamines, leukotriene antagonists, mast cell stabilizers • Biologics (omalizumab, dupilumab) • anti-IgE therapy • Allergen avoidance (medications such as opioids and, certain antibiotics and analgesic agents) • Immunotherapy • Anaphylaxis: epinephrine • Advanced clonal mast cell activation disease: tyrosine kinase inhibitors • Bone disease: osteopenia, bone fractures—bisphosphonates, Interferon alfa-2a

Delayed-type hypersensitivity (DTH) Eosinophilic/T2 inflammation	• Skin (atopic or contact dermatitis) • Eosinophilic lung disease • Eosinophilic gastrointestinal disease (eosinophilic esophagitis, gastroenteritis)	• hEDS/HSD • EDS (unspecified subtypes)	• CBC with differential • Elevated blood eosinophil count • Eosinophilic cationic protein • Organ specific assessment (e.g., biopsy, urine eosinophils, sputum eosinophils)	• Oral medications: immunosuppressants • Biologics therapy • Allergen avoidance • Immunotherapy • Anaphylaxis: epinephrine
Primary immunodeficiency (PID)/dysfunction	• Severe combined immunodeficiency (SCID) • Antibody deficiencies • Complement deficiencies, mannose binding lectin • Neutropenia • Lymphocytopenia • IPEX syndrome • Chronic granulomatous disease • Omenn syndrome • Connective tissue (filaggrin deficiency)	• hEDS/HSD • EDS (unspecified subtypes) • Peridontal EDS	• CBC with differential • Serum, IgG, IgA, IgM • IgG subclasses • Lymphocyte subset analysis • Pathogen protection (pneumococcal haemophilus influenza, measles, mumps, rubella, varicella) • Complement levels • Genetic testing	• Prophylactic antibiotics • Immunizations • Supplemental immunoglobulin • Monitor for concurrent autoimmune/malignant disorders • Curative treatment (HSCT and gene therapy)

continued

ANNEX TABLE 5-7
Continued

Manifestations		HDCTs (Selected)	Common Diagnostic Techniques	Potential Treatments
Autoinflammatory disorders	- 3 cryopyrin-associated periodic syndromes - Schnitzler syndrome - Familial cold autoinflammatory syndrome - Periodic fever syndromes - Vascultides - X-linked lymphoproliferative disease - 27 and IL-2-inducible T cell kinase deficiency - Nijmegen breakage syndrome - Defects in nucleic acid disposal - Immuno-osteodysplasias - SAMHD1 deficiency - Aicardi-Goutières syndrome	- hEDS/HSD - EDS (other types, unspecified)	- CBC - Blood biochemistries - Sedimentation rate - Hepatitis studies - Urinalysis - Complement studies - Autoantibody testing (antinuclear antibody [ANA], anti-double-stranded DNA, anti-Ro, anti-L, anti-Smith, ribonuclear protein antibody, antineutrophil cytoplasmic antibody [ANCA], rheumatoid factor) - Chest X-ray - Pulmonary function studies - Screening for cardiac involvement	- Oral immunosuppressants - Biologics therapies

		hEDS /HSD EDS (unspecified subtypes)		
DTH: Gastrointestinal disorders	Hypersensitivity gastroenteritis (see above)			
	Eosinophilic esophagitis/ gastroenteritis		• Esophagogastroduodenoscopy (EGD) • Colonoscopy • IgE—Foods, aeroallergens (immunoCAP, percutaneous allergen testing) • 6- or 8-food elimination diet • Fecal leukocyte stain • Calprotectin	• Dietary elimination of suspected culprit foods • Oral medications (corticosteroids, proton pump inhibitors • Biologics (anti-IgE)
	Inflammatory bowel disease (ulcerative colitis, Crohn's disease)		• Biopsy on colonoscopy • Fecal calprotectin	• Dietary elimination • Oral medications • Biologics therapies
	Celiac disease		• Blood test • Endoscopy	• Complete elimination of gluten from the diet

continued

ANNEX TABLE 5-7 Continued

Manifestations	HDCTs (Selected)	Common Diagnostic Techniques	Potential Treatments
DTH: Endocrinopathies	Addison's disease • hEDS/HSD • EDS (unspecified subtypes)	• ACTH, morning cortisol • Advanced imaging	• Mineral corticoid replacement and emergency protocol of intravenous fluid replacement and rescue of 100 mg hydrocortisone
	Thyroiditis (Hashimoto's disease)	• Serum TSH, T3, T4 • Antithyroid	• If euthyroid, monitor • Hypothyroidism: thyroid replacement therapy
	• Autoimmune progesterone anaphylaxis • Asthma • Urticaria • Dermatitis	• Percutaneous testing to progesterone • Liver function tests • Thyroid function tests • Urinalysis • RAST for foods and latex • ANA, rheumatoid factor, ESR • Complement studies • tryptase • 24-hour urine for histamine	• Desensitization using progesterone • Oral agents • Anaphylaxis treatment: epinephrine autoinjectors
DTH: Cutaneous disorders	Contact dermatitis • hEDS/HSD • EDS (unspecified subtypes)	• Patch testing • IgE- allergen testing • Primary immunodeficiency disorders (PIDD) screen • Immunodeficiency evaluation	• Contact allergen avoidance • Oral medications • Topical agents • Biologics therapy

Hereditary angioedema (swelling): skin, oropharynx	• hEDS/HSD • EDS (unspecified subtypes)	• Complement studies C1-INH, C4, CH50	Acute attacks: • Intravenous C1-esterase inhibitor replacement • Fresh frozen plasma Prophylaxis—long term: • Intravenous, subcutaneous C1-INH concentrate • Androgens • Tranexamic acid

continued

ANNEX TABLE 5-7 Continued

Manifestations		HDCTs (Selected)	Common Diagnostic Techniques	Potential Treatments
DTH: Neurological disorders	Autoimmune neuropathies/ encephalopathies	• hEDS/HSD • EDS (unspecified subtypes)	• Sinus questionnaire • Asthma screening questionnaire • Food allergy/intolerance questionnaire • Cervical-spine instability evaluation • Occult tethered cord evaluation • CSF leak • Urodynamics study	
	Chronic immune demyelinating neuropathy		• Autoantibody serologies anti-ribosomal anti-endothelial cell, anti-ganglioside, anti-dsDNA, anti-2A/2B subunits of N-methyl-D-aspartate receptors (NMDAR), and anti-phospholipid antibodies	
	Multiple sclerosis		• Clinical • Laboratory testing • Lumbar puncture: CSF analysis • Advanced imaging • Electrodiagnostic testing	

	Postural orthostatic tachycardia syndrome/ neuronal mediated hypotension	• Clinical • Laboratory testing • Lean test/tilt table (assess cervical spine)	• Medications • Physical therapy • Occupational therapy • Environmental modifications
	Small fiber neuropathy	• Clinical • Laboratory testing • Small fiber neuropathy symptom inventory questionnaire (SFN-SIQ) • Sural sensory nerve action potential (SNAP) amplitude and conduction velocity • Skin biopsy	• Medications • Physical therapy • Occupational therapy • Environmental modifications
DTH: Musculoskeletal and rheumatological disorders	• hEDS/HSD • EDS (unspecified subtypes) Arthritides • Rheumatoid arthritis • Sjogren's syndrome • Mixed connective tissue disease • Dermatomyositis/ polymyositis • Scleroderma	• X-rays of affected joints • Blood testing: CBC with differential, complete metabolic panel, autoantibodies, complement studies ESR, CRP • Atopic and PIDD evaluations • Infection (Epstein-Barr virus, ASO+Dnase, viral hepatitis)	• Oral medications • Diet restriction • Biologics

continued

ANNEX TABLE 5-7
Continued

NOTE: ACTH = adrenocorticotropic hormone; CRP = C-reactive protein; CSF = cerebrospinal fluid; EDS = Ehlers-Danlos syndromes; ESR = erythrocyte sedimentation rate; HDCT = heritable disorder of connective tissue; HSCT = hematopoietic stem cell transplantation; HSD = hypermobility spectrum disorder; IPEX = immune dysregulation, polyendocrinopathy, enteropathy, X-linked; RAST = radioallergosorbent test.

SOURCES: Abonia et al., 2013; Arkwright and Gennery, 2011; Cazzato et al., 2016; Cheung and Vadas, 2015; Dang et al., 2019; Hamilton, 2018; Hamilton et al., 2021; Khan, 2013; Leganger et al., 2022; Louisias et al., 2013; Luskin et al., 2021; Lyons et al., 2016; Morgan et al., 2007; Shin et al., 2010; Theoharides et al., 2015; Whitmore and Theoharides, 2011.

ANNEX TABLE 5-8
Selected Gastrointestinal Manifestations Associated with Heritable Disorders of Connective Tissue

Manifestations	HDCTs (Selected)	Common Diagnostic Techniques	Potential Treatments
Gastrointestinal (GI) bleeding	• EDS (unspecified subtypes) • Vascular EDS (vEDS) • LDS	• Upper- and lower-GI endoscopy • Advanced imaging • Stool test	• Medication management • Surgical intervention
Visceroptosis	• EDS (unspecified subtypes)	• Advanced imaging	• Surgical intervention
Intussusception/volvulus	• EDS (unspecified subtypes)	• Ultrasound (children) • Computed tomography (CT) scan (adults)	• Surgical intervention
Diverticulitis	• EDS (multiple subtypes) • vEDS • MFS	• Advanced imaging • Colonoscopy	• Medical management
Organ rupture (e.g., bowel, liver, spleen)	• vEDS	• Advanced imaging	• Surgical intervention
Median arcuate ligament syndrome	• EDS (unspecified subtypes)	• Duplex ultrasonography • Advanced imaging • Endoscopy	• Surgical intervention

continued

ANNEX TABLE 5-8 Continued

Manifestations	HDCTs (Selected)	Common Diagnostic Techniques	Potential Treatments
Superior mesenteric artery syndrome	• EDS (unspecified subtypes) • LDS	• Duplex ultrasonography • Advanced imaging	• Surgical intervention
Eventration of the diaphragm	• EDS (unspecified subtypes)	• Diagnostic imaging • Pulmonary function testing	• Physical therapy • Respiratory rehabilitation • Surgical intervention
Immune-mediated GI disorders	• HDS • EDS (unspecified subtypes) • MFS	• Clinical • Testing based on presentation	• Nutritional consultation • Medication management • Physical therapy • Surgical intervention
Gastroparesis	• EDS (unspecified subtypes) • LDS	• Barium swallow X-ray • Barium egg swallow • Radioisotope gastric emptying scan • Gastric manometry • Wireless motility capsule • Autonomic nervous system testing • Autoimmune testing	• Nutritional consultation • Medication management • Physical therapy

Inflammatory bowel diseases: • Crohn's disease • Ulcerative colitis • Microscopic colitis • Other mucosal inflammatory disorders	• EDS (unspecified subtypes) • LDS	• Biopsy by endoscopy • Fecal calprotectin • Stool samples • CBC • Food allergy testing	• Nutritional consultation • Medication management • Physical therapy • Surgical intervention
Celiac disease	• EDS (unspecified subtypes)	• Blood test • Endoscopy • Stool samples • Food allergy testing	• Nutritional consultation • Medication management
Eosinophilic gastrointestinal disease	• EDS (unspecified subtypes) • LDS	• Biopsy • Stool samples • CBC • Food allergy testing	• Nutritional consultation • Medication management • Endoscopic procedures

NOTE: CBC = complete blood count; EDS = Ehlers-Danlos syndrome; HDCT = heritable disorder of connective tissue; LDS = Loeys-Dietz syndrome; MFS = Marfan syndrome.

SOURCES: Brooks et al., 2021; Castori et al., 2015b; de Leeuw et al., 2012; Dordoni et al., 2013; Fikree et al., 2017; Frank et al., 2019; Guerrerio et al., 2016; Hassan et al., 2002; Huynh et al., 2019; Inayet et al., 2018; Iwama et al., 1989; Kahn et al., 1988; Kucera and Sullivan, 2017; Laszkowska et al., 2016; Leganger et al., 2016; Lybil and Genie, 2019; MacCarrick et al., 2014; Malyuk et al., 2022; Nelson et al., 2015a; Reinstein et al., 2012; Suster et al., 1984; Yasuda et al., 2013.

ANNEX TABLE 5-9
Selected Cutaneous Manifestations Associated with Heritable Disorders of Connective Tissue

Manifestations		HDCTs (Selected)	Common Diagnostic Techniques	Potential Treatments
Structural	Poor wound healing; failure of surgical wound closure	• Classical EDS (cEDS) • Hypermobile EDS (hEDS) • Kyphoscoliotic EDS (kEDS) • BCS • Musculocontractural (mcEDS) • LDS	• Full skin examination—assess for hyperextensibility of the skin, wound healing defects, atrophic or abnormal scarring • Beighton scoring scale—assess for hypermobility of a joint, in which a score of 5 or more indicates generalized joint hypermobility • Molecular genetic testing • Skin biopsy	• Perform skin closure in two layers (cutaneous and subcutaneous) without excessive tension • Use generous sutures, deep stitches, and Steri-Strips as reinforcement devices • Leave sutures twice as long as normally recommended
	Capillary fragility; ecchymoses	• vEDS • cEDS • hEDS • kEDS • BCS • mcEDS • LDS	• Clinical	• Vitamin C • Protective devices • Environmental modification

Inflammatory	Inflammatory dermatoses Atopic dermatitis	• cEDS • hEDS • BCS • LDS	• Environmental and food allergen-specific IgE testing • Eosinophilic cationic protein • Skin biopsy	• Environmental modification • Topical or systemic immunosuppressants • Barrier emollients • Biologics—Dupilumab
	Urticaria/ angioedema	• hEDS/HSD • cEDS • LDS	• Allergen-specific IgE testing • Serum tryptase, urine histamine • CBC with differential • Serum immunoglobulins • ANA, ESR • CH50, C3+C4, C1-inhibitor • Chronic urticaria panel anti-IgE or anti-FcReI IgG	• Conservative management • Environmental modification • Medications (oral and topical) • Biologics

continued

ANNEX TABLE 5-9 Continued

Manifestations		HDCTs (Selected)	Common Diagnostic Techniques	Potential Treatments
Neuropathic	Complex regional pain syndrome Reflex sympathetic dystrophy syndrome	• hEDS/HSD • cEDS	• Clinical	• Medications • Physical therapy • Occupational therapy • Environmental modifications
	Erythromelalgia • Gerhardt disease • Mitchell disease • Weir-Mitchell disease	• hEDS/HSD • cEDS	• Photographs of the affected areas during symptoms are helpful (e.g., photos of red feet or hands during symptoms—the redness is almost unique to erythromelalgia when associated with the history) • Exercise or immersion of an affected region in hot water for a certain period (e.g., approximately 10–30 minutes) to provoke a flare so a diagnosis may be made	• Topical lidocaine, capsaicin, diclofenac gel 1%, brimonidine, and compounded gabapentin ointment 6% • Oral therapies include aspirin, gabapentin, amitriptyline, cyroheptadine, pregabalin, diltiazem, and venlafaxine • Misoprostol • Systemic glucocorticoids, intravenous gamma globulin
	Diaphoresis or hyperhidrosis	• hEDS/HSD • cEDS	• Clinical • Sweat test • Diagnosis of underlying condition	• Management of underlying condition • Medications (oral, topical, injectable) • Environmental modifications • Surgical intervention

NOTE: ANA = antinuclear antibody; BCS = brittle cornea syndrome; EDS = Ehlers-Danlos syndrome; ESR = erythrocyte sedimentation rate; HDCT = heritable disorder of connective tissue; HSD = hypermobility spectrum disorder; LDS = Loeys-Dietz syndrome; MFS=Marfan syndrome.

SOURCES: American Academy of Dermatology Association, 2022; Bechara et al., 2007; Castori, 2012; Catala-Pétavy et al., 2009; Kalava et al., 2013; Malfait et al., 2017; Oaklander and Klein, 2013; Tang et al., 2015.

ANNEX TABLE 5-10
Selected Genitourinary Manifestations Associated with Heritable Disorders of Connective Tissue

Manifestations		HDCTs (Selected)	Common Diagnostic Techniques	Potential Treatments
Pelvic floor disorders	Stress urinary incontinence Urge urinary incontinence Urinary retention and voiding dysfunction	• MFS • Hypermobile EDS (hEDS)/HSD • EDS (other subtypes)	• Medical history and physical exam that may include pelvic and rectal exam • Urine analysis • Urinary stress tests • Urodynamic tests, including video urodynamics • Cystoscopy	• Dependent on type of urinary incontinence • Behavioral training • Pelvic floor physical therapy (PFPT) • Medications (i.e., anticholinergics, mirabegron, alpha blockers, topical estrogen) • Electrical stimulation • Medical devices (i.e., pessary) • Interventional therapies (i.e., Botox) • Surgical intervention
	Urinary problems secondary to vascular and neurologic complications		• Same as above but may also include X-rays and advanced imaging (e.g., MRI, CT)	• As above but also includes catheterization, surgeries that include urinary diversion, bladder resection, and sphincter resection
	Pelvic organ prolapse (bowel, uterus, bladder)	• MFS • LDS • hEDS/HSD • EDS (other subtypes)	• Medical history and physical examination • Dynamic MRI • Perineal ultrasound	• PFPT • Surgical intervention

Vulvodynia and dyspareunia	• hEDS/HSD • Classical EDS (cEDS) • Vascular EDS (vEDS)	• Medical history and physical exam that includes the cotton swab test	• PFPT • Psychological interventions • Medications (antinociceptive agents, anti-inflammatory agents, neuromodulating medications, hormonal agents, and muscle relaxants) • Vestibulectomy
Chronic pelvic pain	• hEDS/HSD • vEDS • cEDS	• Pelvic exam • Ultrasonography • Advanced imaging • Laparoscopy	• Topical medications • PFPT • Psychological interventions • Oral medications
Uterine disorders — Menorrhagia	• vEDS • cEDS • hEDS/HSD	• Detailed history and physical examination • Laboratory investigations • Ultrasonography with instillation of saline solution • Hysteroscopy and biopsy • Advanced imaging	• Medical management (including hormonal management as tolerated) • Surgical management
Dysmenorrhea		• Detailed medical, psychosocial, and gynecologic history • Physical examination (age dependent) • Ultrasonography	• Medications (nonsteroidal anti-inflammatories, hormonal treatments as tolerated based on diagnosis)

continued

ANNEX TABLE 5-10
Continued

Manifestations		HDCTs (Selected)	Common Diagnostic Techniques	Potential Treatments
Renal abnormalities	Cysts	MFS vEDS	Ultrasonography Advanced imaging	Management is based on symptomology Renal cyst aspiration (usually with sclerotherapy) Laparoscopic decortication
	Focal glomerulosclerosis	MFS	Laboratory evaluation Renal biopsy	Medical management
	Interstitial cystitis	hEDS/HSD	Urine analysis Cystoscopy Immune dysfunction (immune deficiency—complement, mannose binding lectin)	Diet restrictions Oral agents (histamine blockade, tricyclic agents, prophylactic antibiotics) Intravesical treatments (dimethyl sulfoxide, Botox, bicarbonate-lidocaine-heparin-hydrocortisone)
Pregnancy-related diagnoses	Preterm delivery/premature rupture of membranes	hEDS EDS (other subtypes)	Pelvic exam Transvaginal ultrasound for cervical length Uterine monitoring Fetal fibronectin	Progesterone prophylaxis (consider) Short-term treatment for fetal lung maturity and neurologic protection (steroids, magnesium sulfate, antibiotics)
	Cervical insufficiency	EDS (unspecified subtypes)	Pelvic exam Transvaginal ultrasonography	Cerclage Progesterone prophylaxis (consider)
	Aortic root dissection	MFS LDS vEDS Arthrochalasia EDS	Medical and physical examination Echocardiogram	Surgical management

Uterine rupture	• vEDS • EDS (other subtypes) • LDS	• Physical examination • Imaging if appropriate	• Surgical management
Obstetrical hemorrhage	• MFS • LDS • vEDS • cEDS • Classical-like EDS	• Physical and laboratory examinations	• Medical and surgical management

NOTE: CT = computed tomography; EDS = Ehlers-Danlos syndrome; HDCT = heritable disorder of connective tissue; HSD = hypermobility spectrum disorder; LDS = Loeys-Dietz syndrome; MFS = Marfan syndrome.

SOURCES: Bas et al., 2015; Berglund and Björck, 2012; Blagowidow, 2021; Carley and Schaffer, 2000; Carr et al., 1994; Castori et al., 2012; Cauldwell et al., 2019a,b; Chan et al., 2019; Chow et al., 2007; De Martino et al., 2019; De Toma et al., 2000; Demirdas et al., 2017; Donnez, 2011; Drera et al., 2011; Gilliam et al., 2020; Glayzer et al., 2021; Gupta et al., 2010; Henderson et al., 2017; Hentzen et al., 2018; Hernandez and Dietrich, 2020; Hugon-Rodin et al., 2016; Hurst et al., 2014; Jabs and Child, 2016; Jesudas et al., 2019; Kho and Shields, 2020; Kliethermes et al., 2016; Lind and Wallenburg, 2002; Makatsariya et al., 2020; Practice bulletin no. 176: Pelvic organ prolapse, 2017; Ritelli et al., 2013; Rosen et al., 2019; Russo et al., 2018; Sorokin et al., 1994; van de Laar et al., 2011; van de Laar et al., 2012; Wallace et al., 2019.

ANNEX TABLE 5-11
Selected Vision, Hearing, and Speech Manifestations Associated with Heritable Disorders of Connective Tissue

Manifestations	HDCTs (Selected)	Common Diagnostic Techniques	Potential Treatments
Vision			
Disorders of cornea	Thinning and steepening		
	• Classical EDS (cEDS) • Hypermobile EDS (hEDS) • Kyphoscoliotic EDS (kEDS) • BCS • Musculocontractural (mcEDS) • LDS	• Pachymetry • Cornea topography	• Refractive prosthesis (e.g., contact lens, spectacle)
	Microcornea Sclerocornea Cornea plana Prone to rupture Acute hydrops		
	• kEDS	• Slit lamp exam	• Refractive correction • Low-vision rehabilitation • Hyperosmotic agents • Patch graft for impending rupture
	Microcornea		
	• mcEDS	• Slit lamp exam	• Refractive correction • Low-vision rehabilitation
	Megalocornea Keratoconus Keratoglobus Prone to rupture		
	• BCS	• Slit lamp exam • Pachymetry • Corneal topography	• Lubrication • Amniotic graft • Cornea crosslinking • Corneal graft (partial or full thickness) • Conjunctival flap

Disorders of conjunctiva	• Dry eye	• cEDS • hEDS	• Schirmer's test • Tear osmolarity • Slit lamp exam • Tear break-up time	• Artificial lubrication • Punctal occlusion • Tear quality improvement medications
	• Conjunctivochalasis	• cEDS • hEDS • Classical-like EDS (clEDS)	• Slit lamp exam • Schirmer's test • Tear break-up time • Tear osmolarity	• Conjunctivoplasty • Artificial lubrication • Punctal occlusion • Tear quality improvement medications
	• Subconjunctival hemorrhage	• clEDS	• Slit lamp exam	• Wait for hemorrhage to clear
	• Blue sclera	• mcEDS • cEDS • hEDS • vEDS • kEDS • BCS	• Gross examination	• Counseling for psychological effects of unusual cosmesis • Scleral patch graft (if scleral ectasia)

continued

ANNEX TABLE 5-11
Continued

Manifestations		HDCTs (Selected)	Common Diagnostic Techniques	Potential Treatments
Disorders of lens/iris	• Cataract	• MFS	• Slit lamp exam	• Refraction/retinoscopy • Cataract extraction
	• Ectopia lentis/ dislocation	• MFS	• Slit lamp exam • Ultrasound biomicroscopy	• Refraction • Lensectomy
	• Iris coloboma	• mcEDS	• Slit lamp exam • Anterior segment UBM or OCT	• Glare reduction by spectacles, specialty contact lenses, window tint, screen guards • Iris prosthesis • Iridoplasty
	• Iris transillumination	• MFS	• Slit lamp exam	• Glare reduction by spectacles, specialty contact lenses, window tint, screen guards

Disorders of eyelid/face/orbit	• Floppy eyelid	• cEDS	• Manual exam of eyelid	• Nocturnal lubrication • Plastic surgery
	• Proptosis (from cavernous-carotid fistula)	• vEDS	• CTA/MRA and CTV/MRV • Hertel's exophthalmometry	• Endovascular embolization
	• Hypertelorism	• Arthrochalasia EDS (aEDS) • mcEDS • LDS • MFS	• Pupillary distance measurement	• Observation • Plastic surgery, when indicated for functional or aesthetic reasons

continued

ANNEX TABLE 5-11
Continued

Manifestations		HDCTs (Selected)	Common Diagnostic Techniques	Potential Treatments
Disorders of optic nerve/ brain	• Amblyopia	• MFS • LDS • EDS (unspecified subtypes)	• Refraction • Slit lamp exam • Possibly brain imaging	• Treatment of underlying cause • Occlusion of better-seeing eye by patching or pharmacological penalization
	• Glaucoma (including angle closure)	• Dermatosparaxis EDS (dEDS) • mEDS • BCS • Spondylodysplastic EDS (spEDS) • MFS	• Slit lamp exam • Tonometry • Pachymetry • OCT • Perimetry	• Topical medication • Oral medication (in acute setting) • Glaucoma surgery
	• Strabismus	• mcEDS • MFS • LDS	• Orthoptic examination	• Refractive correction • Prism glasses • Strabismus surgery
	• Optic atrophy • Hypoplastic optic nerve • Optic nerve coloboma	• mcEDS	• Slit lamp exam • Perimetry • Color vision testing • B-scan ultrasonography • OCT	• Treatment for reversible causes of atrophy • Observation
	• Convergence insufficiency	• EDS (unspecified subtype)	• Orthoptic examination	• Orthoptic exercises

• Papilledema (from Chiari) • Downbeat nystagmus (from Chiari)	• hEDS • LDS	• Dilated fundoscopic exam • B-scan ultrasonography • Fluorescein angiography • Perimetry • Optic nerve OTC • MRI	• ICP-lowering medication • Memantine for nystagmus • Surgical decompression of Chiari
• Visual field loss (from glaucoma or dissection from carotid, vertebral or basilar artery)	• dESD • mcEDS • BCS • spEDS • MFS	• Dilated fundoscopic exam • OCT • Perimetry • Bruit in eye/neck/face • Advanced imaging (e.g., MRI, CT) • MRA/CTA brain/neck	• IOP-lowering medication • IOP-lowering surgery • Low-vision rehabilitation • Surgical repair of dissection
• Horner syndrome (carotid dissection)	• vEDS	• Carotid sonogram • Angiography	• Surgical reconstruction

continued

ANNEX TABLE 5-11
Continued

Manifestations		HDCTs (Selected)	Common Diagnostic Techniques	Potential Treatments
Disorders of retina	Retinal detachment	• Cardiac-valvular EDS (cvEDS) • hEDS • dEDS • kEDS • BCS • mcEDS • MFS	• Refraction • Dilated fundoscopic exam • OCT • B-scan ultrasonography	• Laser retinopexy for retina tear • Surgical repair by scleral buckle or vitrectomy
	Fragile retina vessels	• kEDS • vEDS	• Dilated fundoscopic exam	• Precautionary measured
	High myopia	• hEDS • mcEDS • MFS	• Dilated fundoscopic exam • Refraction • OTC • Wide field imaging • Fluorescein angiography	• Refractive correction with glasses or contact lenses • Phakic or aphakic intraocular lenses
Hearing				
Disorders of hearing	Sensorineural hearing impairment	• EDS (unspecified subtype) • kEDS (FKBP14, FKBP22 subtypes) • mEDS • Stickler syndrome • MFS • LDS	• Advanced imaging • Clinical • Diagnostic pure tone audiometry • Speech audiometry • Bone conduction testing	• Medication • Environmental modification • Hearing aids • Personal sound amplification products • Auditory rehabilitation

	Conductive hearing impairment	EDS (unspecified subtype) MFS LDS	• Advanced imaging • Clinical • Diagnostic pure tone audiometry • Speech audiometry • Bone conduction testing	• Hearing aids • Medication • Surgical intervention • Environmental modification
	Mixed sensorineural and conductive hearing impairment	EDS (unspecified subtype) MFS LDS	• Advanced imaging • Clinical • Diagnostic pure tone audiometry • Speech audiometry • Bone conduction testing	• Medication • Environmental modification
	Tinnitus	EDS (unspecified subtype)	• Advanced imaging • Clinical • Audiological exam	• Treatment of underlying condition • Environmental modification • Physical therapy • Behavioral therapy
Speech				
Disorders of speech	Temporomandibular joint dysfunction Laryngeal dysfunction Vocal fatigue	EDS (unspecified subtype)	• Advanced imaging • Clinical	• Speech and language therapy • Physical therapy • Medications • Surgical intervention

NOTE: BCS = brittle cornea syndrome; CT= computed tomography; CTA = computed tomography angiography; EDS = Ehlers-Danlos syndrome; HDCT = heritable disorder of connective tissue; HSD = hypermobility spectrum disorder; IOP = intraocular pressure; ICP = intracranial pressure; LDS = Loeys-Dietz syndrome; MFS = Marfan syndrome; MRA = magnetic resonance angiography; MRI = magnetic resonance imaging; MRV = magnetic resonance venography; OCT = optical coherence tomography; UBM = ultrasound biomicroscopy.

SOURCES: ASHA, 2005; Braverman et al., 2020; Gao et al., 2021; Hamberis et al., 2020; Hear.com, n.d.; Islam et al., 2020; Jeon et al., 2022; Kanigowska et al., 2006; NASEM, 2016, p. 82; NORD, 2017a; Perez-Roustit et al., 2019; Rezar-Dreindl et al., 2019; Roeser et al., 2000; Romano et al., 2002; Segev et al., 2006; University of California San Fransico Health, n.d.

ANNEX TABLE 5-12
Selected Neuropsychiatric Conditions Potentially Connected with Heritable Disorders of Connective Tissue

Conditions	HDCTs (Selected)	Common Diagnostic Techniques	Potential Treatments
Cognitive dysfunction/mild cognitive impairment	• EDS (all types) • HSD • MFS	*Structured interviews:* • Structured clinical interview for DSM (SCID) • Mini international neuropsychiatric interview (MINI) *Performance-based measures:* • Number span forward (attention) and backward (working memory) • Trail Making Test parts A and B (processing speed and executive functioning, respectively) • Phonemic and category fluency (language) • Hopkins Verbal Learning Test-Revised (memory encoding, recall, and recognition)	• Management of associated disorders (e.g., neurologic, immunologic) • Lifestyle measures (e.g., exercise, diet, sleep, avoiding alcohol and drugs, enhance leisure activities)
Depression	• EDS (all types) • HSD • MFS	*Structured interviews:* • SCID • MINI *Self-reported measures:* • Hamilton Depression Rating Scale • Beck Depression Inventory • Hospital Anxiety and Depression Scale	• Medication management • Psychotherapy • Brain stimulation therapies

Anxiety disorders	• hEDS/HSD • MFS	*Structured interviews:* • SCID • MINI *Self-reported measures:* • Beck Anxiety Inventory • Hospital Anxiety and Depression Scale • Panic and Agoraphobia Scale (Bandelow, 1999)	• Psychotherapy • Medication management • Support groups • Stress management techniques • Occupational therapy • Physical therapy

continued

ANNEX TABLE 5-12 Continued

Conditions	HDCTs (Selected)	Common Diagnostic Techniques	Potential Treatments

Intellectual disability	• SGS	*Performance-based measures:*
		• Differential Abilities Scale-II (Elliott, 2007) (children and adolescents)
		• Kaufman Assessment Battery for Children, Second Edition Normative Update (Kaufman and Kaufman, 2018) (children and adolescents)
		• Leiter International Performance Scale, Third Edition (Roid et al., 2013)
		• Wechsler Adult Intelligence Scale, Fourth Edition (Wechsler, 2008)
		• Wechsler Abbreviated Scales of Intelligence, Second Edition (Wechsler, 2011)
		• Wechsler Intelligence Scale for Children, Fifth Edition (Wechsler, 2014)
		• Wechsler Preschool and Primary Scale of Intelligence, Fourth Edition (Wechsler, 2012)
		• Reynolds Intellectual Assessment Scales, Second Edition (Reynolds and Kamphaus, 2015)
		• Kaufman Brief Intelligence Test, Second Edition (Kaufman and Kaufman, 2004)
			• Occupational therapy
			  o Self-care (e.g., grooming, dressing, feeding, bathing)
			  o Employment activities and skills
			  o Leisure activities (e.g., knitting, playing games)
			  o Domestic activities (e.g., cooking, cleaning, laundry)
			• Speech therapy
			  o Improves communication skills
			  o Improves receptive and expressive languages skills
			  o Improves speech articulation
			  o Improves vocabulary
			• Physical therapy
			  o Enhances quality of life by maximizing mobility and self-locomotion
			  o Provides adaptive solutions to mobility problems
			  o Increases sensory integration
			• Adapted Dialectical Behavior Therapy
			• Pain Management
			• Family support

Personality disorder	• hEDS/HSD • MFS	*Self-reported measures:* • Borderline Personality Disorder Checklist • International Personality Disorder Examination • Personality Assessment Inventory	• Psychotherapy • Medication management • Support groups • Stress management techniques • Occupational therapy
Sleep disorders	• hEDS/HSD • MFS	• Sleep study *Structured interviews:* • SCID • MINI *Self-reported measures:* • Epworth Sleepiness Scale	• Psychotherapy • Medication management • Support groups • Insomnia management techniques • Occupational therapy • Physical therapy
Eating disorders	• hEDS/HSD • MFS	• Evaluation of gastrointestinal symptoms and disordered eating *Structured interviews:* • SCID • MINI *Self-reported measures:* • Eating Disorder Examination • Eating Attitudes Test (26)	• Nutritional • Psychotherapy • Medication management • Support groups • Stress management techniques • Occupational therapy
Attention-deficit/ hyperactivity disorder (ADHD)	• hEDS/HSD • MFS	*Structured interviews:* • SCID • MINI *Self-reported measures:* • Adult ADHD Self-Report Scale • Barrat Impulsiveness Scale	• Medication management • Psychotherapy and psychosocial interventions • Support groups • Stress management techniques • Occupational therapy • Physical therapy

continued

ANNEX TABLE 5-12
Continued

NOTE: ADL = activities of daily living; EDS = Ehlers-Danlos syndrome; HDCT = heritable disorder of connective tissue; hEDS = hypermobile EDS; HSD = hypermobility spectrum disorder; MFS = Marfan syndrome; SGS = Shprintzen-Goldberg syndrome.

SOURCES: Arnold et al., 2015; Baeza-Velasco et al., 2016, 2017, 2018, 2021, 2022a,b; Becker et al., 2021; Berglund et al., 2015; Bulbena-Cabré et al., 2021; Cederlöf et al., 2016; Cicerone et al., 2019; Doğan et al., 2011; Domany et al., 2018; Eccles et al., 2014; Greally, 2020; Hershenfeld et al., 2016; Hofman et al., 1988; Huang et al., 2020; Kandola and Stubbs, 2020; Kandola et al., 2018; Lambez et al., 2020; Langhinrichsen-Rohling et al., 2021; Lannoo et al., 1996; Moss et al., 2018; Nijs et al., 2018; NORD, 2017b; Oppizzi and Umberger, 2018; Pasquini et al., 2014; Reisberg et al., 1982; Ross et al., 2013; Shiari et al., 2013; Smith et al., 2013; Tsui et al., 2017; Wasim et al., 2019; Wells et al., 2020; Zhang and Yuan, 2019.

ANNEX TABLE 5-13
Global Functioning Associated with Heritable Disorders of Connective Tissue

Domain	Potential Reasons for Limitation or Symptom	Selected Assessments	Selected Assistive Technologies and Relevant Accommodations
Full-body functioning (physical)	• Pain (see annex tables 5-3, musculoskeletal; 5-4, neurological; 5-8, gastrointestinal; and 5-10, genitourinary) • Weakness • Fatigue/deconditioning • Joint instability (see Annex Table 5-3, musculoskeletal table) • Orthostatic intolerance/dysautonomia • Balance dysfunction • Cardiovascular and respiratory impairments (see annex tables 5-5 and 5-6, cardiovascular and respiratory) • Neurological compromise (see Annex Table 5-4, neurological table) • See Annex Table 5-14 (physical functioning) for additional reasons • Gastrointestinal dysfunction (see Annex Table 5-8, gastrointestinal table)	*Performance-based measures:* • Bruininks-Oseretsky Test of Motor Proficiency, 2nd Edition (BOT-2)* (Bruininks and Bruininks, 2005) (pediatric population) • Bruininks Motor Ability Test (BMAT)* (Bruininks and Bruininks, 2012) (adult version of BOT-2) • Functional capacity evaluation (Chen, 2007; Fore et al., 2015; Genovese and Galper, 2009; Jahn et al., 2004; Kuijer et al., 2012; Soer et al., 2008) • Exercise testing to include aerobic capacity and neuromuscular performance (Liguori and American College of Sports Medicine, 2021) *Self-reported measures:* • Composite Autonomic Symptom Score-31 (COMPASS-31) (Sletten et al., 2012)	• These will be determined by the specific activity that is limiting full-body functioning (see annex tables 5-14 and 5-15 for physical and vision, hearing, and speech functioning)

continued

ANNEX TABLE 5-13 Continued

Domain	Potential Reasons for Limitation or Symptom	Selected Assessments	Selected Assistive Technologies and Relevant Accommodations
Work-related functioning, activities of daily living (ADLs), and instrumental activities of daily living (IADLs)	• Pain • Fatigue/deconditioning • Weakness • Joint instability • Brain fog • Orthostatic intolerance/dysautonomia • Neurological compromise	*Performance-based measures:* • ADL Profile (head injury and stroke) (Dutil et al., 1990) • ADL-Focused Occupations-Based Neurobehavioral Evaluation (Gardarsdóttir and Kaplan, 2002) • Assessment of Motor and Processing Skills (Fisher and James, 2012; Shirley Ryan AbilityLab, 2019) • Bay Area Functional Performance Evaluation (Houston et al., 1989) • Executive Function Performance Test (Baum et al., 2008) • Functional Independence Measure (Ottenbacher et al., 1996) • Katz ADL Scale (elderly and chronically ill) (Katz, 1983; Katz and Akpom, 1976) • Kohlman Evaluation of Living Skills (IADLs—psychiatric geriatric) (Burnett et al., 2009; Kohlman-Thomson, 1992) *Observation and interview-based measures:* • Multiple Errands Test (brain injury, stroke—executive functioning) (Morrison et al., 2013) • Performance Assessment of Self-Care Skills (Chisholm et al., 2014)	• Orthoses (e.g., splints, braces) • Built-up handles for items used at home for ADLs (e.g., toothbrush, fork, and others) • Reachers to assist with reaching and manipulating objects and avoid bending • Reorganization of home to facilitate pain-free activities • Compression clothing • Assistive devices (e.g., walker, cane, wheelchair) • Devices with large numbers (e.g., telephone, medication box)

Self-reported measures:
- Work Disability Functional Assessment Battery (WD-FAB) Physical Function (Meterko et al., 2015; Meterko et al., 2019)
- Work Ability Index (Ilmarinen, 2007; Tuomi et al., 1998)
- Sheehan Disability Scale (Sheehan, 1983)
- Social and Occupational Functioning Assessment Scale (Rybarczyk, 2011)
- Mental Illness Research, Education, and Clinical Center (MIRECC) version of the Global Assessment of Functioning scale (Niv et al., 2007)
- Barthel Index (Quinn et al., 2011)
- Frenchay Activities Index (IADLs) (Schuling et al., 1993)
- The Lawton IADL Scale (Graf, 2008)
- Manual Ability Measure (neurological and musculoskeletal conditions) (Chen and Bode, 2010)

Caregiver-reported measures:
- Cleveland Scale of Activities of Daily Living (dementia) (Patterson and Mack, 2001)

continued

ANNEX TABLE 5-13 Continued

Domain	Potential Reasons for Limitation or Symptom	Selected Assessments	Selected Assistive Technologies and Relevant Accommodations
Pain	• Musculoskeletal disorders (see musculoskeletal table) • Neurological compromise (see neurological and musculoskeletal tables) • Gastrointestinal dysfunction (see gastrointestinal table) • Mast cell activation dysfunction/mast cell activation disease (see immunologic table) • Poor sleep quality	*Self-reported measures:* • Visual Analog Scale (VAS) for Pain (Bijur et al., 2001) • Numeric Pain Rating Scale (Shirley Ryan AbilityLab, 2013c) • Patient-Reported Outcomes Measurement Information System (PROMIS)—Pain Interference Instruments (HealthMeasures, 2021) • Functional Disability Inventory (Claar and Walker, 2006; Walker and Greene, 1991) (pediatric population)	• Orthoses (e.g., braces, splints) • Compression clothing • Assistive devices (e.g., crutches, wheelchair, reachers) • Psychological support for pain management • Mind-body arts, such as yoga, Pilates, tai chi • Reorganization of the home to decrease unnecessary movement, reaching, etc., that can exacerbate pain

Fatigue			
	- Poor sleep quality
- Chronic pain
- Deconditioning
- Orthostatic intolerance/dysautonomia
- Nutritional deficiencies
- Anxiety and/or depression (see mental disorders table)
- Neuromuscular disorders (see musculoskeletal and neurological tables)
- Cardiovascular and respiratory disorders (see cardiovascular and respiratory tables) | *Performance-based measures:*
- Polysomnography
- Exercise testing to include aerobic capacity and neuromuscular performance (Liguori and American College of Sports Medicine, 2021)

Self-reported measures:
- Brief Fatigue Inventory [BFI]
- Fatigue Severity Scale [FSS]
- Fatigue Symptom Inventory
- Multidimensional Assessment of Fatigue
- Fatigue Impact Scale (modified)
- Multidimensional Fatigue Symptom Inventory
- Multidimensional Fatigue Symptom Inventory Short Form
- Profile of Mood States-Brief, Fatigue subscale PedsQL
- Multi-Dimensional Fatigue Scale
- Profile of Fatigue
- Functional Assessment Chronic Illness Therapy Checklist Individual Strength
- Patient-Reported Outcomes Measurement Information System—Fatigue
- Pittsburgh Sleep Quality Assessment (Buysse et al., 1989)
- VAS to Evaluate Fatigue Severity | - Orthoses (e.g., braces, splints)
- Compression clothing
- Assistive devices (e.g., crutches, wheelchair, reachers)
- Psychological support
- Mind-body arts, such as yoga, Pilates, tai chi |

*Multidimensional assessment: Balance, coordination, dexterity, functional mobility, gait, strength, upper-extremity, function, vestibular.

ANNEX TABLE 5-14
Functional Implications for Physical Activities of Conditions Associated with Heritable Disorders of Connective Tissue

Activity	Potential Reasons for Activity Limitation	Selected Functional Assessments	Selected Assistive Technologies and Reasonable Accommodations
Sitting Note: especially prolonged sitting	• Pain (see musculoskeletal, neurological, gastrointestinal, and global functioning tables) • Instability of cervical or lumbar spine, pelvis, knees (see musculoskeletal table) • Weakness (see musculoskeletal and neurological tables) • Balance dysfunction affecting trunk (see neurological table) • Fatigue/deconditioning (see global functioning table) • Neurological compromise (see neurological table) • Orthostatic intolerance/dysautonomia (see neurological and global functioning tables)	*Physical performance measures:* • Functional Capacity Evaluation (FCE) or specific function testing by a trained health care provider (e.g., physical or occupational therapist) • Berg Balance Scale (Shirley Ryan AbilityLab, 2020a) • Function in Sitting Test (for people who are unable to perform standing balance testing) (Samuel Merritt University, n.d.) *Self-reported outcome measures:* • Roland-Morris Disability Questionnaire (RMDQ) (Chansirinukor et al., 2005; Stevens et al., 2016) • Oswestry Disability Index (ODI) (Shirley Ryan AbilityLab, 2013d) • Neck Disability Index (NDI) (Shirley Ryan AbilityLab, 2015b) • Multidimensional Assessment of Fatigue (Shirley Ryan AbilityLab, 2020b) • Fatigue Severity Scale (Shirley Ryan AbilityLab, 2016)	• Orthoses (e.g., braces, splints) • Worksite modification, especially ergonomic chairs and adjustable workstations that can raise and lower • Reorganization of worksite to minimize need to sit or allow alternating between sitting and other positioning • Reorganization of job requirements to minimize need to sit or allow alternating between sitting and other positioning • Rest breaks • Compression clothing • Telework, work from home

Standing Note: especially prolonged standing, but intermittent standing and ability to get to standing may also be affected; using assistive devices can be very stressful to upper-extremity (UE) joints	• Pain • Instability of lower-extremity (LE) joints or UE joints if assisted devices required • Weakness • Balance dysfunction • Fatigue/deconditioning • Neurological compromise • Orthostatic intolerance/dysautonomia	*Physical performance measures:* • Sensory Organization Test (NeuroCom SMART EquiTest) (Shirley Ryan AbilityLab, 2013f) • Modified Balance Error Scoring System (M-BESS) (Iverson and Koehle, 2013) • Star Excursion Balance Test performance (Hegedus et al., 2015) • Romberg (Shirley Ryan AbilityLab, 2013e) • Berg Balance Scale • 30-second sit-to-stand, or 5x or 10x stand tests (Shirley Ryan AbilityLab, 2013a) • Foot Posture Index-6 • FCE or specific function testing by a trained health care provider *Self-reported outcome measures:* • Lower Extremity Functional Scale (LEFS) (Shirley Ryan AbilityLab, 2013b) • Foot and Ankle Ability Measures (FAAM) (Shirley Ryan AbilityLab, 2015a) • RMDQ • ODI • NDI • The Activities-specific Balance Confidence (ABC) Scale (Powell and Myers, 1995) • Composite Autonomic Symptom Score (COMPASS 31) questionnaire • WOMAC, KOOS, KOOS-PS, or other knee outcome measures (Collins et al., 2011)	• Ability to sit or stand at will • Rest breaks • Compression clothing • Orthoses • Assistive devices (e.g., crutches, walker, wheelchair) • Handrails or devices to assist with balance • Reorganization of worksite to minimize need to stand and allow for changes in positioning • Reorganization of job requirements to minimize need to stand and allow for changes in positioning • Telework, work from home

continued

ANNEX TABLE 5-14 Continued

Activity	Potential Reasons for Activity Limitation	Selected Functional Assessments	Selected Assistive Technologies and Reasonable Accommodations
Walking Note: may be impaired for long or short distances, over uneven ground or different surfaces; using assistive devices can be very stressful to UE joints	• Pain • Instability of spinal or LE or UE joints if assistive devices required; includes subluxations • Fatigue/deconditioning • Weakness • Balance dysfunction • Orthostatic intolerance/dysautonomia • Neurological compromise • Cardiac dysfunction • Respiratory dysfunction	*Physical performance measures:* • 6-minute walk test • 10-meter walk test (Physiopedia, n.d.) • Functional Gait Assessment • Sensory Organization Test (NeuroCom SMART EquiTest) • M-BESS • FCE or specific function testing by a trained health care provider • Berg Balance Scale • 30-second, 5x, or 10x sit-to-stand test • Foot Posture Index-6 *Self-reported outcome measures:* • LEFS • FAAM • RMDQ • ODI • NDI • ABC Scale • WOMAC, KOOS , KOOS-PS, or other knee outcome measures	• Orthoses • Assistive devices • Reorganization of worksite and/or adaptations to the worksite or how the work is performed to minimize mobility needs • Handrails or devices to assist with balance and walking • Reorganization of job requirements to minimize mobility needs • Rest breaks • Compression clothing • Telework, work from home

Activity	Potential issues	Assessment measures	Accommodations/interventions
Strenuous physical activity Note: potentially includes all other activities in this table, plus running and impact activities	• Exercise intolerance • Pain • Instability in any joint • Fatigue/deconditioning • Weakness • Balance dysfunction • Orthostatic intolerance/dysautonomia • Neurological compromise • Cardiac dysfunction (see cardiovascular table) • Respiratory dysfunction (see respiratory table)	*Physical performance measures:* • Exercise testing • Sensory Organization Test (NeuroCom SMART EquiTest) *Self-reported outcome measures:* • LEFS • Disabilities of the Arm, Shoulder and Hand (DASH) questionnaire and QuickDASH (Aasheim and Finsen, 2013; Beaton et al., 2001; Bilberg et al., 2012; Dixon et al., 2008; Jester et al., 2005; Kennedy et al., 2013)	• Potentially anything listed in this table for other activities
Lifting from floor to waist or overhead	• Pain • Instability in any joint • Fatigue/deconditioning • Weakness • Balance dysfunction • Orthostatic intolerance/dysautonomia • Neurological compromise • Cardiac dysfunction (see cardiovascular table) • Aortic dysfunction (see cardiovascular table)	*Physical performance measures:* • FCE or specific function testing by a trained health care provider *Self-reported outcome measures:* • DASH and QuickDASH • Patient-Reported Outcomes Measurement Information System (PROMIS) Upper-Extremity Questionnaire (Overbeek et al., 2015) • Patient-Rated Elbow Evaluation (PREE) • Patient-Rated Wrist Evaluation (PRWE) (MacDermid et al., 1998; Packham and MacDermid, 2013) • Michigan Hand Outcomes Questionnaire (MHQ) (Chung et al., 1998; Shauver and Chung, 2013) • Western Ontario Shoulder Instability Index (WOSI) (Johannessen et al., 2016)	• Mechanical lifting equipment • Reachers • Adjustable high-low table • Adjustable high-low seating • Reorganization of worksite to minimize lifting needs • Reorganization of job requirements to minimize lifting needs • Rest breaks • Orthoses

continued

ANNEX TABLE 5-14 Continued

Activity	Potential Reasons for Activity Limitation	Selected Functional Assessments	Selected Assistive Technologies and Reasonable Accommodations
Carrying Note: usually requires ability to stand, lift, and walk	• Pain • Instability in any joints • Weakness • Balance dysfunction • Fatigue/deconditioning • Orthostatic intolerance/dysautonomia • Neurological compromise	*Physical performance measures:* • FCE or specific function testing by a trained health care provider • M-BESS • Sensory Organization Test (NeuroCom SMART EquiTest) • Foot Posture Index-6 *Self-reported outcome measures:* • ABC Scale • DASH and QuickDASH • PROMIS Upper-Extremity Questionnaire • PREE • PRWE • MHQ • WOSI	• Orthoses • Assistive devices • Reorganization of worksite to minimize need to carry, such as a counter of some kind that could allow pushing an item instead of carrying it • Reorganization of job requirements to minimize need to carry • Devices to help with lifting and/or carrying (e.g., carts, mechanical lifts) • Crossbody bags for carrying item • Rest breaks • Compression clothing
Pushing or pulling Note: includes UE and LE; for UE, usually requires ability to stand and walk (or move wheelchair) with at least one hand free for pushing/pulling	• Pain • Instability in any joints • Weakness • Balance dysfunction • Fatigue/deconditioning • Orthostatic intolerance/dysautonomia • Neurological compromise	*Physical performance measures:* • FCE or specific function testing by a trained health care provider • Sit-and-reach test (Pescatello et al., 2014; Wells and Dillon, 1952) *Self-reported outcome measures:* • DASH and QuickDASH • PROMIS Upper-Extremity Questionnaire • PREE • PRWE • MHQ • WOSI	• Orthoses • Reorganization of worksite to minimize need to push/pull • Reorganization of job requirements to minimize need to push/pull • Manual devices to help with moving materials (e.g., carts, trolleys) • Powered devices to help with moving materials • Rest breaks • Compression clothing

Reaching Note: may require standing	• Pain • Instability in any joints • Weakness • Balance dysfunction • Fatigue/deconditioning • Orthostatic intolerance/dysautonomia • Neurological compromise	*Physical performance measures:* • FCE or specific function testing by a trained health care provider • Sit-and-reach test *Self-reported outcome measures:* • DASH and QuickDASH • PROMIS Upper-Extremity Questionnaire • PREE • PRWE • MHQ • WOSI	• Orthoses • Reorganization of worksite to minimize need to push/pull • Reorganization of job requirements to minimize need to push/pull • The use of reachers to assist with reaching for objects • Manual devices to help with moving materials (e.g., carts, trolleys) • Powered devices to help with moving materials • Rest breaks • Compression clothing
Reaching overhead Note: requires neck extension; may require standing	• Pain • Instability of UE or spine joints • Weakness • Balance dysfunction • Fatigue • Orthostatic intolerance • Neurological compromise	*Physical performance measures:* • FCE or specific function testing by a trained health care provider • Sit-and-reach test *Self-reported outcome measures:* • DASH and QuickDASH • PROMIS Upper-Extremity Questionnaire • PREE • PRWE • MHQ • WOSI	• Orthoses • Reorganization of worksite to minimize need to reach • Reorganization of job requirements to minimize need to reach • The use of reachers to assist with reaching for objects • Devices to help with reaching (e.g., grabbers) • Rest breaks • Compression clothing
Reaching at or below the shoulder Note: may require standing	• Pain • Instability in any joints • Weakness • Balance dysfunction • Fatigue/deconditioning • Orthostatic intolerance/dysautonomia • Neurological compromise	*Physical performance measures:* • FCE or specific function testing by a trained health care provider • Sit-and-reach test *Self-reported outcome measures:* • WOSI	• Orthoses • Reorganization of worksite to minimize need to reach • Reorganization of job requirements to minimize need to reach • The use of reachers to assist with reaching for objects • Rest breaks • Compression clothing

continued

ANNEX TABLE 5-14 Continued

Activity	Potential Reasons for Activity Limitation	Selected Functional Assessments	Selected Assistive Technologies and Reasonable Accommodations
Gross manipulation Note: requires ability to sit and/or stand	• Pain • Instability in spine or UE joints • Weakness • Balance dysfunction • Fatigue/deconditioning • Orthostatic intolerance/dysautonomia • Neurological compromise • Coordination deficit	*Physical performance measures:* • FCE or specific function testing by a trained health care provider • Sequential Occupational Dexterity Assessment (SODA) (van Lankveld et al., 1996) *Self-reported outcome measures:* • DASH and QuickDASH • PROMIS Upper-Extremity Questionnaire • PRWE • MHQ • WOSI	• Orthoses • Ergonomic tools • The use of reachers to assist with reaching and manipulating objects • Reorganization of worksite to minimize need for gross manipulation • Reorganization of job requirements to minimize need for gross manipulation • Rest breaks • Compression clothing
Fine manipulation	• Pain • Instability in cervical or UE joints • Weakness • Balance dysfunction • Fatigue/deconditioning • Orthostatic intolerance/dysautonomia • Neurological compromise • Coordination deficit	*Physical performance measures:* • FCE or specific function testing by a trained health care provider • Nine-hole peg board test • SODA *Self-reported outcome measures:* • Functional Dexterity Test (Shirley Ryan AbilityLab, 2017) • PRWE • MHQ	• Orthoses • Wrist weights • Ergonomic tools • Add built up handles to items used at work, such as pencils/pens, tools, and other items used in the workplace and at home to minimize the need for fine manipulation • Reorganization of worksite to minimize need for fine manipulation • Reorganization of job requirements to minimize need for fine manipulation • Rest breaks • Compression clothing

Activity	Impairments	Measures	Interventions
Foot/leg controls	• Pain • Instability in lumbar or LE joints • Weakness • Balance dysfunction • Fatigue/deconditioning • Orthostatic intolerance/dysautonomia • Neurological compromise	*Physical performance measures:* • FCE or specific function testing by a trained health care provider *Self-reported outcome measures:* • LEFS • FAAM	• Orthoses • Ergonomic tools • Reorganization of worksite to minimize need for foot/leg controls • Reorganization of job requirements to minimize need for foot/leg controls • Rest breaks • Compression clothing
Climbing Note: may include stairs, ramps, ladders, scaffolding, ropes, etc. Normal ambulation devices might not be usable for climbing.	• Pain • Instability any joints • Weakness • Balance dysfunction • Fatigue/deconditioning • Orthostatic intolerance/dysautonomia • Neurological compromise	*Physical performance measures:* • FCE or specific function testing by a trained health care provider • Sensory Organization Test (NeuroCom SMART EquiTest) • M-BESS *Self-reported outcome measures:* • ABC Scale • LEFS • WOMAC, KOOS, KOOS-PS, or other knee outcome measures	• Orthoses • Assistive devices • Reorganization of worksite to minimize need to climb • Handrails, grab bars, or other devices to assist with balance • Reorganization of job requirements to minimize need to climb • Rest breaks • Compression clothing

continued

ANNEX TABLE 5-14 Continued

Activity	Potential Reasons for Activity Limitation	Selected Functional Assessments	Selected Assistive Technologies and Reasonable Accommodations
Low work, including stooping, crouching, kneeling, crawling or lying on the ground Note: includes need to get up and down from the ground	• Pain • Instability any joints • Weakness • Balance dysfunction, including vestibular issues • Fatigue/deconditioning • Orthostatic intolerance/dysautonomia • Neurological compromise	*Physical performance measures:* • FCE or specific function testing by a trained health care provider *Self-reported outcome measures:* • LEFS • WOMAC, KOOS, KOOS-PS, or other knee outcome measures	• Orthoses • Kneepads • Assistive devices (e.g., reachers, scooters, rolling sit-carts, high-low chairs/stools) • Reorganization of job requirements or work environment to minimize need for low work • Reorganization of worksite to minimize need for low work • Raise the level where work is done • Handrails or devices to assist with getting up and down • Rest breaks • Compression clothing

NOTE: KOOS = Knee Injury and Osteoarthritis Outcome Score; WOMAC = Western Ontario and McMaster Universities Osteoarthritis Index.

ANNEX TABLE 5-15
Functional Implications for Vision, Hearing, and Speaking Activities of Conditions Associated with Heritable Disorders of Connective Tissue

Activity	Potential Reasons for Activity Limitation	Selected Functional Assessments	Selected Assistive Technologies and Reasonable Accommodations
Near visual acuity	• Uncorrected refractive error • Accommodative insufficiency • Glare • Cataract • Dislocated lens • Cornea scarring • Keratoconus • Dry Eye • Retina scarring • Amblyopia	• Snellen Chart • Bailey-Lovie Chart • Brightness acuity testing	• Over-the-counter reading glasses, prescription glasses or contact lenses, occasionally prism glasses • Low-vision devices • Auditory replacements for vision tasks • Glare-reducing equipment
Distance (far) visual acuity	• Uncorrected refractive error • Cataract • Dislocated lens • Cornea scarring • Keratoconus • Dry eye • Retina scarring • Amblyopia	• Snellen Chart • Bailey-Lovie Chart • Brightness acuity testing	• Prescription glasses or contact lenses • Low-vision devices • Orientation and mobility training
Binocular function	• Reduced stereopsis • Strabismus • Deficient pursuits • Vergence infacility • Deficient saccades	• Orthoptic examination • Titmus stereo test • Howard-Dolman test • Infrared oculography	• Computerized orthoptic therapy • Prism glasses • Strabismus surgery • Sectoral occlusion

continued

ANNEX TABLE 5-14 Continued

Activity	Potential Reasons for Activity Limitation	Selected Functional Assessments	Selected Assistive Technologies and Reasonable Accommodations
Peripheral vision	• Glaucoma • Retina scarring/detachment • Stroke (including ischemic and hemorrhagic)	• Perimetry	• Low-vision devices • Auditory accessories • Orientation and mobility training
Hearing	• Sensorineural hearing impairment • Conductive hearing impairment • Mixed sensorineural and conductive hearing impairment	*Performance-based measures:* • Pure tone audiometry • Speech recognition in noise testing • Internet- and telephone-based screening *Self-reported outcome measures:* • Hearing Handicap Inventory for Adults (Newman et al., 1990) • Speech, Spatial, and Qualities of Hearing Questionnaire (Gatehouse and Noble, 2004)	• Hearing aids • Personal sound-amplification products • Remote-microphone hearing assistive technology • Captioning • Telecommunications relay service • Other assistive technologies • Environmental modification

| Speaking | • Temporomandibular joint dysfunction
• Laryngeal dysfunction
• Vocal fatigue | • Speech/Phoneme Intelligibility Test (Madonna Rehabilitation Hospitals, n.d.)
• Assessment of Intelligibility in Dysarthric Speech (Yorkston and Beukelman, 1984)
• Frenchay Dysarthria Assessment, Second Edition (Enderby and Palmer, 2008)
• Apraxia Battery for Adults, Second Edition (Dabul, 2000)
• Apraxia of Speech Rating Scale (Strand et al., 2014)
• Communication Participation Item Bank (Baylor et al., 2013)
• Levels of Speech Usage (Baylor et al., 2008)
• Fatigue Severity Scale (Krupp et al., 1989)
• Quality of Communication Life Scale (Paul et al., 2004)
• ASHA Functional Assessment of Communication Skills for Adults (Frattali et al., 2017) | • Assistive technologies
• Environmental modification
• Occupational therapy |
|---|---|---|---|

NOTE: ASHA = American Speech-Language-Hearing Association; EDS = Ehlers-Danlos syndrome.
SOURCES: Giguère et al., 2008; Laroche et al., 2003; McBride et al., 1994; Smits et al., 2004; Watson et al., 2012; Yueh et al., 2003.

ANNEX TABLE 5-16
Functional Implications for Mental Activities of Conditions Associated with Heritable Disorders of Connective Tissue

Activity	Potential Reasons for Activity Limitation	Selected Functional Assessments	Selected Assistive Technologies and Reasonable Accommodations
Understand, remember, and apply information	• Pain • Fatigue • Mild cognitive impairment (sometimes described as "brain fog") • Mood (low, high) • Depression • Anxiety • Cognitive impairment	*Intellectual abilities and general cognition* • Leiter International Performance Scale, Third Edition (Roid et al., 2013) • Repeatable Battery for Assessment of Neuropsychological Status Update (Randolph, 2012) • Montreal Cognitive Assessment (screen) (Nasreddine et al., 2005) • Brief Assessment of Cognition (Keefe et al., 2004; Keefe et al., 2008) • Short Orientation-Memory-Concentration Test of Cognitive Impairment (Katzman et al., 1983) • Cognitive Capacity Screening Examination (Jacobs et al., 1977) • Stanford-Binet Intelligence Scales, Fifth Edition (Roid, 2003) • Wechsler Adult Intelligence Scale, Fourth Edition (Wechsler, 2008) • Wechsler Abbreviated Scales of Intelligence, Second Edition (Wechsler, 2011) • Reynolds Intellectual Assessment Scales, Second Edition (Reynolds and Kamphaus, 2015) • Kaufman Brief Intelligence Test, Second Edition (Kaufman and Kaufman, 2004)	• Short, step-by-step instructions, recorded for play-back on cell phone • Short, step-by-step, written instructions in plain language, on cell phone, pocket cards, or wall signs • Tasks broken down into sequential steps, outlined in simple language, and posted within view at the worksite • Tasks broken down into sequential steps and outlined in simple language via recordings in short, simple, sentences, that provide specific instructions for work tasks • Work performed in a quiet area without distractions • Work performed sitting instead of standing, with breaks as needed • Provision of a job coach

Executive functioning
- Delis-Kaplan Executive Function System (Delis et al., 2001)
- Symbol Digit Modalities Test (Smith, 1973)
- Tower of London-DX, Second Edition (Culbertson and Zillmer, 2005)
- Wisconsin Card Sorting Test (Grant and Berg, 1981)

Attention and working memory
- Conners Continuous Performance Test Third Edition (Conners, 2014)
- The Test of Variables of Attention, Version 9 (Greenberg et al., 2017)
- Wide Range Assessment of Memory and Learning, Second Edition (Sheslow and Adams, 2003)

Self-reported measures:
- Work Disability Functional Assessment Battery (WD-FAB) (Marfeo et al., 2019)
- Beck Anxiety Inventory (BAI)
- Beck Depression Inventory (BDI)
- Hospital Anxiety and Depression Scale
- Autism Spectrum Quotient

continued

ANNEX TABLE 5-16
Continued

Activity	Potential Reasons for Activity Limitation	Selected Functional Assessments	Selected Assistive Technologies and Reasonable Accommodations
Problem solve	• Mild cognitive impairment • Pain • Fatigue • Mood (low, high) • Depression • Anxiety • Hyperactivity • Attention deficit	*Intellectual abilities and general cognition* • See above *Executive functioning* • See above *Self-reported measures:* • BAI • BDI • Hospital Anxiety and Depression Scale	• Short, step-by-step instructions, recorded for play-back on cell phone • Short, step-by-step, written instructions in plain language, on cell phone, pocket cards, or wall signs • Tasks broken down into sequential steps, outlined in simple language, and posted within view at the worksite • Tasks broken down into sequential steps and outlined in simple language via recordings in short, simple, sentences, that provide specific instructions for work tasks • Work performed in a quiet area without distractions • Provision of a job coach

| Concentrate, persist, or maintain pace | - Pain
- Fatigue
- Cognitive impairment
- Mood (low, high)
- Depression
- Anxiety
- Impulsivity
- Hyperactivity
- Attention deficit | *Attention and working memory*
- See above
Processing speed
- Symbol Digit Modalities Test (Smith, 1973)
Self-reported measures:
- Adult ADHD Self-Report Scale
- Barrat Impulsiveness Scale
- BAI
- BDI
- Hospital Anxiety and Depression Scale | - Work performed in a quiet area without distractions
- Use of a noise-canceling headset
- Short, step-by-step instructions, recorded for play-back on cell phone
- Short, step-by-step, written instructions in plain language, on cell phone, pocket cards, or wall signs
- Tasks broken down into sequential steps, outlined in simple language, and posted within view at the worksite
- Tasks broken down into sequential steps and outlined in simple language via recordings in short, simple, sentences, that provide specific instructions for work tasks
- Provision of a job coach |

continued

ANNEX TABLE 5-16
Continued

Activity	Potential Reasons for Activity Limitation	Selected Functional Assessments	Selected Assistive Technologies and Reasonable Accommodations
Interact with others	• Fatigue • Cognitive impairment • Mood (low, high) • Depression • Anxiety • Impulsivity • Hyperactivity • Attention deficit	*Adaptability/personal interactions* *Self-reported measures:* • WD-FAB (Marfeo et al., 2013) • Personal and Social Performance Scale (Morosini et al., 2000) • Sheehan Disability Scale (Sheehan, 1983) • Social and Occupational Functioning Assessment Scale (Rybarczyk, 2011) • Mental Illness Research, Education, and Clinical Center (MIRECC) version of the Global Assessment of Functioning scale (Niv et al., 2007) • Adult ADHD Self-Report Scale • Borderline Personality Disorder Checklist • International Personality Disorder Examination • Personality Assessment Inventory (Morey, 1991) • Panic and Agoraphobia Scale • Autism Spectrum Quotient *Language* • Verbal Tasks from IQ Batteries (Kaufman and Kaufman, 2004; Reynolds and Kamphaus, 2015; Roid, 2003; Wechsler, 2008, 2011, 2012, 2014) • Expressive Vocabulary Test, Third Edition (Williams, 2018) • Peabody Picture Vocabulary Test, Fifth Edition (Dunn, 2018)	• Structured, work-related, and/or social activities • Option to work independently, away from others • Option to work with others in a structured work environment, with or without breaks • Provision of a job coach

Adapt or manage oneself	• Depression • Anxiety • Fatigue • Mood (low, high) • Cognitive impairment	

Adaptive functioning
- Adaptive Behavior Assessment System, Third Edition (Harrison and Oakland, 2015)
- Vineland Adaptive Behavior Scales, Third Edition (Sparrow et al., 2016)

Adaptability/personal interactions
- See above

Attention and working memory
- See above

Processing speed
- See above

Executive functioning
- See above

Self-reported measures:
- Sheehan Disability Scale
- Adult ADHD Self-Report Scale
- Personality Assessment Inventory
- Panic and Agoraphobia Scale
- Autism Spectrum Quotient

- Work performed in a quiet area without distractions
- Structured, work-related, and/or social activities
- Option to work independently, away from others
- Option to work with others in a structured work environment, with or without breaks
- Self-pacing of work performed with short, step-by-step instructions, recorded for play-back on cell phone
- Short, step-by-step, written instructions in plain language, on cell phone, pocket cards, or wall signs
- Tasks broken down into sequential steps, outlined in simple language, and posted within view at the worksite
- Tasks broken down into sequential steps and outlined in simple language via recordings in short, simple, sentences, that provide specific instructions for work tasks, and when breaks can occur
- Provision of a job coach

NOTE: ADHD = attention deficit hyperactivity disorder.

ANNEX TABLE 5-17
Examples of Social Security Administration Listings That May Apply to Individuals with Heritable Disorders of Connective Tissue

Listings*	Notes
1.15 Disorders of the skeletal spine resulting in compromise of a nerve root(s)	Standard imaging may not clearly demonstrate abnormalities. Flexion and extension imaging, or magnetic resonance imaging (upright, if tolerated) may be needed.
1.16 Lumbar spinal stenosis resulting in compromise of the cauda equine	Standard imaging might not detect abnormalities. Specialized imaging such as flexion or extension imaging may be needed. Some individuals may be unable to use mobility devices due to upper-extremity impairments.
1.17 Reconstructive surgery or surgical arthrodesis of a major weight-bearing joint	Individuals with HDCTs are more likely to have a poor outcome with major surgery, especially if the HCDT was not previously recognized or taken into account in performing surgery and after-care. Wound healing is slow in many HDCTs and wound dehiscence may occur despite excellent surgical and postoperative care. Some individuals may be unable to use mobility devices due to upper-extremity impairments. Patients are sometimes unable to fully engage in postoperative therapy because of associated problems such as fatigue, orthostatic intolerance, mast cell activation disease, depression, brain fog, gastrointestinal disorders, or other musculoskeletal issues. Surgical outcomes may therefore be compromised.
1.18 Abnormality of a major joint(s) in any extremity	Frequent episodes of subluxation or dislocation strongly impacting function often influence how consistent people can be in performing work activities. For example, if a person's hip dislocates, they will be unable to stand or walk. Individuals prone to dislocations may be afraid to perform certain activities or even to leave their homes for fear of causing a dislocation. Physical examination and standard imaging might not identify subluxations that only occur with movement or weight bearing. Specific imaging such as dynamic imaging, imaging at end-range, or visualization of soft-tissue damage may be needed. Patients with significant upper-extremity involvement may not be candidates for assistive technology to aid mobility. Consequently, the patient might not have been given a mobility device because he/she would not have been able to effectively use it.

ANNEX TABLE 5-17
Continued

Listings*	Notes
1.21 Soft-tissue injury or abnormality under continuing surgical management	Soft-tissue injuries/pain are very common. Sometimes a single body part is severely involved, but it is also common that there may be many body parts that combine to create severe functional limitations. For example, involvement of bilateral upper-extremity involvement in addition to bilateral lower-extremity involvement may limit capacity to use mobility devices. For example, using a wheelchair may aggravate hand instability and pain, thus incapacitating the hands as well. Surgery is often less successful and more often avoided in patients with than in those without hypermobility. Therefore, the requirement of past surgery is less likely to be met even though a patient may have equally severe functional limitations due to soft-tissue problems. Patients are sometimes unable to fully engage in therapy because of associated problems such as fatigue, depression, brain fog, gastrointestinal disorders, or other musculoskeletal issues.
2.02 Loss of central visual acuity (meeting the specified criteria)	
2.03 Contraction of the visual field in the better eye (meeting the specified criteria)	
2.04 Loss of visual efficiency, or visual impairment, in the better eye (meeting the specified criteria)	
2.07 Disturbance of labyrinthine-vestibular function (including Ménière's disease), characterized by a history of frequent attacks of balance disturbance, tinnitus, and progressive loss of hearing	Might meet vestibular criteria but hearing criteria may not be applicable.
3.03 Asthma	
3.07 Bronchiectasis	
3.14 Respiratory failure	
4.10 Aneurysm of aorta or major branches	
5.08 Weight loss due to any digestive disorder (meeting the specified criteria)	

continued

ANNEX TABLE 5-17
Continued

Listings*	Notes
11.08 Spinal cord disorders	
12.04 Depressive, bipolar, and related disorders	
12.06 Anxiety and obsessive-compulsive disorders	
14.09 Inflammatory arthritis	

*SSA, n.d.-b, provides the criteria for each of the listings included here.

6

Overall Conclusions[1]

This chapter presents eight overall conclusions derived by the committee from evidence provided throughout the report. The first section includes narrative summaries of evidence supporting these overall conclusions. Chapters 2 through 5 of the report each end with a set of chapter-specific findings and conclusions based on the evidence presented in that chapter. The second section of the present chapter includes a selection of those chapter-specific findings and conclusions that support each of the overall conclusions.

OVERALL CONCLUSIONS

Nature of Heritable Disorders of Connective Tissue

Heritable disorders of connective tissue (HDCTs) are a heterogeneous group of inherited disorders that affect connective tissues throughout the body. Connective tissue is an integral component of all organ systems and plays a crucial role in their function. Hence, the physical and mental secondary impairments (i.e., medical diagnoses, syndromes, or comorbid and other health conditions) associated with HDCTs manifest throughout the body and can affect functioning in every body system.

Marfan syndrome (MFS) often manifests in cardiovascular, nervous, respiratory, musculoskeletal, and ocular system impairments. Loeys-Dietz

---

[1] This chapter does not include references. Citations to support the text and conclusions herein are provided in previous chapters of the report.

syndrome (LDS) and congenital contractural arachnodactyly are related hereditary aortopathies that manifest particularly in cardiovascular, cerebrovascular, respiratory, musculoskeletal, craniofacial, ocular, and neurological impairments. Shprintzen-Goldberg syndrome manifests in developmental delays and intellectual disability, as well as impairments associated with the other hereditary aortopathies.

The Ehlers-Danlos syndromes (EDS) are a group of HDCTs that share common elements of joint hypermobility and skin and soft-tissue involvement. Hypermobility spectrum disorders (HSD) are clinically similar to hypermobile EDS (hEDS) with respect to their manifestations and management. EDS/HSD manifest in secondary impairments in any organ system and often in multiple organ systems in a given individual, although the likelihood of specific manifestations depends on the type of EDS. Vascular impairments, which can be life-threatening, are characteristic of vascular EDS (vEDS), for example. As with many other chronic conditions, mental disorders (e.g., depression and anxiety) are also commonly experienced by individuals with EDS. Additional features of pain; fatigue; mild cognitive impairment; dysautonomia; and gastrointestinal, respiratory, neurological, and immune dysfunction are also common among EDS patients but often underappreciated, particularly given their waxing and waning nature in affected individuals.

Physical and mental secondary impairments associated with HDCTs may develop and vary in severity over time. Many manifestations of MFS and the related hereditary aortopathies worsen over time, with some manifestations not appearing until adulthood. The type and severity of EDS manifestations frequently vary both among individuals and throughout an affected individual's lifetime. Secondary impairments associated with EDS often emerge or worsen during puberty. Notably, mortality resulting from unanticipated vascular events was found to have increased 3-fold in males with vEDS under age 20. The severity of HDCTs is linked to the severity of affected individuals' physical and mental secondary impairments, including the combined effects of multiple impairments, as well as the frequency, severity, and predictability of their fluctuations. Secondary impairments in any of the body systems can be severe and affect an individual's physical and mental functioning.

MFS and related hereditary aortopathies have multiple clinical manifestations that, individually or in combination, can cause functional limitations of varying severity, often involving multiple body systems. Increases in the life spans of affected individuals resulting from improvements in management of previously fatal complications (e.g., aortic rupture, spontaneous pneumothorax) are accompanied by concurrent increases in the occurrence and severity of age-related secondary impairments. General physical activity guidelines exist for people with MFS and related disorders, such as avoidance of intense isometric exercise, contact sports that can lead to blows to the head, activities that involve rapid acceleration and deceleration over short distances (sprinting) or rapid changes in pressure (e.g., scuba diving), and exercise to the point of exhaustion.

Individuals with EDS/HSD also exhibit multiple clinical manifestations that, individually or in combination, can affect their functioning with varying degrees of severity. Limitations associated with pain, fatigue, and anxiety may be particularly pronounced. Chronic pain, chronic fatigue, and cognitive dysfunction are some of the most common and potentially disabling manifestations of EDS, especially hEDS/HSD, and MFS. The functional limitations experienced by individuals with HDCTs are also affected by environmental factors (e.g., extreme heat and cold, noise, vibration, wetness, humidity, atmospheric conditions) and physical and mental demands. In addition, physical and mental demands related to school or work may precipitate or exacerbate these limitations.

For these reasons, the committee drew the following overall conclusion:

1. Heritable disorders of connective tissue (HDCTs) comprise a large and varied group of disorders in children and adults that share the common feature of pronounced involvement of connective tissues, usually in multiple organ systems. HDCTs can lead to a variety of physical and mental secondary impairments (i.e., manifestations, medical diagnoses, syndromes, comorbidities, or other health conditions) and associated functional limitations. Impairments can range from minor to severe and even life-threatening and may fluctuate in severity over time in an individual. Functional limitations may be sufficiently severe to interfere with participation in work and school, as well as social and recreational activities, and may include precautions and restrictions on activities to avoid aggravating the condition.

Heritable Disorders of Connective Tissue and Disability

A challenge in assessment of functioning in individuals with HDCTs is capturing the full effect of their impairment(s) on their daily activities, including participation in work and school. This is particularly true when a person has multiple impairments. Numerous validated performance-based and self-reported measures are available for assessing physical and mental functioning in persons with HDCTs, including several that can be used to perform an integrated assessment of an individual's overall physical and mental functioning. Individuals with HDCTs may experience significant variability in their physical and/or mental secondary impairments from day to day or even within a single day. This variability is often unpredictable and may limit the ability to sustain gainful employment.

Upon reviewing SSA's Listing of Impairments–Adult Listings, the committee found that some of the listings include severity criteria for some of the secondary impairments that may be experienced by individuals with MFS, EDS, and other HDCTs. The committee also concluded that other listings, with some modification, could apply to certain secondary impairments experienced by individuals with HDCTs. In addition, the combined effects of the secondary impairments experienced by an individual may limit function with a degree of severity sufficient to preclude the person's ability to participate in work on a "regular and continuing basis" (i.e., 8 hours per day, 5 days per week, or an equivalent work schedule) or, for children, to result in "marked and severe functional limitations." The concept of functional equivalence used by SSA in some disability determinations in children is particularly well suited to evaluating the combined effects on an applicant's functioning of the many and varied impairments that often manifest in HDCTs and other multisystem disorders.

For these reasons, the committee drew the following overall conclusion:

2. **Some of SSA's Adult Listings apply directly to secondary impairments experienced by individuals with HDCTs and could be used to evaluate disability in those individuals. Other listings, with some modification, could apply to certain secondary impairments experienced by individuals with HDCTs.**

Diagnosis

Early diagnosis of HDCTs is important to reduce physical injury, reduce psychological harm to the affected individual and family members, and prevent the risks associated with inappropriate or fragmented medical care. HDCTs are diagnosed through a combination of clinical findings and established clinical criteria, followed by confirmatory molecular genetic testing when specific genes have been identified for the suspected disorder. Some HDCTs, such as hEDS, do not yet have a known genetic marker or test, and the absence of molecular genetic testing should not necessarily rule out the diagnosis if the clinical suspicion remains based on clinical findings. An HDCT diagnosis should be considered for individuals who present with previously undiagnosed complex multisystem disorders; however, diagnosis of some HDCTs, in particular EDS, is often delayed, in some cases for a decade or more. One reason for delayed diagnosis is that because HDCTs can cause a wide variety of physical and mental secondary impairments involving multiple organ systems, patients often are referred to a succession of different specialists. Other factors that may contribute to delays in diagnosis of HDCTs include minimal training in and knowledge about the disorders among health care providers and a corresponding shortage of providers with expertise in diagnosing and managing them.

Delayed diagnosis may exacerbate manifestations of HDCTs or have life-threatening consequences. For example, lack of monitoring for aortic root enlargement in MFS or LDS could lead to aortic dissection and death. Likewise, failure to recognize a characteristic phenotype (e.g., of MFS) in a patient presenting with chest pain could result in delayed diagnosis of aortic dissection, with potentially catastrophic results. When diagnosed early, and with appropriate management, most people with classic MFS have a relatively normal life expectancy. Conversely, in addition to complications from secondary impairments, individuals with undiagnosed EDS may face unanticipated EDS-specific risks and harms, such as tissue fragility and physiologic reactivity resulting from autonomic and immune dysregulation, that attend routine procedures and therapies. Similarly, people with versus those without EDS often have a worse trajectory following trauma or surgery, in terms of both length of recovery and frequency of complications. Affected individuals also report inappropriate assessments and incorrect diagnoses, and many develop a mistrust of medical professionals and negative expectations about future health care encounters, which may lead them to avoid further medical consultations.

For these reasons, the committee drew the following overall conclusion:

3. **Early diagnosis of HDCTs is important to reduce physical injury, reduce psychological harm to the individual and family members, and prevent the risks associated with inappropriate or fragmented medical care.**
    - Diagnosis of HDCTs is often delayed because of
        - the multisystem, complex, and phenotypically variable nature of the disorders;
        - lack of knowledge about HDCTs among health care providers, patients and family members, and other stakeholders;
        - lack of experience with using the syndromic approach to diagnosis, in which diagnosis is based on characteristic groups of symptoms and signs;
        - lack of access to comprehensive, multidisciplinary care teams with expertise in HDCTs (due to a shortage of clinicians, especially in some geographic areas);
        - historical bias and denial among health care providers, patients, and family members about the reality of the lived experience of manifestations of the disorders; and
        - inaccurate expectations that there will be a diagnostic genetic test for every HDCT.

- Delayed or misdiagnosis of individuals with HDCTs can result in
  - inappropriate medical interventions;
  - inability to accurately assess the risks and benefits associated with medical procedures;
  - inability to access necessary reasonable accommodations at work or school;
  - family stress and dysfunction;
  - stress associated with unexplained and repeated evidence of trauma, leading to inappropriate suspicion of child abuse;
  - inappropriate assessments and incorrect diagnoses; and
  - mistrust of health care providers and negative expectations for future health care encounters.
- Timely diagnosis and recognition of the many physical and mental secondary impairments with which HDCTs can present and action to address them, even if in the absence of a specific molecular diagnosis, can dramatically improve individuals' quality of life and functional status, including the ability to participate in work and school.

Management

HDCTs are lifelong disorders for which there presently exist no curative treatments, but appropriate management can reduce the frequency and severity of the disorders' manifestations and resulting functional limitations. Management of HDCTs involves supportive care, early diagnosis and treatment of associated physical and mental secondary impairments, and preventive strategies to lessen or prevent problems that may occur over time. Because of the complex, multisystem nature of HDCTs, high-quality care for individuals with these disorders relies on effective coordination among a team of health care providers across a broad range of disciplines with expertise in the disorders.

For these reasons, the committee drew the following overall conclusion:

4. Although curative treatments for HDCTs do not exist at this time, appropriate understanding and management of the disorders can reduce the frequency and severity of their manifestations and resulting functional consequences. High-quality care for individuals with HDCTs relies on effective coordination among a team of clinicians across a broad range of physical and mental health care disciplines who are knowledgeable about these disorders.

Barriers to Access to Care

Individuals with HDCTs often experience difficulty obtaining appropriate and integrated multidisciplinary care to address the wide range of associated impairments. Barriers to appropriate care include insufficient training in and knowledge about the disorders among health care providers, which contributes to a shortage of clinicians with expertise in their diagnosis and management. In addition, access to multidisciplinary teams and relevant specialists is limited or nonexistent in rural areas; even many university centers lack multidisciplinary teams with expertise in HDCTs.

For these reasons, the committee drew the following overall conclusion:

5. **Access to comprehensive, multidisciplinary care for the diagnosis and management of HDCTs can be limited by geography and other factors, including the availability of care teams with expertise in the disorders.**

Education

Education about HDCTs, including their multisystem manifestations, diagnosis, and management, is important for all health care providers to help increase recognition and earlier diagnosis of the disorders. With appropriate education, a variety of health care providers, including, for example, physicians, nurses, psychologists, neuropsychologists, rehabilitation specialists (e.g., physiatrists; physical, occupational, and speech therapists), nutritionists, and others, should be able to recognize HDCTs and direct affected individuals to the appropriate care providers for management. Clinicians performing procedures or providing anesthesia and periprocedures management need to be aware of the altered procedural and postprocedural risks associated with HDCTs and to have a screening strategy for these disorders. It is also important for individuals with HDCTs and their family members to learn about strategies for preventing or mitigating symptoms, as well as the risks associated with certain activities that may result in physical trauma, such as physically demanding activities or pregnancy and childbirth. Relevant support groups provide valuable education regarding the manifestations and lived experience of the disorders. Increased recognition of the breadth and scope of HDCTs is needed among health care professional education programs, professional organizations, and publishers of quality biomedical research.

For these reasons, the committee drew the following overall conclusions:

6. Education about HDCTs, including their multisystem manifestations, diagnosis, and management, is important for all clinicians to help increase recognition and earlier diagnosis of the disorders and enable the provision of appropriate care.
   - A variety of health care providers should be able to recognize HDCTs and direct affected individuals to the appropriate clinicians for management.
   - Individuals with HDCTs and relevant support groups can provide valuable insight regarding the manifestations and lived experience of the disorders.
   - Increased recognition of the breadth and scope of HDCTs by health care professional education programs, professional organizations, and publishers of quality biomedical research is needed.

7. Education of individuals with the disorders and their families, as well as employers and school staff, is important to improve the quality of life for affected individuals and their families, to facilitate appropriate accommodations at work and school, and to help inform the disability assessment and determination process.

Research Gaps

HDCTs can be difficult to diagnose, and the true prevalence of many of these disorders is unknown. As noted above, HDCTs are diagnosed through a combination of clinical findings and established clinical criteria, followed by confirmatory molecular genetic testing when specific genes have been identified for the suspected disorder. However, diagnosis of hEDS and HSD is based solely on clinical criteria, since currently no associated causative genes have been identified for either disorder. Understanding of and diagnostic criteria for these disorders continue to evolve. There currently are no curative treatments for MFS and related hereditary aortopathies, EDS, or HSD, making this an important area for research. In addition, more research is needed to improve understanding of the pathophysiological mechanisms of EDS/HSD and the recognition, management, and outcomes of the many secondary impairments associated with these disorders.

The clinical course of HDCTs and their effects on functioning vary greatly among affected individuals. Longitudinal studies of individuals with different HDCTs would increase understanding of the clinical course of the disorders; associated functional limitations; and potentially the impact of interventions, including reasonable accommodations, on participation in work and school.

While the severity of HDCTs is linked to the severity of the affected individual's physical and mental secondary impairments, including the combined effects of multiple impairments, improved understanding and measurement of the effects of impairments and multiple impairments on functioning could advance management of the disorders and improve functional status and quality of life for patients.

For these reasons, the committee drew the following overall conclusion:

8. **Ongoing research on HDCTs is important to advance understanding of the disorders and their effects. In particular, research on care services and interventions for HDCTs and secondary impairments is needed, including**
   - more specific diagnostic criteria and biomarkers;
   - functional and biomeasures of severity;
   - effective treatment for HDCTs and management of their physical and mental manifestations, including comparative treatment trials;
   - the clinical course of the disorders throughout the lifetime of affected individuals;
   - the impact of relevant reasonable accommodations on affected individuals' ability to participate in work and school; and
   - benefits versus risks of participation in common childhood activities (e.g., contact sports, gymnastics, dance).

SELECTED FINDINGS AND CONCLUSIONS IN SUPPORT OF THE COMMITTEE'S OVERALL CONCLUSIONS

Box 6-1 shows the links between the overall conclusions presented above and some of the most relevant chapter-specific findings and conclusions that support them.[2]

---

[2] Not all of the committee's chapter-specific findings and conclusions are included in Box 6-1. Those that are included are numbered according to the chapter in which they appear.

BOX 6-1
Overall Conclusions and Selected Chapter-Specific Findings and Conclusions

1. Heritable disorders of connective tissue (HDCTs) comprise a large and varied group of disorders in children and adults that share the common feature of pronounced involvement of connective tissues, usually in multiple organ systems. HDCTs can lead to a variety of physical and mental secondary impairments (i.e., manifestations, medical diagnoses, syndromes, comorbidities, or other health conditions) and associated functional limitations. Impairments can range from minor to severe and even life-threatening and may fluctuate in severity over time in an individual. Functional limitations may be sufficiently severe to interfere with participation in work and school, as well as social and recreational activities, and may include precautions and restrictions on activities to avoid aggravating the condition.

Findings

2-1. Heritable disorders of connective tissue (HDCTs) are a heterogeneous group of inherited disorders that affect connective tissues in organ systems throughout the body.

2-2. Connective tissues are an integral component of every organ system and play a crucial role in the function of those systems. Hence, the physical and mental secondary impairments associated with HDCTs, which may develop and potentially progress or wax and wane over time, manifest throughout the body and affect functioning in every body system.

3-1. Marfan syndrome (MFS), Loeys-Dietz syndrome (LDS), congenital contractural arachnodactyly (CCA; also known as Beals-Hecht syndrome), and Sphrintzen-Goldberg syndrome (SGS) affect multiple body systems, often with cardiovascular, skeletal, and ocular manifestations.

3-3. Many manifestations of hereditary aortopathies worsen over time, with some not appearing until adulthood.

3-6. As the life spans of patients with these syndromes increase with improvements in management of previously fatal complications (e.g., aortic rupture, spontaneous pneumothorax), concurrent increases are seen in the occurrence and severity of age-related secondary impairments.

3-7. Hereditary aortopathies can affect individuals' everyday physical and mental functioning, often impacting multiple body systems. MFS frequently manifests in cardiovascular, nervous, respiratory, musculoskeletal, and ocular system impairments. LDS and CCA manifest particularly in cardiovascular, cerebrovascular, respiratory, musculoskeletal, craniofacial, ocular, and neurological impairments. SGS manifests in developmental delays and intellectual disability as well as impairments associated with the other hereditary aortopathies.

4-1. The Ehlers-Danlos syndromes (EDS) are a group of multisystem, heritable disorders of connective tissue (HDCTs) that share common elements of joint hypermobility and skin and soft tissue involvement. Hypermobility spectrum disorders (HSD) are also multisystem connective tissue disorders

that are clinically similar to hypermobile EDS (hEDS) with respect to their manifestations and management.
4-3. EDS/HSD can manifest in physical and mental secondary impairments in any organ system and often in multiple organ systems in a given individual.
4-4. The type and severity of physical and mental manifestations associated with EDS/HSD often vary both among individuals and throughout an affected individual's lifetime. Epidemiologic evidence supports multi–organ system manifestations, high treatment burden, and high disease burden.

Conclusions

3-1. MFS and related hereditary aortopathies have multiple physical and mental manifestations that, individually or in combination, can cause functional limitations of varying severity. Some manifestations may become apparent only with age, and the severity of manifestations may, and often does, progress with age. Treatment can be successful in reducing impairments in selected cases.
4-1. EDS and HSD have multiple clinical manifestations that, individually or in combination, can cause functional limitations of varying severity. Some manifestations may become apparent only with age, and the types and severity of manifestations may vary throughout an affected individual's lifetime.

2. Some of SSA's Adult Listings apply directly to secondary impairments experienced by individuals with HDCTs and could be used to evaluate disability in those individuals. Other listings, with some modification, could apply to certain secondary impairments experienced by individuals with HDCTs.

Findings

2-9. The clinical course of HDCTs is highly variable and can be impacted not only by the disease-specific manifestations of each unique syndrome, but also by individuals' physical and mental secondary impairments, as well as environmental factors and physical and psychological demands.
2-10. The severity of HDCTs is linked to the severity of affected individuals' physical and mental secondary impairments, including the combined effects of multiple impairments, as well as the frequency, severity, and predictability of their fluctuations.
3-1. Marfan syndrome (MFS), Loeys-Dietz syndrome (LDS), congenital contractural arachnodactyly (CCA; also known as Beals-Hecht syndrome), and Sphrintzen-Goldberg syndrome (SGS) affect multiple body systems, often with cardiovascular, skeletal, and ocular manifestations.
3-3. Many manifestations of hereditary aortopathies worsen over time, with some not appearing until adulthood.
3-6. As the life spans of patients with these syndromes increase with improvements in management of previously fatal complications (e.g., aortic rupture, spontaneous pneumothorax), concurrent increases are seen in the occurrence and severity of age-related secondary impairments.

continued

**BOX 6-1
Continued**

3-7. Hereditary aortopathies can affect individuals' everyday physical and mental functioning, often impacting multiple body systems. MFS frequently manifests in cardiovascular, nervous, respiratory, musculoskeletal, and ocular system impairments. LDS and CCA manifest particularly in cardiovascular, cerebrovascular, respiratory, musculoskeletal, craniofacial, ocular, and neurological impairments. SGS manifests in developmental delays and intellectual disability, as well as impairments associated with the other hereditary aortopathies.

3-8. Pregnancy can be a high-risk condition in some individuals with hereditary aortopathies.

4-1. The Ehlers-Danlos syndromes (EDS) are a group of multisystem, heritable disorders of connective tissue (HDCTs) that share common elements of joint hypermobility and skin and soft tissue involvement. Hypermobility spectrum disorders (HSD) are multisystem connective tissue disorders that are clinically similar to hypermobile EDS (hEDS) with respect to their manifestations and management.

4-3. EDS/HSD can manifest in physical and mental secondary impairments in any organ system and often in multiple organ systems in a given individual.

4-4. The type and severity of physical and mental manifestations associated with EDS/HSD often vary both among individuals and throughout an affected individual's lifetime. Epidemiologic evidence supports multi–organ system manifestations, high treatment burden, and high disease burden.

4-13. EDS/HSD can affect individuals' everyday physical and mental functioning, particularly as a result of limitations associated with pain, fatigue, and anxiety.

4-14. Secondary impairments in any of the body systems can be severe and affect the functioning of individuals with EDS/HSD.

4-15. Physical and mental secondary impairments associated with EDS/HSD often manifest or worsen during puberty, especially in females. Males with vascular EDS (vEDS) are at higher risk for complications during puberty.

4-16. Pregnancy can be a high-risk condition in some individuals with EDS; women with vEDS have an increased risk of uterine rupture or peripartum hemorrhage.

5-1. The number, type, and severity of the physical and mental secondary impairments experienced by an individual with a heritable disorder of connective tissue (HDCT) drive the person's functioning and potential disability.

5-3. Both physical and mental conditions can precipitate or exacerbate decrements in physical and mental functioning in individuals with HDCTs.

5-4. Chronic pain, chronic fatigue, and mild cognitive impairment are some of the most common and potentially disabling manifestations of the Ehlers-Danlos syndromes (EDS), especially hypermobile EDS (hEDS), hypermobility spectrum disorders (HSD), and Marfan syndrome (MFS).

5-6. Pain can interfere with all types of physical activities that may be entailed in work or school, including sedentary activities. Pain also has an effect on cognitive functioning.

5-7. Fatigue associated with EDS and MFS can result in a number of physical and mental functional impairments that affect daily activities, including participation in work and physical activities.

5-8. Mild cognitive impairment can adversely affect participation in school, work, and social activities.

5-13. Physical activity guidelines and restrictions for individuals with HDCTs need to be tailored to the specific person.

5-14. General physical activity guidelines exist for people with MFS and related disorders, such as avoidance of intense isometric exercise, contact sports that can lead to blows to the head, activities that involve rapid acceleration and deceleration over short distances (sprinting) or rapid changes in pressure (e.g., scuba diving), and exercise to the point of exhaustion.

5-17. Individuals with HDCTs may experience significant variability in their physical and/or mental secondary impairments from day to day or even within a single day. This variability is often unpredictable and may limit the ability to sustain gainful employment.

Conclusions

3-1. MFS and related hereditary aortopathies have multiple physical and mental manifestations that, which individually or in combination, can cause functional limitations of varying severity. Some manifestations may become apparent only with age, and the severity of manifestations may, and often does, progress with age. Treatment can be successful in reducing impairments in selected cases.

4-1. EDS and HSD have multiple clinical manifestations that, individually or in combination, can cause functional limitations of varying severity. Some manifestations may become apparent only with age, and the types and severity of manifestations may vary throughout an affected individual's lifetime.

5-1. Given that individuals with HDCTs typically experience physical and mental secondary impairments in multiple body systems, it is important to assess the collective effect of all their physical and mental impairments on their ability to function in daily life, including at work and in school.

3. Early diagnosis of HDCTs is important to reduce physical injury, reduce psychological harm to the individual and family members, and prevent the risks associated with inappropriate or fragmented medical care.

Findings

2-9. The clinical course of HDCTs is highly variable and can be impacted not only by the disease-specific manifestations of each unique syndrome, but also by individuals' physical and mental secondary impairments, as well as environmental factors and physical and psychological demands.

2-10. The severity of HDCTs is linked to the severity of affected individuals' physical and mental secondary impairments, including the combined effects of multiple impairments, as well as the frequency, severity, and predictability of their fluctuations.

continued

**BOX 6-1
Continued**

5-1. The number, type, and severity of the physical and mental secondary impairments experienced by an individual with an HDCT drive the person's functioning and potential disability.

5-9. A challenge in assessment of functioning is capturing the full effect of individuals' impairments on their daily activities, including at work and in school. This is particularly true when a person has multiple impairments.

5-10. Numerous validated performance-based and self-reported measures are available for assessing physical and mental functioning, including several that can be used to perform an integrated assessment of an individual's overall physical and mental functioning.

5-16. Some of the listings in SSA's Listing of Impairments—Adult Listings include severity criteria for some of the secondary impairments that may be experienced by individuals with HDCTs such as MFS, EDS, and related disorders.

5-17. Individuals with HDCTs may experience significant variability in their physical and/or mental secondary impairments from day to day or even within a single day. This variability is often unpredictable and may limit the ability to sustain gainful employment.

Conclusions

5-2. Accurately assessing the full effect of an individual's impairment(s) is especially important for SSA disability determinations. This is particularly true when a person has multiple impairments that individually do not rise to the level of severity required by SSA but collectively may do so. The concept of functional equivalence used by SSA in some disability determinations in children is particularly well suited to evaluating the combined effects on an applicant's functioning of the many and varied impairments that often manifest in HDCTs and other multisystem disorders.

5-5. Some of SSA's Listing of Impairments—Adult Listings apply directly to secondary impairments experienced by individuals with HDCT syndromes and could be used to evaluate disability in those individuals. Other listings, with some modification, could apply to individuals with certain secondary impairments associated with their HDCTs.

5-6. The combined effects of an individual's physical and/or mental secondary impairments may limit function with a degree of severity sufficient to preclude the ability to participate in work on a "regular and continuing basis" (8 hours per day, 5 days per week, or an equivalent work schedule) or, for children, to cause "marked and severe functional limitations."

4. **Although curative treatments for HDCTs do not exist at this time, appropriate understanding and management of the disorders can reduce the frequency and severity of their manifestations and resulting functional consequences. High-quality care for individuals with HDCTs relies on effective coordination among a team of clinicians across a broad range of physical and mental health care disciplines who are knowledgeable about these disorders.**

Findings

2-9. The clinical course of HDCTs is highly variable and can be impacted not only by the disease-specific manifestations of each unique syndrome, but also by individuals' physical and mental secondary impairments, as well as environmental factors and physical and psychological demands.

3-4. No curative treatments currently exist for MFS, LDS, CCA, SGS, or other hereditary aortopathies. Management of these disorders involves early diagnosis and aggressive monitoring and treatment of manifestations in multiple organ systems, including treatment of associated physical and mental secondary impairments present at the time of identification and measures to reduce or prevent problems that may occur with age.

4-8. There are currently no curative treatments for EDS or HSD. Management of the disorders involves early diagnosis and recognition; monitoring; and treatment of the manifestations in multiple organ systems, including treatment of associated physical and mental secondary impairments present at the time of identification and preventive measures to lessen or prevent problems that may develop over time.

4-12. Delayed diagnosis may result in a lack of or inappropriate management that may exacerbate physical and mental manifestations of EDS/HSD. Unanticipated risks and harms may attend routine procedures and therapies that carry EDS/HSD-specific risks, such as tissue fragility and physiologic reactivity resulting from autonomic and immune dysregulation.

4-13. EDS/HSD can affect individuals' everyday physical and mental functioning, particularly as a result of limitations associated with pain, fatigue, and anxiety.

4-14. Secondary impairments in any of the body systems can be severe and affect the functioning of individuals with EDS/HSD.

4-15. Physical and mental secondary impairments associated with EDS/HSD often manifest or worsen during puberty, especially in females. Males with vEDS are at higher risk for complications during puberty.

4-17. Following trauma or surgery, individuals with versus those without EDS/HSD often have a worse trajectory in terms of both length of recovery and frequency of complications.

Conclusions

2-2. Early diagnosis of HDCTs is important to reduce physical injury, reduce psychological harm to affected individuals and their family members, and prevent the risks associated with inappropriate medical care.

2-3. Appropriate multisystem assessments are important at the time of HDCT diagnosis and at intervals across a person's life.

2-4. Appropriate multidisciplinary understanding and management of HDCTs can reduce the frequency and severity of their manifestations and resulting functional limitations.

continued

**BOX 6-1
Continued**

3-2. Management of MFS and related hereditary aortopathies requires a multidisciplinary approach and involves early diagnosis of the multisystem findings associated with these syndromes, treatment of associated physical and mental secondary impairments, and measures to reduce or prevent problems that may present with aging.

4-2. Development of a screening tool to identify EDS/HSD could provide timely diagnosis of the disorder and help mitigate the negative effects of delayed diagnosis and EDS/HSD-specific risks that may attend routine procedures and therapies.

4-3. Management EDS/HDS requires a multidisciplinary approach and involves early diagnosis of the multisystem findings, treatment of associated physical and mental secondary impairments, and measures to reduce or prevent problems that may present over time.

4-6. Health care providers need to be aware of the EDS/HSD-specific risks that may attend routine procedures and therapies.

5. Access to comprehensive, multidisciplinary care for the diagnosis and management of HDCTs can be limited by geography and other factors, including the availability of care teams with expertise in the disorders.

Findings

2-6. HDCTs are lifelong disorders for which no curative treatments currently exist. Management involves supportive care, treatment of associated secondary impairments, and preventive measures to mitigate or prevent problems that may occur or worsen over time.

2-9. The clinical course of HDCTs is highly variable and can be impacted not only by the disease-specific manifestations of each unique syndrome, but also by individuals' physical and mental secondary impairments, as well as environmental factors and physical and psychological demands.

3-4. No curative treatments currently exist for MFS, LDS, CCA, SGS, or other hereditary aortopathies. Management of these disorders involves early diagnosis and aggressive monitoring and treatment of manifestations in multiple organ systems, including treatment of associated physical and mental secondary impairments present at the time of identification and measures to reduce or prevent problems that may occur with age.

3-5. Management of MFS and related hereditary aortopathies is lifelong and involves specialists across multiple physical and mental health disciplines.

4-8. There are currently no curative treatments for EDS or HSD. Management of the disorders involves early diagnosis and recognition; monitoring; and treatment of the manifestations in multiple organ systems, including treatment of associated physical and mental secondary impairments present at the time of identification and preventive measures to lessen or prevent problems that may develop over time.

4-10. Individuals with vEDS have a decreased life expectancy, with a median survival age of 46 for males and 54 for females.

4-12. Delayed diagnosis may result in a lack of or inappropriate management that may exacerbate physical and mental manifestations of EDS/HSD. Unanticipated risks and harms may attend routine procedures and therapies that carry EDS/HSD-specific risks, such as tissue fragility and physiologic reactivity resulting from autonomic and immune dysregulation.

4-13. EDS/HSD can affect individuals' everyday physical and mental functioning, particularly as a result of limitations associated with pain, fatigue, and anxiety.

4-14. Secondary impairments in any of the body systems can be severe and affect the functioning of individuals with EDS/HSD.

4-17. Following trauma or surgery, individuals with versus those without EDS/HSD often have a worse trajectory in terms of both length of recovery and frequency of complications.

Conclusions

2-1. Consideration of a diagnosis of an HDCT is warranted for individuals who present with previously undiagnosed complex multisystem disorders.

2-2. Early diagnosis of HDCTs is important to reduce physical injury, reduce psychological harm to affected individuals and their family members, and prevent the risks associated with inappropriate medical care.

2-3. Appropriate multisystem assessments are important at the time of HDCT diagnosis and at intervals across a person's life.

2-4. Appropriate multidisciplinary understanding and management of HDCTs can reduce the frequency and severity of their manifestations and resulting functional limitations.

3-1. MFS and related hereditary aortopathies have multiple physical and mental manifestations that, individually or in combination, can cause functional limitations of varying severity. Some manifestations may become apparent only with age, and the severity of manifestations may, and often does, progress with age. Treatment can be successful in reducing impairments in selected cases.

3-2. Management of MFS and related hereditary aortopathies requires a multidisciplinary approach and involves early diagnosis of the multisystem findings associated with these syndromes, treatment of associated physical and mental secondary impairments, and measures to reduce or prevent problems that may present with aging.

4-2. Development of a screening tool to identify EDS/HSD could provide timely diagnosis of the disorder and help mitigate the negative effects of delayed diagnosis and EDS/HSD-specific risks that may attend routine procedures and therapies.

4-3. Management of EDS/HSD requires a multidisciplinary approach and involves early diagnosis of the multisystem findings, treatment of associated physical and mental secondary impairments, and measures to reduce or prevent problems that may present over time.

4-6. Health care providers need to be aware of the EDS/HSD-specific risks that may attend routine procedures and therapies.

continued

**BOX 6-1
Continued**

6. Education about HDCTs, including their multisystem manifestations, diagnosis, and management, is important for all clinicians to help increase recognition and earlier diagnosis of the disorders and enable the provision of appropriate care.

Findings

2-1. Heritable disorders of connective tissue (HDCTs) are a heterogeneous group of inherited disorders that affect connective tissues in organ systems throughout the body.

2-2. Connective tissues are an integral component of every organ system and play a crucial role in the function of those systems. Hence, the physical and mental secondary impairments associated with HDCTs, which may develop and potentially progress or wax and wane over time, manifest throughout the body and affect functioning in every body system.

2-4. Because HDCTs can cause a wide variety of physical and mental secondary impairments involving multiple organ systems, affected individuals often are referred to a succession of different specialists, resulting in delayed diagnosis of the underlying HDCT.

2-6. HDCTs are lifelong disorders for which no curative treatments currently exist. Management involves supportive care, treatment of associated secondary impairments, and preventive measures to mitigate or prevent problems that may occur or worsen over time.

3-5. Management of MFS and related hereditary aortopathies is lifelong and involves specialists across multiple physical and mental health disciplines.

4-1. The Ehlers-Danlos syndromes (EDS) are a group of multisystem, heritable disorders of connective tissue (HDCTs) that share common elements of joint hypermobility and skin, and soft tissue involvement. Hypermobility spectrum disorders (HSD) are HDCTs that are clinically similar to hypermobile EDS (hEDS) with respect to their manifestations and management.

4-11. Diagnosis and management of EDS and HSD involve specialists across multiple physical and mental health disciplines.

Conclusions

2-3. Appropriate multisystem assessments are important at the time of HDCT diagnosis and at intervals across a person's life.

2-4. Appropriate multidisciplinary understanding and management of HDCTs can reduce the frequency and severity of their manifestations and resulting functional limitations.

3-2. Management of MFS and related hereditary aortopathies requires a multidisciplinary approach and involves early diagnosis of the multisystem findings associated with these syndromes, treatment of associated physical and mental secondary impairments, and measures to reduce or prevent problems that may present with aging.

4-3. Management EDS/HDS requires a multidisciplinary approach and involves early diagnosis of the multisystem findings, treatment of associated physical and mental secondary impairments, and measures to reduce or prevent problems that may present over time.

7. **Education of individuals with the disorders and their families, as well as employers and school staff, is important to improve the quality of life for affected individuals and their families, to facilitate appropriate accommodations at work and school, and to help inform the disability assessment and determination process.**

Findings

2-3. HDCTs can be difficult to diagnose, and the true prevalence of many of these disorders is unknown.

2-4. Because HDCTs can cause a wide variety of physical and mental secondary impairments involving multiple organ systems, affected individuals often are referred to a succession of different specialists, resulting in delayed diagnosis of the underlying HDCT.

2-5. HDCTs are diagnosed through a combination of clinical findings and established clinical criteria, followed by confirmatory molecular genetic testing when specific genes have been identified for the suspected disorder.

2.7 Individuals with HDCTs often experience difficulty with obtaining appropriate and integrated multidisciplinary care to address the wide range of physical and mental impairments associated with these disorders.

2-8. Access to comprehensive, multidisciplinary care for the diagnosis and management of HDCTs can be limited by geography and other factors, including the availability of care teams with expertise in the disorders.

3-5. Management of MFS and related hereditary aortopathies is lifelong and involves specialists across multiple physical and mental health disciplines.

4-7. Diagnosis of hEDS and HSD is based solely on clinical criteria, since neither has a known genetic test. Understanding of and diagnostic criteria for hEDS and HSD continue to evolve.

4-11. Diagnosis and management of EDS and HSD involve specialists across multiple physical and mental health disciplines.

Conclusion

2-4. Appropriate multidisciplinary understanding and management of HDCTs can reduce the frequency and severity of their manifestations and resulting functional limitations.

8. **Ongoing research on HDCTs is important to advance understanding of the disorders and their effects. In particular, research on care services and interventions for HDCTs and secondary impairments is needed, including**

continued

**BOX 6-1
Continued**

- more specific diagnostic criteria and biomarkers;
- functional and biomeasures of severity;
- effective treatment for HDCTs and management of their physical and mental manifestations, including comparative treatment trials;
- the clinical course of the disorders throughout the lifetime of affected individuals;
- the impact of relevant reasonable accommodations on affected individuals' ability to participate in work and school; and
- benefits versus risks of participation in common childhood activities (e.g., contact sports, gymnastics, dance).

Findings

2-3. HDCTs can be difficult to diagnose, and the true prevalence of many of these disorders is unknown.

2-5. HDCTs are diagnosed through a combination of clinical findings and established clinical criteria, followed by confirmatory molecular genetic testing when specific genes have been identified for the suspected disorder.

2-6. HDCTs are lifelong disorders for which no curative treatments currently exist. Management involves supportive care, treatment of associated secondary impairments, and preventive measures to mitigate or prevent problems that may occur or worsen over time.

3-4. No curative treatments currently exist for MFS, LDS, CCA, SGS, or other hereditary aortopathies. Management of these disorders involves early diagnosis and aggressive monitoring and treatment of manifestations in multiple organ systems, including treatment of associated physical and mental secondary impairments present at the time of identification and measures to reduce or prevent problems that may occur with age.

4-5. The pathophysiologic relationship between EDS/HSD and many of their manifestations and comorbid conditions are unclear, and the evidence linking them is primarily associative.

4-6. Diagnosis of EDS/HSD is based on established clinical criteria, and most, though not all, types can be confirmed through genetic testing.

4-7. Diagnosis of hEDS and HSD is based solely on clinical criteria, since neither has a known genetic test. Understanding of and diagnostic criteria for hEDS and HSD continue to evolve.

4-8. There are currently no curative treatments for EDS or HSD. Management of the disorders involves early diagnosis and recognition; monitoring; and treatment of the manifestations in multiple organ systems, including treatment of associated physical and mental secondary impairments present at the time of identification and preventive measures to lessen or prevent problems that may develop over time.

4-9. The prognosis and clinical course of EDS/HSD depend on individual patient factors, which vary greatly among affected individuals and are often related to the severity of disease-associated physical and mental secondary impairments, as well as the EDS/HSD type.

5-5. A complex relationship exists among pain, fatigue, postural orthostatic tachycardia syndrome, and mast cell activation disease.

Conclusions

4-2. Development of a screening tool to identify EDS/HSD could provide timely diagnosis of the disorder and help mitigate the negative effects of delayed diagnosis and EDS/HSD-specific risks that may attend routine procedures and therapies.

4-4. More research is needed on the pathophysiological mechanisms of EDS/HSD and their comorbid conditions and the implications for appropriate management and outcomes of the many secondary impairments associated with EDS/HSD.

4-5. Longitudinal studies of individuals with different types of EDS/HSD would increase understanding of the clinical course of the disorders; their effects on physical and mental functioning; and potentially the impact of interventions, including reasonable accommodations, on participation in work and school.

4-6. Health care providers need to be aware of the EDS/HSD-specific risks that may attend routine procedures and therapies.

Appendix A

Public Session Agendas

MEETING 2: PUBLIC SESSION
Hosted by the Committee on Selected Heritable Disorders of Connective Tissue and Disability
May 11, 2021
Virtual via Zoom

Agenda
Public Session I
10:05–11:15 p.m. Eastern Daylight Time

10:05 a.m.	**Welcome and Introductions** *Paul Volberding, Committee Chair* *Steven Rollins, Deputy Associate Commissioner, Office of Disability Policy, SSA*
10:10 a.m.	**Social Security Administration Presentations Relevant to the Committee's Task** *Andrea Bento, Policy Analyst, Office of Medical Policy/ Office of Disability Policy, SSA*
10:30 a.m.	**Questions and Discussion**
11:15 a.m.	**Adjourn Public Session I**

Public Session II
12:15–2:00 p.m. Eastern Daylight Time

12:15 p.m.   **Gastrointestinal Conditions in Heritable Disorders of Connective Tissue**
Laura A. Pace, M.D., Ph.D.
Center for Genomic Medicine
University of Utah

12:30 p.m.   **Questions and Discussion**

12:50 p.m.   **Orthostatic Intolerance in Heritable Disorders of Connective Tissue**
Peter C. Rowe, M.D.
Director, Children's Center Chronic Fatigue Clinic
Sunshine Natural Wellbeing Foundation Professor and
    Professor of Pediatrics
Johns Hopkins Children's Center

1:05 p.m.   **Questions and Discussion**

1:25 p.m.   **Mental Health Conditions Associated with Heritable Disorders of Connective Tissue**
Antonio Bulbena-Vilarrasa, M.D., Ph.D., M.Sc. (Cantab)
Distinguished Professor of Psychiatry
Chair, Department of Psychiatry and Forensic Medicine
Universitat Autònoma de Barcelona

1:40 p.m.   **Questions and Discussion**

2:00 p.m.   **Adjourn Public Session II**

MEETING 3: PUBLIC SESSION

Hosted by the Committee on Selected Heritable
Disorders of Connective Tissue and Disability
July 9, 2021
Virtual via Zoom

Agenda
10:15–11:15 a.m. Eastern Daylight Time

10:15 a.m.	**Welcome and Introductions** *Paul Volberding, Committee Chair* *Steven Rollins, Deputy Associate Commissioner, Office of Disability Policy, SSA*
10:20 a.m.	**Panel Discussion: Perspectives on Living with Heritable Disorders of Connective Tissue** *Maggie Buckely, M.B.A., B.C.P.A., Patient Advocate* *Jon Rodis, M.B.A., National Disability and Medical Advocate for Rare Disorders* *Alissa Zingman, M.D., MPH, Founder and CEO of P.R.I.S.M.*
10:45 a.m.	**Questions and Discussion**
11:15 a.m.	**Adjourn**

Appendix B

Commissioned Paper

THE FUNCTIONAL IMPACT OF ORTHOSTATIC
INTOLERANCE IN EHLERS-DANLOS SYNDROME

Peter C. Rowe, M.D.
Professor of Pediatrics; Sunshine Natural Wellbeing Foundation Professor of Chronic Fatigue and Related Disorders; Director, Chronic Fatigue Clinic, Johns Hopkins Children's Center
Department of Pediatrics, Johns Hopkins University School of Medicine, Baltimore, MD, USA

Prepared for the National Academies of Sciences, Engineering, and Medicine's Committee on Selected Heritable Disorders of Connective Tissue and Disability

Correspondence: Dr. Peter C. Rowe, Division of Adolescent/Young Adult Medicine, 200 N Wolfe St, Room 2077, Baltimore, MD, USA 21287; TEL: 410-955-9229, FAX: 410-614-1178. prowe@jhmi.edu

INTRODUCTION

This manuscript addresses the impact of orthostatic intolerance on overall function in those with heritable connective tissue disorders, primarily Ehlers-Danlos syndrome (EDS) and hypermobility spectrum disorders. After discussing the symptoms, physiology, and diagnostic testing for the common forms of orthostatic intolerance, we describe the association between orthostatic intolerance and other disabling conditions, including heritable disorders of connective tissues. We then review the therapeutic measures to attenuate the impact of circulatory dysfunction on daily activities for affected children and adults, moving on to discuss the determinants of the ability to work or attend school. We present some of the techniques for measuring work- and school-related function in those with orthostatic intolerance, and interventions, procedures, and accommodations to mitigate the impact of orthostatic intolerance. Research has identified a strong relationship between joint hypermobility/EDS, orthostatic intolerance, and myalgic encephalomyelitis/chronic fatigue syndrome (ME/CFS) (Barron et al., 2022; De Wandele et al., 2014a,b; Roma et al., 2018b; Rowe et al., 1999). As a result, we will draw on observations from the ME/CFS literature to inform the discussion of treatment and accommodations in the heritable disorders of connective tissue.

ORTHOSTATIC INTOLERANCE: SYMPTOMS, PHYSIOLOGY, DIAGNOSIS

Orthostatic intolerance refers to a heterogeneous group of circulatory disorders in which individuals develop symptoms upon assuming and maintaining upright posture, improving (although not necessarily resolving completely) after they return to a recumbent posture (Gerrity et al., 2002–2003; Low et al., 2009). Hemodynamic abnormalities in orthostatic intolerance can include classical or delayed orthostatic hypotension, neurally mediated hypotension (NMH), and postural tachycardia syndrome (POTS) (Freeman et al., 2011; Goldstein et al., 2002; Low et al., 2009; Rosen and Cryer, 1982; Schondorf and Low, 1993; Sheldon et al., 2015; Stewart et al., 2018). More recently it has become evident that a relatively large proportion of individuals with orthostatic intolerance lack these abnormal heart rate and blood pressure responses to upright posture, but have substantial reductions in brain blood flow when upright (van Campen et al., 2020a).

The most common symptoms of chronic orthostatic intolerance are shown in Table B-1. These clinical features are largely due to two principal physiological changes in response to orthostatic stress: (1) reduced cerebral blood flow and (2) the compensatory adrenergic response to reduced cerebral blood flow (Low et al., 2009). Many of the symptoms in Table B-1 overlap with features seen in EDS, including fatigue, cognitive problems, headaches, exercise intolerance, and anxiety. Patients with orthostatic intolerance can experience lengthy delays before diagnosis, and thus a similarly lengthy delay in initiating therapy. For example, one large survey of POTS patients identified a median diagnostic delay of 24 months (Shaw et al., 2019). Orthostatic intolerance syndromes are relevant for those with connective tissue laxity because treatment of their circulatory conditions

APPENDIX B

TABLE B-1
Symptoms of Orthostatic Intolerance

Due to ↓ CBF	Due (largely) to the Hyperadrenergic Response to ↓ CBF
Lightheadedness	Dyspnea
Syncope	Chest discomfort
Diminished concentration	Palpitations
Headache	Tremulousness
Blurred vision	Anxiety
Fatigue	Diaphoresis
Exercise intolerance	Nausea

NOTE: CBF = cerebral blood flow.

is often associated with amelioration of symptoms and improved overall function.

Some symptoms of orthostatic intolerance, such as lightheadedness, improve promptly on lying down. Once provoked, other symptoms, such as fatigue and brain fog, can persist for hours to days. The initial papers by Sir Thomas Lewis on vasovagal syncope in the 1920s described a soldier who had fainted, had a clear vasovagal reaction to venipuncture, and was fatigued and tremulous for the next 36 hours (Lewis, 1932), indicating a debt of fatigue persisting after the individual had assumed a recumbent posture. While the mechanism for the protracted symptoms is unclear, such an episode establishes the potential for recurrent orthostatic stress in daily life to be associated with chronic symptoms.

Physiologic Responses to Upright Posture

For adults, the assumption of an upright posture is associated with a gravitational redistribution of approximately 500–1000 mL of blood to the dependent vasculature (Smit et al., 1999; Smith et al., 1994). Adolescents are thought to experience a similar change. In response to the gravitational pooling, less blood returns to the heart, which leads to a decrease in cardiac output, reduced stretching of baroreceptors, and ultimately a reduction in blood flow to the brain. The vasomotor center in the brain stem responds by increasing sympathetic neural outflow and by reducing vagal tone. These changes lead to improved vasoconstriction and as much as a 30–40 beats-per-minute (bpm) increase in heart rate, returning sufficient venous blood

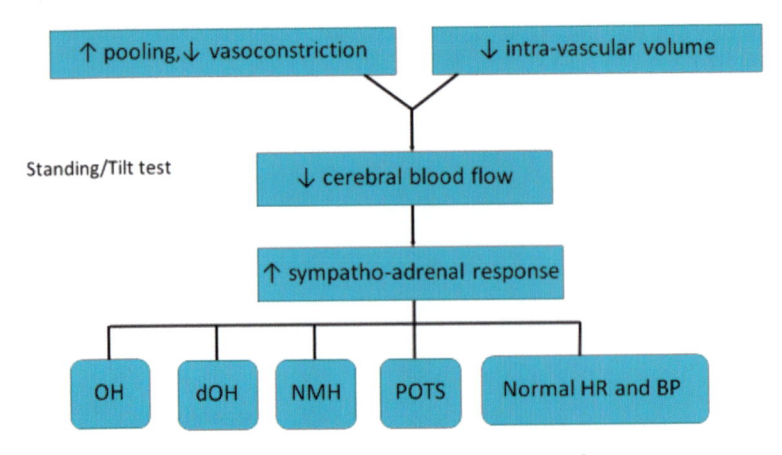

FIGURE B-1 Pathophysiologic factors in orthostatic intolerance.
NOTE: BP = blood pressure; dOH = delayed orthostatic hypotension; HR = heart rate; NMH = neurally mediated hypotension; OH = orthostatic hypotension; POTS = postural tachycardia syndrome.

to maintain blood pressure and cerebral perfusion (Medow et al., 2008; Rowell, 1992; Wieling and Shepherd, 1992).

Figure B-1 illustrates the principal physiological contributors to orthostatic intolerance—namely, excessive gravitational pooling of blood, often related to a defect in vasoconstriction; low blood volume; and an increased sympathetic nervous system and adrenal catecholamine response to the orthostatic reduction in cerebral blood flow. Pathophysiologic contributors to decreased vasoconstriction and increased peripheral pooling of blood include the duration of quiet upright posture, increased compliance of the blood vessel wall in response to hydrostatic pressure, the presence of venous varicosities, obstruction to venous return, and vasodilating substances.

Low blood volume has been observed in a variety of conditions of orthostatic intolerance, including POTS and ME/CFS (Hurwitz et al., 2010; Okamoto et al., 2012; Streeten and Bell, 1998); although, because of its high cost, the measurement of blood volume using nuclear medicine techniques is not readily available outside of research settings. Low blood volume has been associated with lower renin-to-aldosterone ratios and with reductions in antidiuretic hormone (Okamoto et al., 2012; Wyller et al., 2010). Decreased plasma volume, which can result from physical inactivity, can exacerbate symptoms of orthostatic intolerance and interfere further with daily function (Fortney et al., 1996; Takenaka et al., 2002). When individuals who have increased peripheral pooling of blood and/or low blood volume assume an upright posture, they experience a greater decrease in the return of blood to the heart and a markedly increased catecholamine response (Benditt et al., 2003; Rosen and Cryer, 1982).

Goldstein and colleagues (2003) have proposed that the relative balance of epinephrine to norepinephrine can influence the pattern of circulatory response. Individuals with POTS have higher norepinephrine levels, likely related to norepinephrine-mediated vasoconstriction, thereby helping to maintain blood pressure longer, while contributing to the heart rate stimulation that defines POTS. In contrast, those with recurrent neurally mediated syncope have higher epinephrine levels during tilt, in part related to epinephrine's vasodilatory effect on the skeletal muscle vasculature, and resultant hypotension. These two conditions, however, are not mutually exclusive, as patients who develop POTS during the first 10 minutes upright can develop NMH as the orthostatic stress becomes more prolonged, usually 5–59 minutes after the initial orthostatic tachycardia (Kanjwal et al., 2011; Rowe et al., 2001; Sandroni et al., 1996).

Forms of Orthostatic Intolerance

Orthostatic Hypotension

Classical orthostatic hypotension (cOH) requires a sustained reduction in blood pressure of at least 20 mm Hg systolic or 10 mm Hg diastolic during the first 3 minutes after assuming an upright posture (Freeman et al., 2011). This condition is more common in older adults, especially those with comorbid diabetes mellitus or Parkinson's disease (Freeman et al., 2018). While less common in children, cOH can be identified in pediatric patients during febrile illnesses, with voluntary or involuntary fluid and caloric restriction, excessive histamine release, adrenal insufficiency, hemorrhage, or as a response to certain medications. Delayed orthostatic hypotension (dOH) is defined by the same changes in blood pressure as cOH, but occurs after the first 3 minutes upright (Freeman et al., 2011).

Postural Tachycardia Syndrome

Increasingly recognized as a common form of orthostatic intolerance in those with EDS, POTS is more common in females than males; is more common after than before the onset of puberty; and often follows an apparent infectious illness, immunization, trauma, or surgery (Fedorowski, 2019; Grubb, 2008; Vernino et al., 2021). POTS should only be diagnosed (1) in the presence of an increase in heart rate of ≥ 30 bpm in adults (≥ 40 bpm in those under age 20) from lowest supine to peak standing over the first 10 minutes upright, and (2) in the absence of orthostatic hypotension in the first 3 minutes upright. Some have suggested a heart rate of >120 bpm during the first 10 minutes upright as an additional criterion (Fedorowski, 2019). Approximately 40 percent of healthy adolescents would be misclassified as having POTS using the adult heart rate increment of 30 bpm (Singer et al., 2012). At all ages, the diagnosis of POTS is based on more than just the heart rate and also requires the individual to have chronic orthostatic symptoms. Heart rate elevation alone is insufficient for a diagnosis of POTS in individuals who are dehydrated or are being treated with vasodilating medications. Conversely, at the time of orthostatic testing, concurrent consumption of substances that increase plasma volume, such as salt tablets, or agents used to treat orthostatic intolerance (e.g., serotonin reuptake inhibitors, oral contraceptives, stimulant medications, beta adrenergic antagonists, or other medications) can obscure the diagnosis of POTS.

Inappropriate Sinus Tachycardia

As the name suggests, this condition is diagnosed when the patient is in sinus rhythm, but has a heart rate higher than 100 bpm at rest. Symptoms of inappropriate sinus tachycardia are similar to those in POTS (Sheldon et al., 2015).

Neurally Mediated Hypotension

NMH is a reflex form of hypotension, and while its physiology is synonymous with vasovagal syncope or neurocardiogenic syncope (Bou-Holaigah et al., 1995; Grubb, 2005; Rowe et al., 1995), NMH is a more accurate description of the phenotype. Many with NMH experience the same characteristically abrupt drop in blood pressure during tilt testing as those with vasovagal syncope, and they can experience chronic daily orthostatic symptoms *without* having completely lost consciousness. In both children and adults, NMH occurs after the 3-minute cutoff for orthostatic hypotension and is characterized by at least a 25 mm Hg reduction in systolic blood pressure. At the time of presyncope or hypotension, affected individuals can develop a relative slowing of the heart rate that can progress to junctional bradycardia or even asystole. This disorder can be identified during standing, but more commonly requires prolonged period (> 10 minutes) of upright tilt-table testing, which typically provokes characteristic orthostatic symptoms (Wieling et al., 2004). When orthostatic testing lasts less than 10 minutes, this form of hypotension can be missed (Bou-Holaigah et al., 1995). NMH is more common in females than in males and in younger adults and adolescents than in older people; often, the family history is positive (Grubb, 2005).

As has been reviewed elsewhere (Grubb, 2005; Jhanjee et al., 2009; van Dijk et al., 2021; van Lieshout et al., 1991; Wieling et al., 2004), the pathophysiology of NMH involves reduced venous return, which then initiates a series of neural responses that result in withdrawal of sympathetic tone and a relatively unopposed vagal response. These responses lead to slowing of the heart rate and vasodilation, which can result ultimately in a profound drop in blood pressure or syncope if the individual remains upright. Markedly elevated epinephrine levels are present prior to syncope (Benditt et al., 2003; Jardine et al., 1997). Precipitating factors for NHM can include prolonged standing; warm environments (such as hot weather, hot showers, or hot tubs); pain; venipuncture; the sight of blood; or sudden stretching of mechanoreceptors in the gastrointestinal tract, bladder, and lungs. These phenomena can occur individually or in combination (Grubb, 2005; Jhanjee et al., 2009; van Lieshout et al., 1991; Wieling et al., 2004). Although many patients with NMH experience only isolated episodes of syncope that are separated by long periods of normal function, NMH physiology can be associated with chronic, daily orthostatic symptoms. Patients referred for evaluation of recurrent syncope report chronic fatigue, as well as impaired quality of life (Kenney and Graham, 2001; Legge et al., 2008; Rose et al., 2000). Among patients evaluated for chronic orthostatic intolerance, approximately 25 percent have neurocardiogenic syncope without POTS (Goldstein et al., 2005). Thus, POTS cannot be regarded as the only form of chronic orthostatic intolerance.

Low Orthostatic Tolerance

This condition is characterized by the presence of frequent orthostatic symptoms without the heart rate and blood pressure changes that characterize OH, NMH, or POTS (IOM, 2015). Recent research has shown that many of these patients have reductions in cerebral blood flow as measured either by transcranial Doppler ultrasound (which measures cerebral blood flow velocity) or by Doppler ultrasound of the internal carotids and vertebral arteries, which measures total blood flow to the brain (Novak, 2018; van Campen et al., 2020a).

Testing for Orthostatic Intolerance

There is no gold standard test for orthostatic intolerance, but head-up tilt table tests and standing tests are the primary types of testing used in clinical practice. The methods for conducting each type of test vary. We do not know all the pathophysiological contributors to such symptoms as lightheadedness, and some classical "orthostatic" symptoms can be reproduced by postural maneuvers, such as passive straight leg raising, that do not involve upright posture (Rowe et al., 2016).

Head-Up Tilt Table Testing

Modern head-up tilt table testing is conducted using a motorized table with a footboard for weight-bearing (Benditt et al., 1996). The test begins with the patient lying supine and loosely restrained by belts that prevent injury if loss of consciousness ensues. In our center, the period of supine rest lasts 15 minutes, but some investigators have positioned patients supine for up to 60 minutes. Next, the tilt table is gradually raised to a 60–70 degree angle. Higher tilt table angles during testing can provoke syncope more readily in healthy controls. Depending on which form of orthostatic intolerance is being evaluated, the duration of upright tilt can vary between institutions. Ten minutes of upright posture is sufficient to detect OH and POTS, but upright tilt for 45–60 minutes is often required for detection of dOH and NMH.

A variety of methodological factors can affect tilt response (Benditt et al., 1996; Moya et al., 2009; Sheldon, 2005), including the pretest sodium intake, the duration of the pretest fast, the ambient temperature in the laboratory, the time of day for the study, and whether the patient is permitted to remain on medications that have hemodynamic effects. Test factors can include the degree of patient movement permitted, whether there is invasive instrumentation (higher rates of syncope can be seen if arterial catheters are placed), the use of pharmacologic agents to provoke hypotension (e.g., isoproterenol [Natale et al., 1995], nitroglycerine), and the way an abnormal test is defined. Past studies often required reproduction of syncope as the end-point of testing. However, OH, POTS, and NMH can be identified before syncope occurs, and the table can be returned to the horizontal position.

In most laboratories, heart rate and blood pressure are monitored using beat-to-beat measurements, although in some centers only intermittent blood pressure measurements are made, for example, every 1–2 minutes for 5–10 minutes, then every 5 minutes unless presyncopal symptoms are identified. Measurement of end-tidal CO_2 for detecting orthostatic hypocapnia is a helpful adjunctive technique (Naschitz et al., 2000; Natelson et al., 2007; Novak, 2018; Razumovsky et al., 2003; van Campen et al., 2020a). During both supine and upright phases, at approximately 5-minute intervals, patients are asked to rate changes in symptoms on a 0–10 scale (lightheadedness, fatigue, headache, mental fogginess, warmth, shortness of breath, nausea, and pain).

Head-up tilt testing is not necessary in all individuals with orthostatic symptoms. Among those in whom the clinical history is consistent with reflex or neurally mediated syncope, and the heart is structurally normal, head-up tilt testing is no longer thought to be necessary for diagnosis (Benditt et al., 1996; Moya et al., 2009; Sheldon, 2005; Strickberger et al.,

2006). Among the most impaired individuals with ME/CFS or EDS, upright tilt can provoke postexertional exacerbation in symptoms during and for at least a week after the tilt test (van Campen et al., 2021b). In the most impaired individuals, brief orthostatic vital signs obtained in supine, seated, and standing positions over 1–3 minutes in some instances, or a 20-degree tilt angle, are sufficient as an indication of orthostatic intolerance. In those who have symptoms provoked during the tilt testing, and who might be at risk for postexertional malaise in the following days, our experience is that this symptom flare can be ameliorated by administration of 1–2 L of warmed normal saline immediately after the end of the period upright (IOM, 2015).

Standing Tests

Two closely related forms of standing tests are used in the orthostatic intolerance literature: active standing (Plash et al., 2013; Streeten et al., 2000) and passive standing, in which the individual leans against a wall (Hyatt et al., 1975; Roma et al., 2018a). Standing tests can be conducted in a clinical office, and thus are cheaper and more readily available than tilt table tests. No specialist consultation or specialized equipment is required. The period of supine rest before standing varies between studies, but in most instances a consistent baseline heart rate and blood pressure can be obtained within 5–15 minutes. Although the duration of upright posture can be as long as 60 minutes (Streeten et al., 2000), most centers perform a 10-minute standing test to identify POTS and to ascertain worsening symptoms during orthostasis. As with 10-minute tilt testing, this duration of standing will miss many instances of dOH and NMH. Symptoms are recorded immediately before standing and at intervals of 1–2 minutes when upright. Some studies during the COVID-19 pandemic have been conducted at home, but it is important that the test be witnessed given the potential for injury to occur if individuals have a rapid onset of syncope. We discourage the postural counter-maneuvers that can improve venous return to the heart during quiet standing (e.g., fidgeting, shifting weight, and contracting the leg muscles). While helpful in day-to-day life, these constitute partial treatment during the diagnostic test. Box B-1 provides the instructions and reporting form for conducting the passive standing test used in the Johns Hopkins Chronic Fatigue Clinic.

Few investigations have compared the available orthostatic testing methods. Among the studies that have compared tilt testing and active standing, none have examined prolonged upright posture (Hyatt et al., 1975; Plash et al., 2013). During the first 5 minutes upright, similar heart rate changes occur during active standing and tilt testing (Hyatt et al., 1975). Beyond the first 5 minutes, however, passive tilt provokes a larger

BOX B-1
Methods and Reporting Form for the Passive Standing Test

PASSIVE STANDING TEST:

The following is a modification of the passive standing test (Hyatt et al., 1975) that has been used in the Chronic Fatigue Clinic at Johns Hopkins Hospital since the mid-1990s.

The standing test begins with the subject lying supine, with an automated blood pressure (BP) cuff set to record BP and heart rate (HR) at 1-minute intervals. The subject is supine for 5 minutes. The baseline HR and BP are measured and recorded each minute for 5 minutes supine. At the 4–5 minute point, record the intensity of the patient's current symptoms (on a 0–10 scale).

The patient is then instructed to stand, with the heels 2–6 inches away from the wall, and with the upper back leaning against the wall in a comfortable but **motionless position** for a maximum of 10 minutes. Each minute, HR and BP are recorded and the patient is asked about symptoms, for a maximum of 10 minutes upright. At the conclusion of the standing period, the patient is instructed to lie supine again, while the BP, HR, and symptom intensity are measured for a further 2 minutes.

Specific instructions are as follows:

> "We'd like you to stand as still as possible for up to 10 minutes. During the standing test you must be as motionless as possible in order to get an accurate result. Therefore, try not to wiggle your toes or fingers, scratch your nose, or move your arms or legs. We will monitor for any movements and will remind you not to move or wiggle. We want you to tell us if you are feeling anything different or uncomfortable during the test. Be as specific as possible. **We need to know if you feel you can't stay standing any longer, and if this is the case you can sit down.** It is not necessary to remain standing for the entire 10 minutes, but we'd like to measure how long you can do this. Each minute we will check your blood pressure and heart rate with an automatic measuring device."

COMMENTS: If the subject reports any changes in symptoms, list these in the comments column of the Standing Test Data Sheet (see below), corresponding to the time recorded for the BP and HR. Also note if and when the subject had to sit down before the completion of 10 minutes upright and mention whether the BP was performed sitting or while still standing.

DEFINITIONS:

<u>Postural tachycardia syndrome (POTS):</u> an increase in heart rate of at least 30 beats per minute (bpm) in adults or at least 40 bpm in adolescents (ages 12–19) from the lowest supine value to the maximum heart rate during the 10 minutes of standing, in the absence of orthostatic hypotension. POTS requires the presence of chronic orthostatic symptoms—including lightheadedness, visual blurring or dimming, fatigue, exercise intolerance, headaches, cognitive difficulties (problems with concentration and memory, often termed "brain fog"), shortness of breath, chest pain, and nausea—and these are often reproduced during the standing test.

The increment in heart rate should be calculated from the lowest HR supine (either pre- or posttest, provided the patient has not had syncope or presyncope) and the peak HR standing.

<u>Classical orthostatic hypotension (cOH):</u> a reduction in systolic BP of ≥ 20 mm or in diastolic BP ≥ 10 mm in the first 3 minutes.

<u>Delayed orthostatic hypotension (dOH):</u> a reduction in systolic BP of ≥ 20 mm or in diastolic BP ≥ 10 mm after the first 3 minutes.

<u>Neurally mediated hypotension (NMH):</u> at least a 25 mm Hg decrease in systolic BP from baseline supine values, with no associated increase in heart rate, together with the emergence of presyncopal symptoms.

Low orthostatic tolerance: the presence of prominent orthostatic symptoms without the heart rate and blood pressure changes that characterize cOH, dOH, NMH, or POTS.

Modified from Freeman et al., 2011 and Bou-Holaigah et al., 1995.

continued

**BOX B-1
Continued**

STANDING TEST DATA SHEET

Name: _____ Date of Test: _____

Medications in last 2 weeks: _____

_____

	Heart Rate	Blood Pressure	Comments/Symptom ratings
SUPINE			
1 min			
2 min			
3 min			
4 min			
5 min			
STANDING			
1 min			

change in heart rate in those with POTS than does active standing (Plash et al., 2013). While application of lower-body negative pressure with the patients in a supine position can approximate the physiology of upright testing, it is usually only used in research settings (Wyller et al., 2008). While perhaps desirable in clinical settings for patient flow, shorter periods of passive standing or head-up tilt will miss diagnosing a proportion of those who meet POTS criteria after 10 minutes of testing; therefore, a full 10-minute period upright is recommended (Roma et al., 2018a).

2 min				
3 min				
4 min				
5 min				
6 min				
7 min				
8 min				
9 min				
10 min				
SUPINE				
1 min				
2 min				

Abbreviations:

ACRO = acrocyanosis, **COG** = cognitive difficulties, **FTG** = fatigue, **HA** = headache, **HOT** = warmth/hot flash, **LH** = lightheadedness, **NAU** = nausea, **PALL** = pallor, **PN** = muscle pain/ache, **SOB** = trouble breathing, **SW** = sweating.

ASSOCIATION OF ORTHOSTATIC INTOLERANCE WITH OTHER DISABLING CONDITIONS

Myalgic Encephalomyelitis/Chronic Fatigue Syndrome

Among those with ME/CFS or the related condition fibromyalgia, orthostatic stress consistently provokes fatigue and other symptoms (IOM, 2015; Martinez-Lavin, 2006; van Campen et al., 2020a). In pediatric ME/CFS, rates of orthostatic intolerance exceed 96 percent of affected participants (IOM, 2015; Stewart et al., 1999). Differences in cardiovascular responses between ME/CFS patients and healthy controls can be detected with as little as 20 degrees of upright stress (van Campen 2020c; Wyller et al., 2007). In our experience, approximately 50–60 percent of those meeting criteria for pediatric ME/CFS also meet criteria for joint hypermobility, defined in those studies as a Beighton score of at least 4 (Barron et al., 2002; Roma et al., 2019). In adults with ME/CFS, past studies reported a variable prevalence of orthostatic intolerance.

Combining 14 controlled studies evaluated in a 2015 review of the evidence by the Institute of Medicine (IOM, 2015), 484 adults with ME/CFS had been evaluated with orthostatic stress tests lasting more than 10 minutes. Of these, 202 (42 percent) developed hypotension during the test, compared with 15 percent among healthy controls. The percentage of abnormalities across studies varied markedly, from 0 to 96 percent, suggesting wide variability in testing methods and patient selection (IOM, 2015).

More recently, van Campen and colleagues (2018) demonstrated that total cerebral blood inflow could be measured reliably using a Doppler technique that captures flow through each internal carotid and each vertebral artery, with image acquisition for the four vessels taking approximately 3 minutes. Adding the flows through each of the four vessels (necessary in part because of unilateral vessel dominance in some patients) provides a measure of total cerebral blood flow (van Campen et al., 2018). Based on reductions of cerebral blood flow >2 standard deviations from the mean reduction of 7 percent seen in controls between supine and 30 minutes upright, a > 13 percent reduction of cerebral blood flow is defined as abnormal.

Applying the same Doppler technology to measure cerebral blood flow during tilt testing in adults with ME/CFS, van Campen and colleagues (2020a) studied 429 adults with ME/CFS and 44 healthy controls. In response to 30 minutes of head-up tilt table testing, 247 (58 percent) of the ME/CFS participants had a normal heart rate and blood pressure response, as did all of the healthy controls, while 62 (14 percent) with ME/CFS developed dOH and 120 (28 percent) met criteria for POTS (van Campen et al., 2020a). This study was unable to evaluate those with neurally mediated syncope because the blood pressure drop was too rapid to allow for 3 minutes of image acquisition. Figure B-2 shows the percent reduction in cerebral blood flow from the supine values at mid-tilt and end-tilt: healthy individuals experienced a 7 percent reduction in brain blood flow compared with a 26 percent reduction in the ME/CFS patients overall. In subgroups of ME/CFS, those with dOH had a 28 percent reduction, and those with POTS had a 29 percent reduction. Importantly, among the 58 percent with a normal hemodynamic response (no dOH or POTS)—who in the absence of the Doppler measures might have been diagnosed as having nothing wrong—there was a 24 percent reduction in cerebral blood flow, representing over a three-fold greater reduction in brain blood flow than the

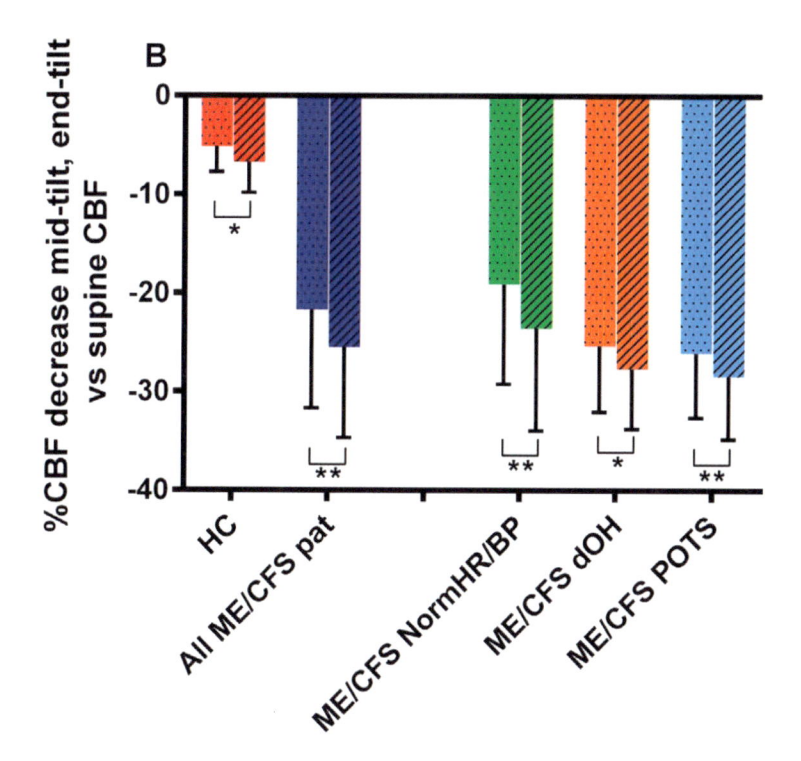

FIGURE B-2 Changes in cerebral blood flow during 30 minutes of head-up tilt compared to supine values in 44 healthy controls and 429 adults with ME/CFS. The dotted column is mid-tilt and the hatched column is end-tilt.
NOTE: BP = blood pressure; CBF = cerebral blood flow; dOH = delayed orthostatic hypotension; HC = healthy controls; HR = heart rate; ME/CFS = myalgic encephalomyelitis/chronic fatigue syndrome; POTS = postural tachycardia syndrome.
SOURCE: van Campen et al., 2020a. This work is licensed under the Creative Commons Attribution-NonCommercial-NoDerivatives 4.0 International License. To view a copy of this license, visit http://creativecommons.org/licenses/by-nc-nd/4.0.

healthy controls. In total, 90 percent of adults with ME/CFS experienced a significant reduction in cerebral blood flow (van Campen et al., 2020a). There was a significant correlation between summed orthostatic symptoms and the degree of cerebral blood flow reduction at mid-tilt. The implication from this study is that limiting the diagnosis of orthostatic intolerance to heart rate and blood pressure abnormalities has the potential to misdiagnose the majority of people who have a clinically significant drop in cerebral blood flow. This novel method of confirming orthostatic intolerance by measuring cerebral blood flow has yet to be adopted widely, but it appears to be a more sensitive measure for diagnosis in a variety of patient groups.

In subsequent work, van Campen and colleagues (2020b) have shown that sitting can provoke a clinically important reduction in cerebral blood flow. This has implications for workplace accommodations for those with heritable disorders of connective tissue. In a study of 100 adults with ME/CFS who had severe functional impairment (mostly bed-bound or dependent on others for daily care), cerebral blood flow was similar to that of the 15 healthy controls when tested in a supine position. However, when tested in a seated position, these patients with ME/CFS developed a 24.5 percent reduction in cerebral blood flow compared with a 0.4 percent reduction in healthy controls (van Campen et al., 2020b). Similarly, a separate study of 19 patients severely affected by ME/CFS, all of whom met the criteria for an abnormal cerebral blood flow reduction, a shorter 15-minute tilt test with a reduced 20-degree head-up tilt angle was capable of provoking a significant (27 percent) decline in cerebral blood flow (van Campen et al., 2020c).

Ehlers-Danlos Syndrome

Chronic fatigue is a prevalent symptom and an important determinant of impaired health-related quality of life in EDS (Rombaut et al., 2010). The association between EDS, chronic fatigue syndrome, and orthostatic intolerance was first described in 1999 (Rowe et al., 1999). Over a 1-year period, 12 of 100 consecutively tested adolescents with chronic fatigue syndrome also met criteria for EDS. The median Beighton score was 7 (range, 5–9), and all 12 patients reported joint dislocations, 3 of whom had undergone joint surgery. Genetic and ophthalmologic consultations confirmed that 6 patients satisfied the criteria at the time for classical EDS and 6 satisfied the criteria for hypermobile EDS. All 12 experienced an increase in their usual symptoms during the first 10 minutes of orthostatic testing, and 10 met the criteria for POTS. Of the 12 patients with chronic fatigue syndrome, 9 developed NMH either alone or in combination with POTS. In these 12, their EDS had not been recognized despite a median of 37 months (range, 12–62 months) of fatigue beforehand (Rowe et al., 1999).

Given the overlap among EDS, orthostatic intolerance, and ME/CFS, Barron and colleagues (2002) compared the prevalence of nonsyndromic joint hypermobility in adolescents with ME/CFS and in healthy controls. The ME/CFS group had a 60 percent prevalence of Beighton scores ≥ 4, compared with 24 percent of healthy adolescents ($P < .001$), a rate similar to that reported in other studies of healthy individuals at the same age. The odds ratio for having joint hypermobility if participants had ME/CFS was 3.5 (95% confidence interval [CI], 1.6–7.5; $P < .001$) (Barron et al., 2002). This study provided further corroboration of an association between orthostatic intolerance and joint hypermobility.

De Wandele and colleagues (2014a) performed the largest and most comprehensive study of the association between autonomic dysfunction and heritable disorders of connective tissue. In a convenience sample of 80 patients with hypermobile EDS (hEDS), 11 patients with classical EDS, 7 patients with vascular EDS, and 43 healthy controls (n = 43), 94 percent of those with hEDS reported symptoms of orthostatic intolerance (De Wandele et al., 2014a). Their burden of autonomic symptoms was also higher than that of the other EDS groups and the controls.

De Wandele and colleagues (2014b) also conducted comprehensive autonomic testing on 39 female adults with hEDS and a sex-matched group of 35 similar-aged controls. During head-up tilt testing, the hEDS group developed orthostatic symptoms at an earlier point than the control group. POTS and other forms of orthostatic intolerance were more common in those with hEDS than in controls (41 percent vs. 11 percent for POTS, and 74 percent vs. 34 percent for any form of orthostatic intolerance). Joint hypermobility correlated with a larger heart rate increment and lower blood pressure when upright.

Subsequent work by van Campen and colleagues (2021a) has confirmed that adults who have ME/CFS differ in the degree of cerebral blood flow reduction during orthostatic stress depending on their degree of joint hypermobility. In a case-control study of females matched by age and disease duration, 100 hypermobile ME/CFS patients were compared with 100 patients who had ME/CFS without joint hypermobility. Joint hypermobility was considered to be present if a rheumatologist, geneticist, or rehabilitation specialist had made the diagnosis of either hEDS or joint hypermobility. If patients had not been formally diagnosed with hypermobility, participants were asked whether they were hypermobile or highly flexible, which was then confirmed with a Beighton score. Participants were included in the hypermobility group if the Beighton score was 6 or higher. During tilt testing, those with joint hypermobility were significantly more likely to develop POTS than the nonhypermobile patients and had a significantly larger reduction in cerebral blood flow. As shown in Figure B-3, cerebral blood flow fell by 32 percent in the hypermobile patients compared with 23 percent in those without hypermobility ($P < .0001$), regardless of whether the hemodynamic phenotype involved POTS or was characterized by a normal heart rate and blood pressure response (van Campen et al., 2021a). The larger cerebral blood flow reduction is consistent with the hypothesis that increased blood vessel laxity contributes to increased gravitational pooling of blood in the presence of higher hydrostatic pressure below the heart during upright posture (Barron et al., 2002; Rowe et al., 1999).

Accurate prevalence estimates for orthostatic intolerance among those with EDS are not available, as there have been no population-based studies that have employed measures to evaluate for joint hypermobility or EDS

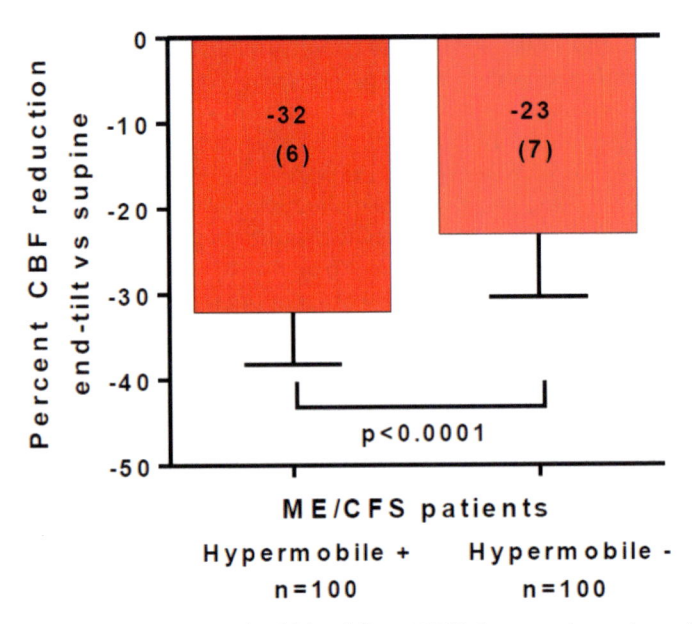

FIGURE B-3 Reductions in cerebral blood flow (CBF) from supine values after 30 minutes of head-up tilt in 100 hypermobile and 100 nonhypermobile adults with myalgic encephalomyelitis/chronic fatigue syndrome (ME/CFS).
SOURCE: Reproduced from van Campen et al., 2021a.

in which all participants have undergone consistent orthostatic testing. In clinic-based reports, which have varying degrees of referral bias, between 41 and 100 percent of people with joint hypermobility or EDS endorse symptoms of orthostatic intolerance on a regular basis (Roma et al., 2018b). The studies with the highest prevalence involve more complete ascertainment of orthostatic symptoms (see, e.g., De Wandele et al, 2014a). Similarly, heart rate and blood pressure abnormalities can be identified in 56–80 percent of joint hypermobility patients; the higher prevalence rates are reported in studies with more prolonged orthostatic testing (Roma et al., 2018b).

TREATMENT OF ORTHOSTATIC INTOLERANCE

While the treatment of orthostatic intolerance begins with nonpharmacologic interventions, in our experience, most individuals with more than mild functional impairments will require medications. Pharmacologic treatment has the potential to ameliorate the impact of orthostatic intolerance, but improvements are not automatic or universally effective.

Nonpharmacologic Measures

Nonpharmacologic treatment for orthostatic intolerance is focused in four main areas. Individuals need to (1) avoid conditions that increase dependent pooling of blood, (2) avoid depletion of salt and water and other causes of low blood volume, (3) use techniques to improve venous return to the heart, and (4) avoid situations that further increase catecholamines.

Avoid conditions that increase dependent pooling of blood

Patients are advised to avoid prolonged sitting by obtaining permission to move around during classroom lectures or longer meetings, and by standing and stretching periodically when seated at a desk. Similarly, they are advised to avoid long lines (e.g., by shopping at nonpeak times, obtaining permission to preboard when traveling). In the home setting, patients can take short, cooler baths and showers; avoid hot tubs and saunas; and avoid sunbathing. Many prefer to study in a horizontal position that reduces gravitational pooling of blood in the legs, and improves brain blood flow. Because large meals and high carbohydrate intake can contribute to a shift of blood volume to the splanchnic circulation, patients often fare better with frequent, smaller meals.

Avoid depletion of salt and water

Adolescents and adults with orthostatic intolerance need to drink 2–3 L of fluid daily, drinking fluids every 1–2 hours during the day. Adequate sodium intake helps retain fluids in the intravascular space, but no specific amount of sodium works for each individual. We recommend salting food according to taste, adding buffered salt tablets if needed, and supplementing with oral rehydration fluids. Among those with orthostatic intolerance, higher-sodium food options include olives, dill pickles, soups, tomato juice, salted nuts, soy sauce, and salsa. An important accommodation needed at school or work is access to salty snacks and fluids throughout the day.

Improve venous return to the heart

Without necessarily understanding why, many individuals with orthostatic intolerance have already adopted postural countermaneuvers that utilize the muscle pump function of the lower limbs to improve venous return. Examples include standing with the legs crossed, shifting weight while standing from one leg to the other, sitting with the knees to the chest, or performing leg muscle contraction exercises before standing (Smit et al., 1997; van Lieshout et al., 1992). Wearing heeled shoes or boots can promote increased calf muscle contraction. We advise against sitting on a high stool with the legs dangling freely, as that position provides no resistance to blood pooling in the legs. Positioning the knees higher than the hips improves afterload and tolerance of sitting. Examples include sitting in a low chair (Smit et al., 1997), resting the feet on a low foot rest, or sitting with one or both legs folded under the buttocks.

Compression garments of various types can be helpful. Waist-high stockings are more effective for compression than are thigh-high, which in turn are more effective than knee-high (Bourne et al., 2021; Heyer, 2014; van Campen et al., 2022). We usually recommend support hose with 20–30 mm Hg compression. While stockings with 30–40 mm Hg compression provide a greater effect, they can be difficult and somewhat impractical to get off and on. For those with joint hypermobility, the effort required to pull up 30–40 mm Hg compression stockings has the potential to cause hand and wrist pain or subluxation; therefore, we usually recommend avoiding this level of compression in the hypermobile population. Some prefer wearing abdominal binders or body shaper garments, both of which can reduce excessive pooling in the splanchnic beds. An older method of improving blood volume is to elevate the bed frame by 10–15 degrees so that the head is higher than the feet. While this is not comfortable for everyone, and theoretically could reduce brain blood flow in severely impaired patients, in those who tolerate the head-up position, it is thought to help by reducing urine formation and retaining more vascular volume fluid at night (MacLean and Allen, 1940; van Lieshout et al., 2000).

Many medications and supplements have the potential to increase vasodilation, including niacin, narcotic analgesics, phenothiazine antiemetics, and antipsychotic medications. Their use may need to be minimized or avoided. Low doses of tricyclic antidepressants can occasionally aggravate hypotension. This class of medications is not absolutely contraindicated, as tricyclic antidepressants are often tolerated and are useful in this population for management of headaches, pain, mast cell activation, and insomnia.

Avoid increasing catecholamines

Catecholamine levels are increased in those with orthostatic intolerance and worsen with upright posture. Because physiological stressors, including pain and emotional distress, can elevate catecholamine levels even higher, stress avoidance can help with symptom management.

It is important to screen for medications that have the potential to increase catecholamines and thereby aggravate orthostatic symptoms. For example, in patients with comorbid asthma, beta-adrenergic agonists (e.g., albuterol) can mimic the effects of epinephrine and contribute to lightheadedness and tremulousness. Caffeine intake (including in coffee or soft drinks) can help symptoms by acting as a vasoconstrictor, but some patients experience adverse effects, such as excessive stimulation or diuretic effects.

Treatment of Other ME/CFS Symptoms and Comorbid Conditions

The second step in managing orthostatic intolerance is to treat other comorbid conditions. This includes managing migraine headaches, allergies, mast cell activation syndrome, anxiety, depression, menstrual dysfunction, and areas of biomechanical dysfunction with physical therapy or osteopathic manual therapy (Rowe, 2016). Temporomandibular joint dysfunction and neurogenic thoracic outlet syndrome are common conditions among those with joint hypermobility and EDS, and are important comorbidities to treat. Patients therefore need permission to miss school or work without penalty in order to incorporate appointments and treatments into their weekly schedule.

Pharmacologic Interventions

The third step in managing orthostatic intolerance is to initiate pharmacologic therapy. While ideally we attempt to identify a single effective medication, rational polytherapy (using medications that have different mechanisms of action) is often required for optimal symptom control. Medications should be introduced one at a time in most instances, starting at low doses and increasing gradually.

Commonly used medications for orthostatic intolerance are listed in Table B-2 by their general mechanism of action (Rowe et al., 2017). Some physicians recommend either a low-dose beta blocker or midodrine as the first-line agent in those with POTS (Johnson et al., 2010). Often, however, the specifics of the patient's condition and existing comorbidities allow an individualized approach. For example, fludrocortisone might be a good first choice if the patient has a relatively low resting blood pressure for age or an increased desire for salt. Beta blockers would need to be used with caution in those with asthma, but would be a reasonable first choice for those with elevated resting heart rates or headaches. Midodrine is an effective treatment for recurrent syncope, but dosing in 4-hour increments makes it less convenient for students to take when in school. Stimulants such as methylphenidate or dextroamphetamine and others can be helpful in as vasoconstrictors, and can help with fatigue and cognitive symptoms. Pyridostigmine bromide can help with gastrointestinal motility as well as with orthostatic intolerance.

Adolescent and young adult females with acne, excessive menstrual blood loss, dysmenorrhea, or perimenstrual exacerbation of orthostatic intolerance symptoms can benefit from hormonal contraceptive therapy

TABLE B-2
Medications for Orthostatic Intolerance

Medication	Usual Adolescent Dose	Comments/Indications
Vasoconstrictors		
Midodrine	2.5 mg every 4 hours while awake. Increase every 3–7 days by 2.5 mg until an optimal dose is achieved. Max 10 mg every 4 hours while awake.	Suggested as first-line therapy for those with baseline hypotension.
Stimulants		
Methylphenidate	Immediate-release form: 5–10 mg BID, increasing gradually to 15–40 mg/day. Sustained-release form: start with 10 mg once daily and increase gradually until an optimal effect is found.	Suggested as first-line therapy for those with prominent cognitive dysfunction or a personal or family history of attention deficit hyperactivity disorder. Common adverse effects can include reduced appetite, insomnia, and agitation.
Dextroamphet-amine	Sustained-release form: 5–10 mg in the morning. Increase by 5–10 mg weekly. Max 15–40 mg daily.	
Volume Expanders		
Sodium chloride	Oral: 1 g tablets with meals. IV: 1–2 L over 1–2 hours.	Oral supplements not always sufficient as the only therapy. IV normal saline is impractical over the longer term but can help restore baseline function after acute infections or as rescue therapy.
Fludrocortisone	0.05 mg daily for 1 week, then 0.1 mg daily. Increase gradually to max of 0.2 mg daily.	Suggested as first-line therapy for those with baseline hypotension or increased salt appetite. Potassium supplementation is recommended to prevent hypokalemia, as fludrocortisone increases urinary potassium losses. Can aggravate acne.
Hormonal contraceptives	Most are fine. Conventional dosage or continuous pills for 84 days (one period every 3 months).	Indicated for females with dysmenorrhea or when fatigue and lightheadedness worsen with menses.

TABLE B-2
Continued

Medication	Usual Adolescent Dose	Comments/Indications
Desmopressin acetate	0.1 mg at bedtime, increasing to 0.2 mg daily.	Suggested for those with nocturia. Hyponatremia can occur.
Sympathetic Tone and Heart Rate Modifiers		
Pyridostigmine bromide	Rapid release: 30 mg daily, increase by 30 mg every 3-7 days to 60 mg BID or TID. Sustained-release: 180 mg daily.	Effective in POTS and neurally mediated hypotension. Also helpful for gastrointestinal motility problems.
Clonidine	0.05 mg at bedtime. Increase after 1 week to 0.1 mg nightly. Occasionally higher doses are tolerated.	Suggested for those with anxiety, problems with attention, hyperhidrosis, or insomnia.
Ivabradine	Start with 2.5 mg BID. Max 10 mg BID.	Suggested for those with elevated baseline heart rate.
Beta adrenergic antagonists		
Atenolol	12.5-25 mg daily, increase by 12.5 mg increments until optimal effect. Usual dose is 25-50 mg. Doses above 1 mg/kg often aggravate fatigue and lightheadedness, so lower doses are usually better tolerated.	Suggested as first-line therapy for those with a relatively elevated resting heart rate, anxiety, or headache. Can exacerbate asthma. Contraindicated for diabetics.
Propranolol	0.5-1 mg/kg body weight 10-20 mg 3-4 times daily.	
SSRI/SNRI		
Sertraline	25-100 mg daily.	Indicated for dysthymia, depression, or anxiety.
Escitalopram	5 mg daily for 2-4 weeks, increase to 10 mg daily up to max of 40 mg daily.	
Duloxetine	20-30 mg daily for 2 weeks, increase to max of 60-90 mg daily.	Useful if myalgias are prominent.

NOTE: BID = twice daily; POTS = postural tachycardia syndrome; TID = three times daily.
SOURCE: Modified from Rowe et al., 2017. This work is licensed under the Attribution 4.0 International License. To view a copy of this license, visit http://creativecommons.org/licenses/by/4.0.

(Boehm et al., 1997). Women whose orthostatic symptoms are aggravated in the perimenstrual period often fare better when treated with continuously active hormonal regimens that induce one menstrual period every 90 days or more. The mechanism by which hormonal contraceptives improve orthostatic symptoms is not entirely clear.

Even in nondepressed patients with NMH refractory to other therapies, selective serotonin reuptake inhibitors (SSRIs) can lead to improvements in orthostatic symptoms (Grubb et al., 1994). Duloxetine (a serotonin and norepinephrine reuptake inhibitor [SNRI]) has been shown in randomized trials to be effective in fibromyalgia (Arnold et al., 2004) and has the potential to be effective for pain, independent of its effect on mood. The SSRI and SNRI medications might also be attractive initial options when symptoms such as anxiety, pain, dysthymia, or premenstrual syndrome are present.

Concurrent use of medications with different mechanisms of action (e.g., a mineralocorticoid, a beta blocker, and a vasoconstrictor) is sometimes necessary in managing severe orthostatic intolerance. Among patients whose orthostatic symptoms are relatively refractory to treatment, it is important to examine whether a comorbid condition is contributing to difficulty in obtaining relief. One example would be instability of the cervical spine, which can be associated with frequent syncope and presyncope that improves after surgical stabilization (Henderson et al., 2021), although the prevalence of this abnormality and the optimal methods of selecting patients for surgery need to be studied.

Intravenous Saline

In some individuals with orthostatic intolerance for whom medications have provided insufficient relief, periodic intravenous infusions of normal saline have helped (Burklow et al., 1999; Moak et al., 2016; Ruzieh et al., 2017). IV saline infusions can be used as "rescue therapy" when orthostatic symptoms become more intense (such as after an infection) or to allow tolerance of an important personal or family event. Because most adolescents and adults with orthostatic intolerance have a lower blood volume, our experience has been that they can withstand a rapid infusion of 2 L of normal saline over 1–2 hours. Infusions improve autonomic tone, tolerance of upright tilt (Burklow et al., 1999), and a more rapid restoration of intravascular volume than is possible orally. We recommend peripheral IV catheters where possible, as these can be removed at the end of the infusion. Placement of peripherally inserted central catheters (PICCs) or central lines increases the risk of thrombosis, local infection, or bacteremia (Moak et al., 2016), so placing an indwelling catheter must be undertaken only when more conservative and safer measures have been exhausted, and after demonstration that the IV fluids improve quality of life and function.

Ivabradine

A variety of medications can be used to combat the vasoconstriction defect, improve blood volume, or affect the release or impact of catecholamines. Ivabradine is a newer medication introduced for the treatment of tachycardia in the setting of congestive heart failure (DiFrancesco, 2010). It slows heart rate by selectively blocking specific channels in the sinoatrial node. Selectively blocking these channels can lower heart rate without other important effects on blood pressure and cardiac or autonomic function.

Ivabradine has been used in the treatment of idiopathic sinus tachycardia and postural tachycardia syndrome, as has been demonstrated by several groups. McDonald and colleagues (2011) reported improvement in fatigue and tachycardia in 55 percent of POTS patients treated with ivabradine. Barzilai and Jacob (2015) reported that ivabradine attenuated orthostatic symptoms and heart rate at rest and during tilt table testing. Ivabradine has also been shown to help with sinus tachycardia–related syncope and inappropriate sinus tachycardia (Sutton et al., 2014).

To illustrate the potential use of ivabradine in this context, Table B-3 shows the resting heart rate and the response to exercise in a young adult patient who had mast cell activation, joint hypermobility, and orthostatic intolerance as comorbid features of her ME/CFS. Her resting heart rate was 115 bpm, consistent with inappropriate sinus tachycardia—a form of circulatory dysfunction that overlaps substantially with POTS. When she tried to exercise, as many advise as a *primary* treatment of orthostatic intolerance, just 2 minutes of activity on an elliptical machine caused an elevation in her heart rate to 180 bpm, associated with provocation of a migraine that lasted 2 days. She was provoking postexertional malaise and harming her

TABLE B-3
Response to Ivabradine in a Young Adult with Joint Hypermobility and Inappropriate Sinus Tachycardia

Dose	Resting HR	Exercise HR
0 mg	115	170-180 in 2 min, w/HA
2.5 mg	110	170-180 in 2 min, w/HA
5 mg BID	90	155, no HA
7.5 mg	80	140, no HA
10 mg BID	72	130s with 30-40 minutes on elliptical; no HA

NOTE: BID = twice daily; HA = headache; HR = heart rate.

overall function by trying to perform too much exercise before her circulatory dysfunction had been treated.

For this patient, increases in ivabradine were associated with gradual lowering of her resting heart rate to 72 bpm. With improvement in circulation, she could exercise for 40 minutes on the elliptical with a rise in heart rate to a more normal 130 bpm, no longer associated with provoking a migraine. She is not cured, but her symptoms are well-managed with ivabradine. Each year, she has a 2-week period during which ivabradine treatment is interrupted by her insurance company's insistence that she have the drug reauthorized. Even though this individual is quite fit, she experiences an immediate resumption of tachycardia and exercise intolerance when the ivabradine is withheld. Parenthetically, this young woman is an occupational therapist who has worked for the past 2 years on a hospital COVID-19 ward, helping on the proning team. She is an example of a hypermobile patient who has responded to treatment and is not inexorably consigned to disability.

Some have argued that the main treatment of orthostatic intolerance and ME/CFS needs to rely on graded increases in exercise, and this position often leads physicians to insist that the patient complete a course of graded exercise therapy before medications will be prescribed (Fu and Levine, 2018). This patient's course illustrates the harm that could arise if there is an excessive emphasis of physical exercise alone to treat orthostatic intolerance. In her situation, exercise was possible only *after* the control of her circulatory dysfunction, not the other way around.

DETERMINANTS OF THE ABILITY TO WORK

In examining determinants of the ability to work in those with orthostatic intolerance, important contributors include the overall severity of an individual's self-reported symptoms, the degree to which those symptoms interfere with activities, and the degree to which the individual is able to be upright without symptoms. Often, symptoms of orthostatic intolerance and ME/CFS can be unpredictable from day to day, influenced by the level of activity or the degree of orthostatic and other physiologic stressors in the preceding days, as these can provoke postexertional malaise (PEM). PEM involves an increase in a variety of symptoms (not just fatigue) after people have increased their usually tolerated physical, cognitive, or orthostatic stress. PEM symptoms can include lightheadedness, cognitive dysfunction, headache, sensitivity to sensory stimuli, and generalized pain. Another provocation of PEM is excessive neuromuscular strain (often termed "adverse neural tension") that involves application of an elongation strain to the spinal cord and peripheral nerves, although this is less well-studied than the other stressors (Rowe et al., 2016).

In earlier work among adults, VanNess and colleagues (2010) evaluated 25 females with ME/CFS and 23 sedentary controls after a maximal cardiopulmonary exercise test (duration 5–15 minutes). At 24 hours, 87 percent of healthy controls—but no patients with ME/CFS—reported a full recovery; by 48 hours, the rate of full recovery had reached 100 percent of the controls and only 4 percent of the patients. A full 60 percent of the patients with ME/CFS reported that it took at least 5 days to recover. Common PEM symptoms included fatigue, lightheadedness, pain, and cognitive dysfunction (VanNess et al., 2010).

Objective correlates of these postexertional symptoms have come from a series of studies by Light and colleagues (2012). After patients with ME/CFS and healthy controls completed a 25-minute period of exercise to 70 percent of their maximal predicted heart rate, symptoms were recorded after 8, 24, and 48 hours. Gene expression changes in peripheral blood mononuclear cells were measured at the same time intervals for a series of pain pathway, adrenergic, and immune genes. The healthy controls had minimal symptom and gene-expression changes after exercise. In contrast, patients with ME/CFS had a distinctive increase in gene expression peaking at 24 hours, coinciding with increases in self-reported symptoms. The adrenergic gene expression was eight- to nine-fold higher by 24 hours after exercise. The patterns of gene expression in the adults with ME/CFS were distinct from those of individuals with other fatiguing illnesses, including multiple sclerosis.

Neuropsychological testing after exercise has also shown a significant increase in symptoms for patients with ME/CFS compared with healthy controls. Healthy controls experienced a pre- to postexercise improvement in cognitive performance, contrasting with worsening performance for patients with ME/CFS (LaManca et al., 1998). Functional magnetic resonance imaging (fMRI) has confirmed greater increase in brain activity during a challenging working memory task from pre- to postexercise in several regions for those with ME/CFS compared with controls (Cook et al., 2007).

These postexercise studies are relevant to the understanding of variability in the ability to work among those with EDS and orthostatic intolerance. They provide objective evidence of changes that correlate with self-reported exacerbations in symptoms, helping to explain why individuals might be able to perform a given activity on one day, only to be impaired for days afterwards.

Patients with joint hypermobility and EDS can have other associated comorbid conditions that also contribute to orthostatic intolerance and reduced cerebral blood flow, including pelvic venous insufficiency (pelvic congestion syndrome, ovarian varices, May-Thurner anomaly, and others) (Knuttinen et al., 2021; Sandman et al., 2021), mast cell activation syndrome (Seneviratne et al., 2017), Chiari malformation and various forms of ligamentous instability at the skull base (including atlantoaxial and craniocervical instability) (Henderson et al., 2021; Milhorat et al., 2007), cervical spinal stenosis (Rowe et al., 2018), and obstruction to cerebral venous drainage (Arun et al., 2022), among other conditions. Variability in the symptoms related to these problems contributes to the variability of overall function and ability to work.

MEASURING WORK- AND SCHOOL-RELATED FUNCTION IN THOSE WITH ORTHOSTATIC INTOLERANCE

Overall function in chronic illness is most readily measured by self-reported, health-related quality-of-life questionnaires, such as the SF-36 (36-item Short Form Survey), EuroQoL (European Quality of Life), or PROMIS (Patient-Reported Outcomes Measurement Information System) measures in adults (Cook et al., 2012; EuroQol, 1990; Ware and Sherbourne, 1992). For pediatric patients, the Functional Disability Inventory or Pediatric Quality of Life (PedsQL) instruments are age specific, reach young-adult age ranges, and are capable of distinguishing healthy from chronically ill individuals (Claar and Walker, 2006; Varni et al., 2001; Walker and Greene, 1991). Brief self-reported measures of general or cognitive fatigue include the PedsQL Mutidimensional Fatigue Inventory (MFI), the Wood Mental Fatigue Inventory, and the Fatigue Severity Scale, among others (Krupp et al., 1989; Varni and Limbers, 2008; Wood et al., 1991).

Few studies have compared objective with self-reported measures of physical function. Van Campen and colleagues (2020d) examined the correlation of the physical functioning scale (PFS) of the SF-36, the percent peak VO_2 (volume oxygen) of a cardiopulmonary stress test, and the number of steps per day using an actometer in 99 female ME/CFS patients in whom the three different measures were completed within 3 months (van Campen et al., 2020d). These measures were significantly and positively correlated (PFS vs. % peak VO_2, PFS vs. steps/day, and steps/day vs. % peak VO_2: all $P < .001$). Despite the close correlation, van Campen and colleagues (2020d) emphasize the limitations of relying completely on these measures given a large variation within individual patients on the three measures. For example, when examining individual variability among those who scored at the 30 percent level of the PFS, individual patients had taken between 1,558 and 4,266 steps per day. The number of steps per day varied between 6,277 and 9,641 for those at a PFS of 60 percent, reflecting substantially different levels of function (van Campen and colleagues, 2020d). The same held true in this study for the peak VO_2 on a cardiopulmonary exercise test versus the actigraphy data. The number of steps per day for individual patients ranged between 1,135 and 4,683 at a peak VO_2 between 50 and 60 percent of normal. The researchers concluded that while the SF-36 PFS can distinguish between diseased and nondiseased individuals, it is less useful to define the disability level for individual patients, especially in light of the variation of the number of steps per day for a certain value of the PFS (van Campen et al., 2020d). This is likely to be the case among those with EDS, as function can be affected not only by orthostatic intolerance and fatigue, but also by joint instability and pain.

On neurocognitive tests, while those with ME/CFS usually demonstrate scores at baseline similar to those of healthy controls (Lange et al., 2005), fMRI studies show that they activate more regions of the brain to obtain the same scores (Cockshell and Mathias, 2010). Abnormalities might appear if the testing is repeated after exercise (Cook et al., 2007) or after the addition of orthostatic stress. For example, among pediatric patients with POTS and ME/CFS, the speed and accuracy of responses is similar when assessed in a supine position, but patients with ME/CFS begin to make more errors and have slower response time as the degree of orthostatic stress increases (Ocon et al., 2012). Similarly, after a period of orthostatic stress, adults with ME/CFS can have impairment of cognitive function. When tested 5 minutes after a period of 30 minutes of head-up tilt, compared with pretilt responses, the proportion of correct responses on an N-back test (which measures attention and working memory) drops from 57 to 41 percent ($P < .0001$). The raw reaction time on the test increased from 950 to 1102 msec ($P < .0001$) (van Campen et al., 2020e). One-week after the tilt test, cognitive scores in adults with ME/CFS had not returned to normal (van Campen et al., 2021b).

These studies illustrate the challenges of objective confirmation of physical and cognitive function in those with ME/CFS. Test responses are likely to vary depending on the activity level on a given day and the extent to which PEM is provoked by orthostatic stress on the days before testing. Given the overlaps in physiology and symptoms, these challenges also are likely to apply to those with heritable disorders of connective tissue. As a corollary to the observation that orthostatic intolerance can be present and correlate with self-reported symptoms, even in the absence of objective heart rate and blood pressure responses to upright tilt, caution is needed in relying exclusively on neuropsychological tests, and self-reported symptoms cannot be ignored.

MITIGATING THE IMPACT OF ORTHOSTATIC INTOLERANCE: MODIFICATIONS AND ACCOMMODATIONS AT WORK AND IN SCHOLASTIC SETTINGS

Accommodations are unlikely to allow those with severe orthostatic intolerance to be able to work or attend school. For example, in a study by Henderson and colleagues (2021) on atlantoaxial instability in 20 individuals with EDS or hypermobility spectrum disorder, 9 had multiple episodes of syncope and presyncope weekly, which would create a risk of injury and be incompatible with steady classroom attendance or employment. Surgical stabilization, however, significantly decreased the frequency of syncope and presyncope. If individuals have orthostatic intolerance and are at risk for syncope, it would be unsafe for them to climb, bend, or stand for long periods of time. A cashier or store clerk, for example, would need to perform activities in a seated position.

Similarly, in those satisfying the definition of severe ME/CFS, a 20 degree upright tilt angle lowered cerebral blood flow by 27 percent, almost a four-fold greater reduction than is seen in healthy individuals (van Campen et al., 2020c). It is reasonable to assume that in such individuals, upright sitting at a desk would provoke clinically significant cognitive dysfunction and other symptoms, making work and study impossible.

Because orthostatic symptoms are worse in the morning when blood volume is at its lowest, those with mild to moderate orthostatic intolerance might benefit from a later start to their day. Individuals with moderate orthostatic intolerance, fatigue, and PEM might benefit from a reduction in their workload. For example, some students can attend school on Mondays and Tuesdays, but adding a third consecutive day provokes enough PEM that they miss the next two school days. They often benefit from a planned day off midweek, which allows enough rest and recovery to permit attendance on Thursdays and Fridays, increasing their attendance from 3 to 4 days weekly.

In those with milder orthostatic intolerance, the ability to perform tasks in an upright position can be improved by frequent breaks to provide an ability to get up and move around, which in turn uses the muscles of the limbs to pump pooled blood back to the heart and brain. A variety of postural countermaneuvers when standing or sitting also improves venous return and blood pressure, including standing with the legs crossed, walking rather than standing still, sitting with the knees up to the chest, bending forward, or sitting in lower chairs to allow the knees to be higher than the hips. Hot environments are detrimental to those with orthostatic intolerance, as heat will shift blood from the central circulation to the skin. Patients with heat intolerance usually need to be in an air-conditioned environment.

Because PEM and postinfectious exacerbations in symptoms can be unpredictable, those with orthostatic intolerance need flexible hours and attendance. Because increased physical activity can provoke further PEM, lifting objects too frequently might aggravate fatigue and PEM, especially as the weight of the items increases. These individuals often need elevator access, and some benefit from a place to lie down at work.

CONCLUDING COMMENTS

Orthostatic intolerance is common in individuals with EDS and hypermobility spectrum disorders and can be associated with heterogeneous blood pressure and heart rate responses to orthostatic stress, including POTS, orthostatic hypotension, and NMH. Importantly, as measured by Doppler techniques, orthostatic reductions in cerebral blood flow can be present even in those with a normal heart rate and blood pressure response to upright posture. Prominent orthostatic intolerance symptoms include lightheadedness or syncope, fatigue, exercise intolerance, cognitive dysfunction, and headaches. Management of orthostatic intolerance requires close attention to the factors that provoke symptoms, a willingness to try several medications before achieving a good fit, and a realization that medications often can help manage symptoms but do not necessarily cure orthostatic intolerance. The response to therapy remains less predictable than is desired. Complicating the management of orthostatic intolerance in EDS is the presence of multiple comorbidities. Measuring the ability to work in those with orthostatic intolerance is challenging, given the potential for prolonged upright posture to be followed by unpredictable postexertional increases in symptoms for days afterwards. Orthostatic intolerance can be a substantial contributor to disability, and those with orthostatic intolerance can have comorbid ME/CFS that further limits function. Practitioners' ability to measure the severity of impairments in daily function is limited. Assessment of disability in those with orthostatic intolerance and comorbid hypermobility spectrum disorders cannot ignore self-reported severity of symptoms.

ACKNOWLEDGMENTS

Some of the text for this manuscript was modified using the Creative Commons practices from the following open access publication:

Rowe, P. C., R. A. Underhill, K. J. Friedman, A. Gurwitt, M. S. Medo, M. S. Schwartz, N. Speight, J. Stewart, R. Vallings, and K. Rowe. 2017. Myalgic encephalomyelitis/chronic fatigue syndrome diagnosis and management in young people: A primer. *Frontiers in Pediatrics* 5:121. https://doi.org/10.3389/fped.2017.00121.

The figures and tables were either created by the author (Figure B-1, Box B-1, and Tables B-1 and B-3) or taken from the open access publication above (Table B-2) or from open access publications by the author and his colleagues Linda van Campen and Frans Visser (Figures B-2 and B-3).

REFERENCES

Arnold, L. M., Y. Lu, L. J. Crofford, M. Wohlreich, M. J. Detke, S. Iyengar, and D. J. Goldstein for the Duloxetine Fibromyalgia Trial Group. 2004. A double-blind, multicenter trial comparing duloxetine with placebo in the treatment of fibromyalgia patients with or without major depressive disorder. *Arthritis & Rheumatism* 50(9):2974-2984. https://doi.org/10.1002/art.20485.

Arun, A., M. Amans, N. Higgins, W. Brinjikji, M. Sattur, S. Satti, P. Nakaji, M. Luciano, T. Huisman, A. Moghekar, V. Pereira, R. Meng, K. Fargen, and F. Hui. 2022. A proposed framework for cerebral venous congestion. *Neuroradiology Journal* 35(1):94-111. https://doi.org/10.1177/19714009211029261.

Barron, D. F., B. A. Cohen, M. T. Geraghty, R. Violand, and P. C. Rowe. 2002. Join hypermobility is more common in children with chronic fatigue syndrome than in healthy controls. *Journal of Pediatrics* 141:421-425. https://doi.org/10.1067/mpd.2002.127496.

Barzilai, M., and G. Jacob. 2015. The effect of ivabradine on the heart rate and sympathovagal balance in postural tachycardia syndrome patients. *Rambam Maimonides Medical Journal* 6:e0028. https://doi.org/10.5041/RMMJ.10213.

Benditt, D., D. Ferguson, B. Grubb, W. Kapoor, J. Kugler, B. Lerman, J. Maloney, A. Ravielle, B. Ross, R. Sutton, M. Wolk, and D. Wood. 1996. *Journal of the American College of Cardiology* 28(1):263-275. https://doi.org/10.1016/0735-1097(96)00236-7.

Benditt, D., C. Ermis, B. Padanilam, N. Samniah, and S. Sakagushi. 2003. Catecholamine response during haemodynamically stable upright posture in individuals with and without tilt-table induced vasovagal syncope. *Europace* 5(1):65-70. https://doi.org/10.1053/eupc.2002.0271.

Boehme, K., K. Kip, B. Grubb, and D. Kosinski. 1997. Neurocardiogenic syncope: Response to hormonal therapy. *Pediatrics* 99(44):623-625. https://doi.org/10.1542/peds.99.4.623.

Bou-Holaigah, I., P. Rowe, J. Kan, and H. Calkins. 1995. The relationship between neutrally mediated hypotension and the chronic fatigue syndrome. *Journal of the American Medical Association* 274(12):961-967. https//doi.org/10.1001/jama.1995.03530120053041.

Bourne, K. M., R. S. Sheldon, J. Hall, M. Lloyd, K. Kogut, N. Sheikh, J. Jorge, J. Ng, D. V. Exner, J. V. Tyberg, and S. R. Raj. 2021. Compression garment reduces orthostatic tachycardia and symptoms in patients with postural orthostatic tachycardia syndrome. *Journal of the American College of Cardiology* 77(3):285-296. https://doi.org/10.1016/j.jacc.2020.11.040.

Burklow, T. R., J. P. Moak, J. J. Bailey, and F. T. Makhlouf. 1999. Cardiac syncope: Autonomic modulation after normal saline infusion. *Journal of the American College of Cardiology* 33(7):2059-2066 https://doi.org/10.1016/S0735-1097(99)00133-3.

Claar, R. L., and L. S. Walker. 2006. Functional properties of pediatric pain patients: Psychometric properties of the Functional Disability Inventory. *Pain* 121(1-2):77-84 https://doi.org/10.1016/j.pain.2005.12.002.

Cockshell, S. J., and J. L. Mathias. 2010. Cognitive functioning in chronic fatigue syndrome: A meta-analysis. *Psychological Medicine* 40(8):1253-1567. https://doi.org/10.1017/S0033291709992054.

Cook, D. B., P. J. O'Connor, G. Lange, and J. Steffener. 2007. Functional neuroimaging correlates of mental fatigue induced by cognition among chronic fatigue syndrome patients and controls. *Neuroimage* 36(1):108-122. https://doi.org/10.1016/j.neuroimage.2007.02.033.

Cook, K. F., A. M. Bamer, D. Amtmann, I. R. Molton, and M. P. Jensen. 2012. Six patient-reported outcome measurement information system short form measures have negligible age or diagnosis-related differential item functioning in individuals with disabilities. *Archives of Physical Medicine and Rehabilitation* 93(7):1289-1291 https://doi.org/10.1016/j.apmr.2011.11.022.

De Wandele, I., P. Calders, W. Peersman, S. Rimbaut, T. DeBaker, F. Malfait, A. De Paepe, and L. Rombaut. 2014a. Autonomic symptom burden in the hypermobility type of Ehlers-Danlos syndrome: A comparative study with two other EDS types, fibromyalgia, and healthy controls. *Seminars in Arthritis and Rheumatism* 44(3):353-361. https:///doi.org/10.1016/j.semarthrit.2014.05.013.

De Wandele, I., L. Rombaut, L. Leybaert, P. Van de Borne, T. De Backer, F. Malfait, A. De Paepe, and P. Calders. 2014b. Dysautonomia and its underlying mechanisms in the hypermobility type of Ehlers-Danlos syndrome. *Seminars in Arthritis and Rheumatism* 44(1):93-100. https://doi.org/10.1016/j.semarthrit.2013.12.006.

DiFrancesco, D. 2010. The role of the funny current in pacemaker activity. *Circulation Research* 106(3):434-446. https://doi.org/10.1161/CIRCRESAHA.109.208041.

EuroQol Group. 1990. EuroQol—A new facility for the measurement of health-related quality of life. *Health Policy* 16(3):199-208. https://doi.org/10.1016/0168-8510(90)90421-9.

Fedorowski, A. 2019. Postural orthostatic tachycardia syndrome: Clinical presentation, aetiology and management. *Journal of Internal Medicine* 285(4):352-366. https://doi.org/10.1111/joim.12852.

Fortney, S., V. Schneider, and J. Greenleaf. 1996. The physiology of bed rest. In *Handbook of physiology*, vol. 2, edited by M. Fregley, and C. Blatters. New York: Oxford University Press. Pp. 889-939.

Freeman, R., W. Wieling, F. B. Axelrod, D. G. Benditt, E. Benarroch, I., Biaggioni, W. Cheshire, T. Chelimsky, P. Cortelli, C. Gibbons, D. Goldstein, R. Hainsworth, M. Hilz, G. Jacob, H. Kaufmann, J. Jordan, L. Lipsitz, B. Levin, P. Low, C. Mathias, S. Raj, D. Robertson, P. Sandroni, I. Schatz, R. Schondorff, J. Stewart, and J. Gert van Dijk. 2011. Consensus statement on the definition of orthostatic hypotension, neutrally mediated syncope and the postural tachycardia syndrome. *Clinical Autonomic Research Society* 21(2):69-72. https://doi.org/10.1007/s10286-011-0119-5.

Freeman, R., A. R. Abuzinadah, C. Gibbons, P. Jones, M. G. Miglis, D. I. Sinn. 2018. Orthostatic hypotension: JACC state-of-the-art review. *Journal of the American College of Cardiology* 72(11):1294-1309. https://doi.org/10.1016/j.jacc.2018.05.079.

Fu, W., and B. Levine. 2018. Exercise and non-pharmacological treatment of POTS. *Autonomic Neuroscience* 215:20-27. https://doi.org/10.1016/j.autneu.2018.07.001.

Gerrity T. R., J. Bates, D. S. Bell, G. Chrousos, G. Furst, T. Hedrick, B. Hurwitz, R. W. Kula, S. M. Levine, R. C. Moore, and R. Schondorf. 2002–2003. Chronic fatigue syndrome: What role does the autonomic nervous system play in the pathophysiology of this complex illness? *Neuroimmunomodulation* 10(3):134-141. https://doi.org/10.1159/000067176.

Goldstein, D., C. Holmes, S. Frank, R. Dendi, R. Cannon, Y. Sharabi, M. Esler, and G. Eisenhofer. 2002. Cardiac sympathetic dysautonomia in chronic orthostatic intolerance syndromes. *Circulation* 106(18):2358-2365. https://doi.org/10.1161/01.CIR.0000036015.54619.B6.

Goldstein, D., C. Holmes, S. Frank, M. Naqibuddin, R. Dendi, S. Snader, and H. Calkins. 2003. Sympathoadrenal imbalance before neurocardiogenic syncope. *American Journal of Cardiology* 91(1):53-58. https://doi.org/10.1016/s0002-9149(02)02997-1.

Goldstein, D. S., B. Eldadah, C. Holmes, S. Pechnik, J. Moak, and Y. Sharabi. 2005. Neurocirculatory abnormalities in chronic orthostatic intolerance. *Circulation* 111(7):839-845. https://doi.org/10.1161/01.CIR.0000155613.20376.CA.

Grubb, B. P. 2005. Neurocardiogenic syncope. *New England Journal of Medicine* 352(10):1004-1010. https://doi.org/10.1056/nejmcp042601.

Grubb, B. P. 2008. Postural tachycardia syndrome. *Circulation* 117(21):2814-2817. https://doi.org/10.1161/circulationaha.107.761643.

Grubb, B. P., D. Samoil, D. Kosinski, K. Kip, and P. Brewster. 1994. Use of sertraline chloride in the treatment of refractory neurocardiogenic syncope in children and adolescents. *Journal of the American College of Cardiology* 24(2):480-484. https://doi.org/10.1016/0735-1097(94)90308-5.

Henderson, F. C., P. C. Rowe, M. Narayanan, R. Rosenbaum, M. Koby, K. Tuchmann, and C. A. Francomano. 2021. Refractory syncope and pre-syncope associated with atlanto-axial instability: Preliminary evidence of improvement following surgical stabilization. *World Neurosurgery.* 149:e854–e865. https://doi.org/10.1016/j.wneu.2021.01.084.

Heyer, G. L. 2014. Abdominal and lower-extremity compression decreases symptoms of postural tachycardia syndrome in youth during tilt table testing. *Journal of Pediatrics* 165(2):395-397. https://doi.org/10.1016/j.jpeds.2014.04.014.

Hurwitz, B. E., V. T. Coryell, M. Parker, P. Martin, A. LaPerriere, N. G. Klimas, G. N. Sfakianakis, and M. S. Bilsker. 2010. Chronic fatigue syndrome: Illness severity, sedentary lifestyle, blood volume and evidence of diminished cardiac function. *Clinical Science (London)* 118(2):125-135. https://doi.org/10.1042/CS20090055.

Hyatt, K. H., L. B. Jacobson, and V. S. Schneider. 1975. Comparison of 70 degrees tilt, LBNP, and passive standing as measures of orthostatic tolerance. *Aviation, Space, and Environmental Medicine* 46(6):801-808.

IOM (Institute of Medicine). 2015. *Beyond myalgic encephalomyelitis/chronic fatigue syndrome: Redefining an illness.* Washington, DC: The National Academies Press.

Jardine, D. L., I. C. Melton, I. G. Crozier, S. I. Bennett, R. A. Donald, and H. Ikram. 1997. Neurohormonal response to head-up tilt and its role in vasovagal syncope. *American Journal of Cardiology* 79(9):1302-1306. https://doi.org/10.1016/S0002-9149(9X)00084-9.

Jhanjee, R. I., Can, and D. Benditt. 2009. Syncope. *Disease-a-Month Series* 55(9):532-585. https://doi.org/j.disamonth.2009.04.004.

Johnson, J. N., K. J. Mack, N. L. Kuntz, C. K. Brands, C. J. Porter, and P. R. Fischer. 2010. Postural orthostatic tachycardia syndrome—A clinical review. *Pediatric Neurology* 42(2):77-85.

Kanjwal, K., M. Sheikh, B. Karabin, Y. Kanjwal, and B. Grubb. 2011. Neurocardiogenic syncope coexisting with postural orthostatic tachycardia syndrome in patients suffering from orthostatic intolerance: A combined form of autonomic dysfunction. *Pacing and Clinical Electrophysiology* 34(5):549-554. https://doi.org/10.1111/j.1540-8159.2010.02994.x.

Kenney, R. A., and L. A. Graham. 2001. Chronic fatigue syndrome symptoms common in patients with vasovagal syncope. *American Journal of Medicine* 110(3):242-243. https://doi.org/10.1016/S0002-9343(00)00704-X.

Knuttinen M-G., K. S. Zurcher, N. Khurana, I. Patel, A. Foxx-Orenstein, L. A. Harris, A. Lawrence, F. Aguilar, M. Sichlau, B. H. Smith, and S. J. Smith. 2021. Imaging findings of pelvic venous insufficiency in patients with postural orthostatic tachycardia syndrome. *Phlebology* 36(1):32-37. https://doi.org/10.1177/0268355520947610

Krupp, L. B., N. G. LaRocca, J. Muir-Nash, and A. D. Steinberg. 1989. The Fatigue Severity Scale: Application to patients with multiple sclerosis and systemic lupus erythematosus. *Archives of Neurology* 46(10):1121-1123. https://doi.org/10.1001/archneur.1989.00520460115022.

LaManca, J., S. Sisto, J. DeLuca, S. Johnson, G. Lange, J. Pareja, S. Cook, and B. Natelson. 1998. Influence of exhaustive treadmill exercise on cognitive functioning in chronic fatigue syndrome. *American Journal of Medicine* 105(3A):59S-65S. https://doi.org/10.1016/s0002-9343(98)00171-5.

Lange, G., J. Steffener, D. B. Cook, B. M. Bly, C. Christodoulou, W-C. Liu, J. Deluca, and B. H. Natelson. 2005. Objective evidence of cognitive complaints in chronic fatigue syndrome: A BOLD fMRI study of verbal working memory. *Neuroimage* 26(2):513-524. https://doi.org/10.1016/j.neuroimage.2005.02.011.

Legge, H., M. Norton, and J. L. Newton. 2008. Fatigue is significant in vasovagal syncope and is associated with autonomic symptoms. *Eurospace* 10(9):1095-1101. https://doi.org/10.1093/europace/eun164.
Lewis, T. 1932. A lecture on vasovagal syncope and the carotid sinus mechanism. *British Medical Journal* 1(3723):873-876. https://doi.org/10.1136/bmj.1.3723.873.
Light, A. R., L. Bateman, D. Jo, R. W. Hughen, T. A. VanHaitsma, A. T. White, and K. C. Light. 2012. Gene expression alterations at baseline and following moderate exercise in patients with chronic fatigue syndrome and fibromyalgia syndrome. *Journal of Internal Medicine* 271(1):64-81. https://doi.org/10.1111/j.1365-2796.2011.02405.x.
Low, P. A., P. Sandroni, M. Joyner, and W. K. Shen. 2009. Postural tachycardia syndrome (POTS). *Journal of Cardiovascular Electrophysiology* 20(3):352-358. https://doi.org/10.1111/j.1540-8167.2009.01407.x.
MacLean, A. R., and E. V. Allen. 1940. Orthostatic hypotension and orthostatic tachycardia: Treatment with the "head-up" bed. *Journal of the American Medical Association* 115(25):2162-2167. https://doi.org/10.1001/jama.1940.02810510038010.
Martinez-Lavin, M. 2006. Biology and therapy of fibromyalgia: Stress, the stress response system, and fibromyalgia. *Arthritis Research and Therapy* 9(4):216. https://doi.org/10.1186/ar2146.
McDonald, C., J. Frith, and J. L. Newton. 2011. Single centre experience of ivabradine in postural orthostatic tachycardia syndrome. *Europace* 13(3):427-430. https://doi.org/10.1093/europace/euq390.
Medow, M. S., J. M. Stewart, S. Sanyal, A. Mumtaz, D. Sica, and W. H. Frishman. 2008. Pathophysiology, diagnosis, and treatment of orthostatic hypotension and vasovagal syncope. *Cardiology in Review* 16(1):4-20. https://doi.org/10.1097/CRD.0b013e31815c8032.
Milhorat, T. H., P. A. Bolognese, M. Nishikawa, N. B. McDonnell, and C. A. Francomano. 2007. Syndrome of occipitoatlantoaxial hypermobility, cranial settling, and Chiari malformation Type I in patients with hereditary disorders of connective tissue. *Journal of Neurosurgery: Spine* 7(6):601-609. https://doi.org/10.3171/SPI-07/12/601.
Moak, J. P., D. Leong, R. Fabian, V. Freedenberg, E. Jarosz, C. Toney, S. Hanumanthaiah, and A. Darbari. 2016. Intravenous hydration for management of medication-resistant orthostatic intolerance in the adolescent and young adult. *Pediatric Cardiology* 37(2):278-282. https://doi.org/10.1007/s00246-015-1274-6.
Moya, A., R. Sutton, F. Ammirati, J. Blanc, M. Brignole, J. Dahm, J-C. Deharo, J. Gajek, K. Gjesdal, A. Krahm, M. Massin, M. Pepi, T. Pezawas, R. Ruiz Grannell, F. Sarasin, A. Ungar, J. Gert van Dijk, E. Walma, and W. Wieling. 2009. Guidelines for the diagnosis and management of syncope. *European Heart Journal* 30(21):2631-2671. https://doi.org/10.1093/eurheartj/ehp298.
Naschitz, J., I. Rosner, M. Rozebaum, L. Gaitini, I. Bistritzki, E. Zuckerman, E. Sabo, and D. Yeshurun. 2000. The capnography head-up tilt test for evaluation of chronic fatigue syndrome. *Seminars in Arthritis and Rheumatism* 30(2):79-86. https://doi.org/10.1053/sarh.2000.9201.
Natale, A., M. Akhtar, M. Jazayeri, A. Dhala, Z. Blanck, S. Deshpande, A. Krebs, and J. Sra. 1995. Provocation of hypotension during head-up tilt testing in subjects with no history of syncope or presyncope. *Circulation* 92(1):54-58. https://doi.org/10.1161/01.CIR.92.1.54.
Natelson, B., R. Intriligator, N. Cherniack, H. Chandler, and J. Stewart. 2007. Hypocapnia is a biological marker for orthostatic intolerance in some patients with chronic fatigue syndrome. *Dynamic Medicine* 6, Article 2. https://doi.org/10.1186/1476-5918-6-2.
Novak, P. 2018. Hypocapnic cerebral hypoperfusion: A biomarker of orthostatic intolerance. *PLoS ONE* 13(9):e0204419. https://doi.org/10.1371/journal.pone.0204419.

Ocon, A. J., Z. R. Messer, M. S. Medow, and J. M. Stewart. 2012. Increasing orthostatic stress impairs neurocognitive functioning in chronic fatigue syndrome with postural tachycardia syndrome. *Clinical Science (London, England: 1979)* 122(5):227-228. https://doi.org/10.1042/CS20110241.

Okamoto, L. E., S. R. Raj, A. Peltier, A. Gamboa, C. Shibao, A. Diedrich, B. K. Black, D. Robertson, and I. Biaggioni. 2012. Neurohumoral and haemodynamic profile in postural tachycardia and chronic fatigue syndromes. *Clinical Science (London, England: 1979)* 122(4):183-192. https://doi.org/10.1042/CS20110200.

Plash, W. B., A. Diedrich, I. Biaggioni, E. M. Garland, S. Y. Paranjape, B. D. Black, W. Dupont, and S. R. Raj. 2013. Diagnosing postural tachycardia syndrome: Comparison of tilt testing compared with standing haemodynamics. *Clinical Science (London, England: 1979)* 124(2):109-114. https://doi.org/10.1042/CS20120276.

Razumovsky, A., K. DeBusk, H. Calkins, S. Snader, K. Lucas, P. Vyas, D. Hanley, and P. C. Rowe. 2003. Cerebral and systemic hemodynamics changes during upright tilt in chronic fatigue syndrome. *Journal of Neuroimaging* 13(1):57-67. https://doi.org/10.1111/j.1552-6569.2003.tb00158.x.

Roma, M., C. Marden, and P. C. Rowe. 2018a. Passive standing tests for the office diagnosis of postural tachycardia syndrome: New methodological considerations. *Fatigue: Biomedicine, Health and Behavior* 6(4):179-192. https://doi.org/10.1080/21641846.2018.1512836.

Roma, M., C. L. Marden L., I. De Wandele, C. A. Francomano, and P. C. Rowe. 2018b. Postural tachycardia syndrome and other forms of orthostatic intolerance in Ehlers-Danlos syndrome. *Autonomic Neuroscience* 215(December):89-96. https://doi.org/10.1016/j.autneu.2018.02.006.

Roma, M., C. L. Marden, M. Flaherty, S. E. Jasion, E. M. Cranston, and P. C. Rowe. 2019. Impaired health-related quality of life in adolescent myalgic encephalomyelitis/chronic fatigue syndrome: The impact of core symptoms. *Frontiers in Pediatrics* 7(February):26. https://doi.org/10.3389/fped.2019.00026.

Rombaut, L., F. Malfait, A. Cools, A. De Paepe, and P. Calders. 2010. Musculoskeletal complaints, physical activity and health-related quality of life among patients with Ehlers-Danlos syndrome hypermobility type. *Disability and Rehabilitation* 32(16):1339-1345. https://doi.org/10.3109/09638280903514739.

Rose, M. S., M. L. Koshman, S. Spreng, and R. Sheldon. 2000. The relationship between health-related quality of life and frequency of spells in patients with syncope. *Journal of Clinical Epidemiology* 53(12):1209-1216. https://doi.org/10.1016/S0895-4356(00)00257-2.

Rosen, S. G., and P. E. Creyer. 1982. Postural tachycardia syndrome. Reversal of sympathetic hyperresponsiveness and clinical improvement during sodium loading. *American Journal of Medicine* 72(5):847-850. https://doi.org/10.1016/0002-9343(82)90559-9.

Rowe, P. C. 2016. Fatigue and the chronic fatigue syndrome. In *Neinstein's adolescent and young adult health care*, 6th ed., edited by L. Neinstein. Philadelphia, PA: Wolters Kluwer.

Rowe, P. C., I. Bou-Holaigah, J. S. Kan, and H. Calkins. 1995. Is neutrally mediated hypotension an unrecognized cause of chronic fatigue? *Lancet* 346(8950):623-624. https://doi.org/10.1016/s0140-6736(95)90525-1.

Rowe, P. C., D. F. Barron, H. Calkins, I. H. Maumenee, P. Y. Tong, and M. T. Geraghty. 1999. Orthostatic intolerance and chronic fatigue syndrome associated with Ehlers-Danlos syndrome. *Journal of Pediatrics* 135(4):494-499. https://doi.org/10.1016/S0022-3476(99)70173-3.

Rowe, P. C., H. Calkins, K. DeBusk, R. McKenzie, R. Anand, G. Sharma, B. Cuccherini, N. Soto, P. Hohman, S. Snader, K. Lucas, M. Wolff, and S. Straus. 2001. *Journal of the American Medical Association* 285(1):52-59. https://doi.org/10.1001/jama.285.1.52.

Rowe, P. C., K. R. Fontaine, M. Lauver, S. E. Jasion, C. L. Marden, M. Moni, C. B. Thompson, and R. L. Violand. 2016. Neuromuscular strain increases symptom intensity in chronic fatigue syndrome. *PLOS One* 11(7):e0159386. https://doi.org/10.1371/journal.pone.0159386.

Rowe, P. C., R. A. Underhill, K. J. Friedman, A. Gurwitt, M. S. Medow, M. S. Schwartz, N. Speight, J. M. Stewart, R. Vallings, and K. S. Rowe. 2017. Myalgic encephalomyelitis/chronic fatigue syndrome diagnosis and management in young people: A primer. *Frontiers in Pediatrics* 5(June):121. https://doi.org/10.3389/fped.2017.00121.

Rowe, P. C., C. L. Marden, S. Heinlein, and C. C. Edwards, II. 2018. Improvement of severe myalgic encephalomyelitis/chronic fatigue syndrome symptoms following surgical treatment of cervical spinal stenosis. *Journal of Translational Medicine* 16(1):21. https://doi.org/10.1186/s12967-018-1397-7.

Rowell, L. 1992. *Human cardiovascular control.* New York: Oxford University Press.

Ruzieh, M., A. Baugh, O. Dasa, R. Parker, J. Perrault, A. Renno, B. Karabin, and B. Grubb. 2017. Effects of intermittent intravenous saline infusions in patients with medication-refractory postural tachycardia syndrome. *Journal of Interventional Cardiac Electrophysiology* 48(3):255-260. https://doi.org/10.1007/s10840-017-0225-y.

Sandman, W., T. Scholbach, and K. Verginis. 2021. Surgical treatment of abdominal compression syndromes: The significance of hypermobility-related disorders. *American Journal of Medical Genetics Part C: Seminars in Medical Genetics* 187(4):570-578. https://doi.org/10.1002/ajmg.c.31949.

Sandroni, P., T. L. Opfer-Gehrking, E. E. Benarroch, W-K. Shen, and P. A. Low. 1996. Certain cardiovascular indices predict syncope in the postural tachycardia syndrome. *Clinical Autonomic Research* 6(4):225-231. https://doi.org/10.1007/BF02291138.

Schondorf, R., and P. Low. 1993. Idiopathic postural orthostatic tachycardia syndrome: An attenuated form of acute pandysautonomia? *Neurology* 43(1):132-137. https://doi.org/10.1212/wnl.43.1_part_1.132.

Seneviratne, S., A. Maitland, and L. Afrin. 2017. Mast cell disorders in Ehlers–Danlos syndrome. *American Journal of Medicine Part C: Seminars in Medical Genetics* 175(1):226-236. https://doi.org/10.1002/ajmg.c.31555.

Shaw, B., L. Stiles, K. Bourne, E. Green, C. Shibao, L. Okamoto, E. Garland, A. Gamboa, A. Diedrich, V. Raj, R. Sheldon, I. Biaggioni, D. Robertson, and S. Raj. 2019. The face of postural tachycardia syndrome—Insights from a large cross-sectional online community-based survey. *Journal of Internal Medicine* 286(4):438-448. https://doi.org/10.1111/joim.12895.

Sheldon, R. 2005. Tilt testing for syncope: A reappraisal. *Current Opinion in Cardiology* 20(1):38-41.

Sheldon, R. S., B. P. Grubb, B. Olshansky, W. K. Shen, H. Calkins, M. Brignole, S. R. Raj, A. D. Krahn, C. A. Morillo, J. M. Stewart, R. Sutton, P. Sandroni, K. J. Friday, D. Tessariol Hachul, M. I. Cohen, D. H. Lau, K. A. Mayuga, J. P. Moak, R. K. Sandhu, and K. Kanjwal. 2015. Heart Rhythm Society expert consensus statement on the diagnosis and treatment of postural tachycardia syndrome, inappropriate sinus tachycardia, and vasovagal syncope. *Heart Rhythm* 12(6):e41-e63. https://doi.org/10.1016/j.hrthm.2015.03.029.

Singer, W., D. M. Sletten, T. L. Opfer-Gehrking, C. K. Brands, P. R. Fischer, and P. A. Low. 2012. Postural tachycardia syndrome in children and adolescents: What is abnormal? *Journal of Pediatrics* 160(2):222-226. https://doi.org.10.1016/j.jpeds.2011.08.054.

Smit, A. A., M. A. Hardjowijono, and W. Wieling. 1997. Are portable folding chairs useful to combat orthostatic hypotension? *Annals of Neurology* 42(6):975-978. https://doi.org/10.1002/ana.410420620.

Smit, A. A., J. R. Halliwell, P. A. Low, and W. Wieling. 1999. Pathophysiologic basis of orthostatic hypotension in autonomic failure. *Journal of Physiology* 519(1):1-10.

Smith, J. J., C. M. Porth, and M. Erickson. 1994. Hemodynamic response to the upright posture. *Journal of Clinical Pharmacology* 34(5):375-386. https://doi.org/10.1002/j.1552-4604.1994.tb04977.x.

Stewart, J. M., M. H. Gewitz, A. Weldon, and J. Munzo. 1999. Patterns of orthostatic intolerance: The orthostatic tachycardia syndrome and adolescent chronic fatigue. *Journal of Pediatrics* 135:(2 Pt 1):218-225. https://doi.org/10.1016/S0022-3476(99)70025-9.

Stewart, J. M., J. R. Boris, G. Chelimsky, P. R. Fischer, J. E. Fortunato, B. P. Grubb, G. L. Heyer, I. T. Jarjour, M. S. Medow, M. T. Numan, P. T. Pianosi, W. Singer, S. Tarbell, T. C. Chelimsky, and Pediatric Writing Group of the American Autonomic Society. 2018. Pediatric disorders of orthostatic intolerance. *Pediatrics* 141(1):e20171673. https://doi.org/10.1542/peds.2017-1673.

Streeten, D. H. P., and D. S. Bell. 1998. Circulating blood volume in chronic fatigue syndrome. *Journal of Chronic Fatigue Syndromes* 4(1):3-11. https://doi.org/10.1300/J092v04n01_02.

Streeten, D. H., D. Thomas, and D. S. Bell. 2000. The roles of orthostatic hypotension, orthostatic tachycardia, and subnormal erythrocyte volume in the pathogenesis of the chronic fatigue syndrome. *American Journal of Medical Science* 320(1):1-8. https://doi.org/10.1097/00000441-200007000-0000.

Strickberger, S., D. Benson, I. Biaggioni, D. Callans, M. Cohen, K. Ellenbogen, A. Epstein, P. Friedman, J. Goldberger, P. Heidenreich, G. Klein, B. Knight, C. Morillo, R. Myerburg, and C. Sila. 2006. AHA/ACCF scientific statement on the evaluation of syncope: From the American Heart Association Councils on Clinical Cardiology, Cardiovascular Nursing, Cardiovascular Disease in the Young, and Stroke; Quality of Care and Outcomes Research Interdisciplinary Working Group; American College of Cardiology Foundation; and Heart Rhythm Society. *Journal of the American College of Cardiology* 47(2):473-484. https://doi.org/10.1016/j.jacc.2005.12.019.

Sutton, R., T. V. Salukhe, A-C. Franzen-Mcmanus, A. Collins, P. B. Lim, and D. P. Francis. 2014. Ivabradine in treatment of sinus tachycardia mediated vasovagal syncope. *Europace* 16(2):284-288. https://doi.org/10.1093/europace/eut226.

Takenaka, K., Y. Suzuki, K. Uno, M. Sato, T. Komuro, Y. Haruna, H. Kobayashi, K. Kawakubo, M. Sonoda, M. Asakawa, K. Nakahara, and A. Gunji. 2002. Effects of rapid saline infusion on orthostatic intolerance and autonomic tone after 20 days bed rest. *American Journal of Cardiology* 89(5):557-561. https://doi.org/10.1016/s0002-9149(01)02296-2.

van Campen, C., F. Verheugt, and F. C. Visser. 2018. Cerebral blood flow changes during tilt table testing in healthy volunteers, as assessed by Doppler imaging of the carotid and vertebral arteries. *Clinical Neurophysiology Practice* 3(March):91-95. https://doi.org/10.1016/j.cnp.2018.02.004.

van Campen, C. M. C., F. W. A. Verheugt, P. C. Rowe, and F. C. Visser, 2020a. Cerebral blood flow is reduced in ME/CFS during head-up tilt testing even in the absence of hypotension or tachycardia: A quantitative, controlled study using Doppler echography. *Clinical Neurophysiology Practice* 5(February):50-58. https://doi.org/10.1016/j.cnp.2020.01.003.

van Campen, C., P. C. Rowe, and F. C. Visser. 2020b. Reductions in cerebral blood flow can be provoked by sitting in severe myalgic encephalomyelitis/chronic fatigue syndrome patients. *Healthcare* 8(4):394. https://doi.org/10.3390/healthcare8040394.

van Campen, C., P. C. Rowe, and F. C. Visser, 2020c. Cerebral blood flow is reduced in severe ME/CFS patients during mild orthostatic stress testing: An exploratory study at 20 degrees of head-up tilt testing. *Healthcare* 8(2):169. https://doi.org/10.3390/healthcare8020169.

van Campen, C., P. C. Rowe, F. Verheugt, and F. C. Visser. 2020d. Physical activity measures in patients with myalgic encephalomyelitis/chronic fatigue syndrome: Correlations between peak oxygen consumption, the physical functioning scale of the SF-36 questionnaire, and the number of steps from an activity meter. *Journal of Translational Medicine* 18(1):228. https://doi.org/10.1186/s12967-020-02397-7.

van Campen, C., P. C. Rowe, F. Verheugt, and F. C. Visser. 2020e. Cognitive function declines following orthostatic stress in adults with myalgic encephalomyelitis/chronic fatigue syndrome (ME/CFS). *Frontiers in Neuroscience: Autonomic Neuroscience* 14(June):688. https://doi.org/10.3389/fnins.2020.00688.

van Campen, C., P. C. Rowe, and F. C. Visser. 2021a. Myalgic encephalomyelitis/chronic fatigue syndrome patients with joint hypermobility show larger cerebral blood flow reductions during orthostatic stress testing than patients without hypermobility: A case control study. *Medical Research Archives* 9(6). https://doi.org/10.18103/mra.v9i6.2494.

van Campen, C., P. C. Rowe, F. Verheugt, and F. C. Visser. 2021b. Numeric rating scales show prolonged post-exertional symptoms after orthostatic testing of adults with myalgic encephalomyelitis/chronic fatigue syndrome. *Frontiers in Medicine* 7(January):602894. https://doi.org/10.3389/fmed.2020.602894.

van Campen, C., P. C. Rowe, and F. C. Visser. 2022. Compression stockings improve cardiac output and cerebral blood flow during tilt testing in myalgic encephalomyelitis/chronic fatigue syndrome (ME/CFS) patients: A randomized crossover trial. *Medicina* 58(1):51. https://doi.org/10.3390/medicina58010051.

van Dijk, J.G, I. A. van Rossum, and R. D. Thijs. 2021. The pathophysiology of vasovagal syncope: Novel insights. *Autonomic Neuroscience: Basic and Clinical* 236:1-11.

van Lieshout, J. J., J. W. Wieling, J. M. Karemaker, and D. L. Eckberg. 1991. The vasovagal response. *Clinical Science (London, England: 1979)* 81(5):575-586. https://doi.org/10.1042/cs0810575.

van Lieshout, J J., A. D. ten Harkel, and W. Wieling. 1992. Physical manoeuvres for combating orthostatic dizziness in autonomic failure. *Lancet* 339(8798):897-898. https://doi.org/10.1016/0140-6736(92)90932-s..

van Lieshout, J. J., A. D. ten Harkel, and W. Wieling. 2000. Fludrocortisone and sleeping in the head-up position limit the postural decrease in cardiac output in autonomic failure. *Clinical Autonomic Research* 10(1):35-42. https://doi.org/10.1007/BF02291388.

VanNess, J. M., S. R. Stevens, L. Bateman, T. L. Stiles, and C. R. Snell. 2010. Postexertional malaise in women with chronic fatigue syndrome. *Journal of Women's Health* 19(2):239-244. https://doi.org/10.1089/jwh.2009.1507.

Varni, J. W., and C. A. Limbers. 2008. The PedsQL™ Multidimensional Fatigue Scale in young adults: Feasibility, reliability and validity in a University student population. *Quality of Life Research* 17(1):105-114.

Varni, J. W., M. Seid, and P. S. Kurtin. 2001. PedsQL 4.0: Reliability and validity of the Pediatric Quality of Life Inventory version 4.0 generic core scales in healthy and patient populations. *Medical Care* 39(8):800-812. https://doi.org/10.1097/00005650-200108000-00006.

Vernino, S., K. M. Bourne, L. E. Stiles, B. P. Grubb, A. Fedorowski, J. M. Stewart, A. C. Arnold, L. A. Pace, J. Axelsson, J. R. Boris, J. P. Moak, B. P. Goodman, K. R. Chémali, T. H. Chung, D. S. Goldstein, A. Diedrich, M. G. Miglis, M. M. Cortez, A. J. Miller, R. Freeman, I. Biaggioni, P. C. Rowe, R. S. Sheldon, C. A. Shibao, D. M. Systrom, G. A. Cook, T. A. Doherty, H. I. Abdallah, A. Darbari, and S. R. Raj. 2021. Postural orthostatic tachycardia syndrome (POTS): State of the science and clinical care from a 2019 National Institutes of Health Expert Consensus Meeting—Part 1. *Autonomic Neuroscience* 235(November):102828. https://doi.org/10.1016/j.autneu.2021.102828.

Walker, L. S., and J. W. Greene. 1991. The functional disability inventory: Measuring a neglected dimension of child health status. *Journal of Pediatric Psychology* 16(1):39-58. https://doi.org/10.1093/jpepsy/16.1.39.

Ware, J. E., Jr., and C. D. Sherbourne. 1992. The MOS 36-item short-form health survey (SF-36) I. Conceptual framework and item selection. *Medical Care* 30(6):473-483.

Wieling, W., and J. T. Shepherd. 1992. Initial and delayed circulatory responses to orthostatic stress in normal humans and in subjects with orthostatic intolerance. *International Angiology* 11(1):69-82.

Wieling, W., K. S. Ganzeboom, and J. P. Saul. 2004. Reflex syncope in children and adolescents. *Heart* 90(9):1094-1100. https://doi.org/10.1136/hrt.2003.022996.

Wood, G. C., R. P. Bentall, M. Göpfert, and R. H. Edwards. 1991. A comparative assessment of patients with chronic fatigue syndrome and muscle disease. *Psychological Medicine* 21(3):619-628. https://doi.org/10.1017/s003329170002225x.

Wyller, V. B., J. P. Saul, J. P. Amlie, and E. Thaulow. 2007. Sympathetic predominance of cardiovascular regulation during mild orthostatic stress in adolescents with chronic fatigue. *Clinical Physiology and Functional Imaging* 27(4):231-238. https://doi.org/10.1111/j.1475-097X.2007.00743.x.

Wyller, V. B., J. P. Saul, L. Walloe, and E. Thaulow. 2008. Sympathetic cardiovascular control during orthostatic stress and isometric exercise in adolescent chronic fatigue syndrome. *European Journal of Applied Physiology* 102(6):623-632. https://doi.org/10.1007/s00421-007-0634-1.

Wyller, V. B., J. A. Evang, K. Godang, K. K. Solhjell, and J. Bollerslev. 2010. Hormonal alterations in adolescent chronic fatigue syndrome. *Acta Paediatrica (Oslo, Norway: 1992)* 99(5):770-773. https://doi.org/10.1111/j.1651-2227.2010.01701.x.

Appendix C

Selected Resources

BOOKS

Beighton, P., ed. 1993. *McKusick's heritable disorders of connective tissue*. 5th ed. St. Louis, MO: Mosby.

Daens, S., and I. Dubois-Brock. 2022. *Transforming Ehlers-Danlos syndrome*. 1st ed. Dilbeek, Belgium: GERSED.

Halper, J., ed. 2021. *Progress in heritable soft connective tissue diseases*. 2nd ed. New York: Springer. https://doi.org/10.1007/978-3-030-80614-9.

Jovin, D., ed. 2020. *Disjointed: Navigating the diagnosis and management of hypermobile Ehlers-Danlos syndrome and hypermobility spectrum disorders*. Hidden Stripes Publications.

Liguori, G., and American College of Sports Medicine. 2021. *ACSM's guidelines for exercise testing and prescription*. 11th ed. Philadephia, PA: Lippincott Williams & Wilkins.

Royce, P. M., and B. Steinmann, eds. 2002. *Connective tissue and its heritable disorders: Molecular, genetic, and medical aspects*. 2nd ed. Wilmington, DE: Wiley-Liss.

BOOK CHAPTERS

Byers, P. H. 2019. Vascular Ehlers-Danlos syndrome. In *GeneReviews®* [Internet], edited by M. P. Adam, H. H. Ardinger, R. A. Pagon, S. E. Wallace, L. J. H. Bean, K. W. Gripp, G. M. Mirzaa, and A. Amemiya. Seattle, WA: University of Washington, Seattle; 1993-2022. Original edition, September 2, 1999. https://www.ncbi.nlm.nih.gov/books/NBK1494/ (accessed January 15, 2022).

Callewaert, B. 2019. Congenital contractural arachnodactyly. In *GeneReviews®* [Internet], edited by M. P. Adam, H. H. Ardinger, R. A. Pagon, S. E. Wallace, L. J. H. Bean, K. W. Gripp, G. M. Mirzaa, and A. Amemiya. Seattle, WA: University of Washington, Seattle; 1993-2022. Original edition, January 23, 2001. https://www.ncbi.nlm.nih.gov/books/NBK1386/ (accessed February 1, 2022).

Dietz, H. C. 2022. *FBN1*-Related Marfan syndrome. In *GeneReviews® [Internet]*, edited by M. P. Adam, H. H. Ardinger, R. A. Pagon, S. E. Wallace, L. J. H. Bean, K. W. Gripp, G. M. Mirzaa, and A. Amemiya. Seattle, WA: University of Washington, Seattle; 1993-2022. Original edition, April 18, 2001. https://www.ncbi.nlm.nih.gov/books/NBK1335/ (accessed May 11, 2022).

Greally, M. T. 2020. Shprintzen-Goldberg syndrome. In *GeneReviews® [Internet]*, edited by M. P. Adam, H. H. Ardinger, R. A. Pagon, S. E. Wallace, L. J. H. Bean, K. W. Gripp, G. M. Mirzaa, and A. Amemiya. Seattle, WA: University of Washington, Seattle; 1993-2022. Original edition, January 13, 2006. https://www.ncbi.nlm.nih.gov/books/NBK1277/ (accessed February 1, 2022).

Levy, H. P. 2018. Hypermobile Ehlers-Danlos syndrome. In *GeneReviews®* [Internet], edited by M. P. Adam, H. H. Ardinger, R. A. Pagon, S. E. Wallace, L. J. H. Bean, K. W. Gripp, G. M. Mirzaa, and A. Amemiya. Seattle, WA: University of Washington, Seattle; 1993-2022. Original edition, October 22, 2004. https://www.ncbi.nlm.nih.gov/books/NBK1279/ (accessed February 16, 2022).

Loeys, B. L., and H. C. Dietz. 2018. Loeys-Dietz syndrome. In *GeneReviews® [Internet]*, edited by M. P. Adam, H. H. Ardinger, R. A. Pagon, S. E. Wallace, L. J. H. Bean, K. W. Gripp, G. M. Mirzaa, and A. Amemiya. Seattle, WA: University of Washington, Seattle; 1993-2022. Original edition, February 28, 2008. https://www.ncbi.nlm.nih.gov/books/NBK1133/ (accessed February 1, 2022).

RESEARCH AND REVIEW ARTICLES

Bier, J. D., W. G. M. Scholten-Peeters, J. B. Staal, J. Pool, M. W. van Tulder, E. Beekman, J. Knoop, G. Meerhoff, and A. P. Verhagen. 2018. Clinical practice guideline for physical therapy assessment and treatment in patients with nonspecific neck pain. *Physical Therapy* 98(3):162-171. https://doi.org/10.1093/ptj/pzx118.

Blanpied, P. R., A. R. Gross, J. M. Elliott, L. L. Devaney, D. Clewley, D. M. Walton, C. Sparks, and E. K. Robertson. 2017. Neck pain: Revision 2017. *Journal of Orthopaedic and Sports Physical Therapy* 47(7):A1-A83. https://doi.org/10.2519/jospt.2017.0302.

Byers, P. H., J. Belmont, J. Black, J. De Backer, M. Frank, X. Jeunemaitre, D. Johnson, M. Pepin, L. Robert, L. Sanders, and N. Wheeldon. 2017. Diagnosis, natural history, and management in vascular Ehlers-Danlos syndrome. *American Journal of Medical Genetics. Part C: Seminars in Medical Genetics* 175(1):40-47. https://onlinelibrary.wiley.com/doi/10.1002/ajmg.c.31553.

Carpal tunnel syndrome: A summary of clinical practice guideline recommendations—Using the evidence to guide physical therapist practice. 2019. *Journal of Orthopaedic and Sports Physical Therapy* 49(5):359-360. https://doi.org/10.2519/jospt.2019.0501.

Castori, M., B. Tinkle, H. Levy, R. Grahame, F. Malfait, and A. Hakim. 2017. A framework for the classification of joint hypermobility and related conditions. *American Journal of Medical Genetics. Part C: Seminars in Medical Genetics* 175(1):148-157. https://onlinelibrary.wiley.com/doi/10.1002/ajmg.c.31539.

Clinical guidance to optimize work participation after injury or illness: Using the evidence to guide physical therapist practice. 2021. *Journal of Orthopaedic and Sports Physical Therapy* 51(8):380-381. https://www.jospt.org/doi/abs/10.2519/jospt.2021.0505.

Côté, P., H. Yu, H. M. Shearer, K. Randhawa, J. J. Wong, S. Mior, A. Ameis, L. J. Carroll, M. Nordin, S. Varatharajan, D. Sutton, D. Southerst, C. Jacobs, M. Stupar, A. Taylor-Vaisey, D. P. Gross, R. J. Brison, C. Paulden, C. Ammendolia, J. D. Cassidy, P. Loisel, S. Marshall, R. N. Bohay, J. Stapleton, and M. Lacerte. 2019. Non-pharmacological management of persistent headaches associated with neck pain: A clinical practice guideline from the Ontario protocol for traffic injury management (OPTIMa) collaboration. *European Journal of Pain* 23(6):1051-1070. https://doi.org/10.1016/j.jphys.2020.05.009.

Daley, D., L. P. Payne, J. Galper, A. Cheung, L. Deal, M. Despres, J. D. Garcia, F. Kistner, N. Mackenzie, T. Perry, C. Richards, and R. Escorpizo. 2021. Clinical guidance to optimize work participation after injury or illness: The role of physical therapists. *Journal of Orthopaedic and Sports Physical Therapy* 51(8):CPG1-CPG102. https://www.jospt.org/doi/10.2519/jospt.2021.0303.

Enseki, K., M. Harris-Hayes, D. M. White, M. T. Cibulka, J. Woehrle, T. L. Fagerson, and J. C. Clohisy. 2014. Nonarthritic hip joint pain. *Journal of Orthopaedic and Sports Physical Therapy* 44(6):A1-A32. https://doi.org/10.2519/jospt.2014.0302.

Erickson, M., M. Lawrence, C. W. S. Jansen, D. Coker, P. Amadio, and C. Cleary. 2019. Hand pain and sensory deficits: Carpal tunnel syndrome. *Journal of Orthopaedic and Sports Physical Therapy* 49(5):CPG1-CPG85. https://doi.org/10.2519/jospt.2019.0301.

Exercise for knee injury prevention: A summary of clinical practice guideline recommendations—Using the evidence to guide physical therapist practice. 2018. *Journal of Orthopaedic and Sports Physical Therapy* 48(9):732-733. https://doi.org/10.2519/jospt.2018.0508.

Finucane, L. M., A. Downie, C. Mercer, S. M. Greenhalgh, W. G. Boissonnault, A. L. Pool-Goudzwaard, J. M. Beneciuk, R. L. Leech, and J. Selfe. 2020. International framework for red flags for potential serious spinal pathologies. *Journal of Orthopaedic and Sports Physical Therapy* 50(7):350-372. https://doi.org/10.2519/jospt.2020.9971.

Knee ligament sprain guidelines: Revision 2017: Using the evidence to guide physical therapist practice. 2017. *Journal of Orthopaedic and Sports Physical Therapy* 47(11):822-823. https://www.jospt.org/doi/full/10.2519/jospt.2017.0510.

Levine, D., B. Work, S. McDonald, N. Harty, C. Mabe, A. Powell, and G. Sanford. 2021. Occupational therapy interventions for clients with Ehlers-Danlos syndrome (EDS) in the presence of postural orthostatic tachycardia syndrome (POTS). *Occupational Therapy in Health Care* 1-18. https://doi.org/10.1080/07380577.2021.1975200.

Lin, I., L. Wiles, R. Waller, R. Goucke, Y. Nagree, M. Gibberd, L. Straker, C. G. Maher, and P. P. B. O'Sullivan. 2020. What does best practice care for musculoskeletal pain look like? Eleven consistent recommendations from high-quality clinical practice guidelines: Systematic review. *British Journal of Sports Medicine* 54(2):79-86. https://doi.org/10.1136/bjsports-2018-099878.

Logerstedt, D. S., D. Scalzitti, M. A. Risberg, L. Engebretsen, K. E. Webster, J. Feller, L. Snyder-Mackler, M. J. Axe, and C. M. McDonough. 2017. Knee stability and movement coordination impairments: Knee ligament sprain revision 2017. *Journal of Orthopaedic and Sports Physical Therapy* 47(11):A1-A47. https://doi.org/10.2519/jospt.2017.0303.

Logerstedt, D. S., D. A. Scalzitti, K. L. Bennell, R. S. Hinman, H. Silvers-Granelli, J. Ebert, K. Hambly, J. L. Carey, L. Snyder-Mackler, M. J. Axe, and C. M. McDonough. 2018. Knee pain and mobility impairments: Meniscal and articular cartilage lesions revision 2018. *Journal of Orthopaedic and Sports Physical Therapy* 48(2):A1-A50. https://doi.org/10.2519/jospt.2018.0301.

MacCarrick, G., J. H. Black, 3rd, S. Bowdin, I. El-Hamamsy, P. A. Frischmeyer-Guerrerio, A. L. Guerrerio, P. D. Sponseller, B. Loeys, and H. C. Dietz, 3rd. 2014. Loeys-Dietz syndrome: A primer for diagnosis and management. *Genetics in Medicine* 16(8):576-587. https://doi.org/10.1038/gim.2014.11.

Malfait, F., C. Francomano, P. Byers, J. Belmont, B. Berglund, J. Black, L. Bloom, J. M. Bowen, A. F. Brady, N. P. Burrows, M. Castori, H. Cohen, M. Colombi, S. Demirdas, J. De Backer, A. De Paepe, S. Fournel-Gigleux, M. Frank, N. Ghali, C. Giunta, R. Grahame, A. Hakim, X. Jeunemaitre, D. Johnson, B. Juul-Kristensen, I. Kapferer-Seebacher, H. Kazkaz, T. Kosho, M. E. Lavallee, H. Levy, R. Mendoza-Londono, M. Pepin, F. M. Pope, E. Reinstein, L. Robert, M. Rohrbach, L. Sanders, G. J. Sobey, T. Van Damme, A. Vandersteen, C. van Mourik, N. Voermans, N. Wheeldon, J. Zschocke, and B. Tinkle. 2017. The 2017 international classification of the Ehlers-Danlos syndromes. *American Journal of Medical Genetics Part C: Seminars in Medical Genetics* 175(1):8-26. https://doi.org/10.1002/ajmg.c.31552.

Martin, R. L., T. E. Davenport, J. J. Fraser, J. Sawdon-Bea, C. R. Carcia, L. A. Carroll, B. R. Kivlan, and D. Carreira. 2021. Ankle stability and movement coordination impairments: Lateral ankle ligament sprains revision 2021. *Journal of Orthopaedic and Sports Physical Therapy* 51(4):CPG1-CPG80. https://doi.org/10.2519/jospt.2021.0302.

Mortier, G. R., D. H. Cohn, V. Cormier-Daire, C. Hall, D. Krakow, S. Mundlos, G. Nishimura, S. Robertson, L. Sangiorgi, R. Savarirayan, D. Sillence, A. Superti-Furga, S. Unger, and M. L. Warman. 2019. Nosology and classification of genetic skeletal disorders: 2019 revision. *American Journal of Medical Genetics Part A* 179(12):2393-2419. https://onlinelibrary.wiley.com/doi/10.1002/ajmg.a.61366.

Oliveira, C. B., C. G. Maher, R. Z. Pinto, A. C. Traeger, C. C. Lin, J. F. Chenot, M. van Tulder, and B. W. Koes. 2018. Clinical practice guidelines for the management of non-specific low back pain in primary care: An updated overview. *European Spine Journal* 27(11):2791-2803. https://doi.org/10.1007/s00586-018-5673-2.

Pyeritz, R. E. 2019. Marfan syndrome: Improved clinical history results in expanded natural history. *Genetics in Medicine* 21(8):1683-1690. https://doi.org/10.1038/s41436-018-0399-4.

Physical therapy after an ankle sprain: Using the evidence to guide physical therapist practice. 2021. *Journal of Orthopaedic and Sports Physical Therapy* 51(4):159-160. https://doi.org/10.2519/jospt.2021.0503.

Practice bulletin no. 176: Pelvic organ prolapse. 2017. *Obstetrics and Gynecology* 129(4):e56-e72. https://doi.org/10.1097/aog.0000000000002016.

Richards, S., N. Aziz, S. Bale, D. Bick, S. Das, J. Gastier-Foster, W. W. Grody, M. Hegde, E. Lyon, E. Spector, K. Voelkerding, and H. L. Rehm, on behalf of the AGMC Laboratory Quality Assurance Committee. 2015. Standards and guidelines for the interpretation of sequence variants: A joint consensus recommendation of the American College of Medical Genetics and Genomics and the Association for Molecular Pathology. *Genetics in Medicine* 17(5):405-423. https://doi.org/10.1038/gim.2015.30.

Savarirayan, R., V. Bompadre, M. B. Bober, T.-J. Cho, M. J. Goldberg, J. Hoover-Fong, M. Irving, S. E. Kamps, W. G. Mackenzie, C. Raggio, S. S. Spencer, and K. K. White. 2019. Best practice guidelines regarding diagnosis and management of patients with type II collagen disorders. *Genetics in Medicine* 21(9):2070-2080. https://doi.org/10.1038/s41436-019-0446-9.

Valent, P., C. Akin, and D. D. Metcalfe. 2017. Mastocytosis: 2016 updated WHO classification and novel emerging treatment concepts. *Blood* 129(11):1420-1427. https://doi.org/10.1182/blood-2016-09-731893.

Vernino, S., K. M. Bourne, L. E. Stiles, B. P. Grubb, A. Fedorowski, J. M. Stewart, A. C. Arnold, L. A. Pace, J. Axelsson, J. R. Boris, J. P. Moak, B. P. Goodman, K. R. Chémali, T. H. Chung, D. S. Goldstein, A. Diedrich, M. G. Miglis, M. M. Cortez, A. J. Miller, R. Freeman, I. Biaggioni, P. C. Rowe, R. S. Sheldon, C. A. Shibao, D. M. Systrom, G. A. Cook, T. A. Doherty, H. I. Abdallah, A. Darbari, and S. R. Raj. 2021. Postural orthostatic tachycardia syndrome (POTS): State of the science and clinical care from a 2019 National Institutes of Health expert consensus meeting—Part 1. *Autonomic Neuroscience* 235:102828. https://doi.org/10.1016/j.autneu.2021.102828.

Willy, R. W., L. T. Hoglund, C. J. Barton, L. A. Bolgla, D. A. Scalzitti, D. S. Logerstedt, A. D. Lynch, L. Snyder-Mackler, and C. M. McDonough. 2019. Patellofemoral pain. *Journal of Orthopaedic and Sports Physical Therapy* 49(9):CPG1-CPG95. https://doi.org/10.2519/jospt.2019.0302.

Yueh, B., N. Shapiro, C. H. MacLean, and P. G. Shekelle. 2003. Screening and management of adult hearing loss in primary care: Scientific review. *Journal of the American Medical Association* 289(15):1976-1985. https://doi.org/10.1001/jama.289.15.1976.

JOURNAL VOLUMES

Special Issue: Ehlers-Danlos syndromes, hypermobility spectrum disorders, and associated co-morbidities: Reports from EDS ECHO. 2021. *American Journal of Medical Genetics. Part C: Seminars in Medical Genetics* 187(4). https://onlinelibrary.wiley.com/toc/15524876/2021/187/4.

Special Issue: The Ehlers-Danlos syndromes: Reports from the International Consortium on the Ehlers-Danlos Syndromes. 2017. *American Journal of Medical Genetics. Part C: Seminars in Medical Genetics* 175(1). https://onlinelibrary.wiley.com/toc/15524876/2017/175/1.

WEBSITES

Marfan and Loeys-Dietz Syndromes

Marfan Foundation, The: Contains information on Marfan syndrome, as well as other hereditary aortopathies and Ehlers-Danlos syndromes. https://www.marfan.org (accessed May 27, 2022).

National Heart, Lung, and Blood Institute: Overview of Marfan syndrome. https://www.nhlbi.nih.gov/health-topics/marfan-syndrome (accessed May 27, 2022).

U.S. National Library of Medicine, MedlinePlus: Overview of Loeys-Dietz syndrome. https://medlineplus.gov/genetics/condition/loeys-dietz-syndrome (accessed May 27, 2022).

U.S. National Library of Medicine, MedlinePlus: Overview of Marfan syndrome. https://medlineplus.gov/genetics/condition/marfan-syndrome (accessed May 27, 2022).

Ehlers-Danlos Syndromes (EDS)

Ehlers-Danlos Society, The: Contains information on and resources pertaining to Ehlers-Danlos syndromes and hypermobility spectrum disorders for patients and families, as well as health care providers and researchers. https://ehlers-danlos.com (accessed May 27, 2022).

National Institutes of Health, National Center for Advancing Translational Sciences, Genetic and Rare Diseases Information Center: Overview of EDS. https://rarediseases.info.nih.gov/diseases/6322/ehlers-danlos-syndromes (accessed May 27, 2022).

U.S. National Library of Medicine, MedlinePlus: Overview of EDS. https://medlineplus.gov/genetics/condition/ehlers-danlos-syndrome (accessed May 27, 2022).

Disability Resources

Job Accommodations Network (JAN). https://askjan.org (accessed May 27, 2022).
- JAN provides guidance on workplace accommodations and disability employment and is funded by a contract from the U.S. Department of Labor, Office of Disability Employment Policy (#1605DC-17-C-0038).
- JAN provides A to Z listings by disability, topic, and limitation. The information is designed to help employers and individuals determine effective accommodations and comply with Title I of the Americans with Disabilities Act (ADA), including ADA information, accommodation ideas, and resources for additional information.
    - A to Z of Disabilities and Accommodations. https://askjan.org/a-to-z.cfm (accessed May 27, 2022).
    - Marfan syndrome. https://askjan.org/disabilities/Marfan-Syndrome.cfm (accessed May 27, 2022).
    - Ehlers-Danlos syndrome. https://askjan.org/disabilities/Ehlers-Danlos-Syndrome.cfm (accessed May 27, 2022).

SchoolToolkit for EDS and JHS: This UK-based initiative outlines how schools have worked to best accommodate students so that they can achieve their highest learning potential. https://theschooltoolkit.org/reasonable-adjustments (accessed May 27, 2022).

Appendix D

Biographical Sketches of Committee Members

Paul A. Volberding, M.D. (*Chair*), is professor emeritus at the University of California, San Francisco (UCSF) School of Medicine; former codirector and principal investigator of the UCSF-Gladstone Center for AIDS Research; and director of the UCSF AIDS Research Institute. Trained in medical oncology, Dr. Volberding became involved in the early AIDS epidemic in San Francisco and has worked primarily in the development of antiretroviral therapy but also in clinical trials in HIV-related malignancies. He is a member of the National Academy of Medicine and currently serves on the National Academies of Sciences, Engineering, and Medicine's Standing Committee of Medical and Vocational Experts for the Social Security Administration's Disability Programs. Dr. Volberding has also chaired numerous National Academies committees, including several for the Social Security Administration—most recently, the Committee on Childhood Cancers and Disability.

Rebecca Bascom, M.D., M.P.H., is professor in the departments of Medicine and Public Health Sciences and active staff at Penn State College of Medicine. She trained at the Johns Hopkins Hospital and School of Public Health in internal medicine, pulmonary and critical care, preventive and occupational medicine, and inhalation toxicology. Dr. Bascom has worked with individuals and employers to devise workplace accommodations when medical conditions impact a worker's ability to do the central duties of their job. She is active in clinical research on pulmonary fibrosis, modified-risk tobacco products, and Ehlers-Danlos syndromes (EDS). Dr. Bascom is a founding member of the EDS Comorbidity Coalition (now called the Community Coalition), and she facilitates Penn State's EDS Patient Research Advisory Group and its Stretch Project, which is funded by the Patient-Centered Outcomes Research Institute and based in the Extension for Community Healthcare. She has previously served as a member of multiple National Academies' committees, including, most recently, the Committee on Assessing Toxicologic Risks to Human Subjects Used in Controlled Exposure Studies of Environmental Pollutants and the Committee on Scientific Standards for Studies on Modified Risk Tobacco Products.

Adam D. Bitterman, D.O., F.A.A.O.S., is assistant professor of orthopaedic surgery at the Donald and Barbara Zucker School of Medicine at Hofstra/Northwell. He is a board certified orthopaedic specialist with a focus in treating conditions of the lower leg. His clinical interests include arthritis of the foot and ankle, deformity correction, Achilles tendon disorders, connective tissue disorders, and sports-related injuries to the ankle and foot. Dr. Bitterman is a graduate of Binghamton University and pursued his medical education at the New York College of Osteopathic Medicine. He completed his orthopaedic surgery residency at North Shore-LIJ Plainview Orthopaedic Consortium before graduating from Rush University Medical Center in Chicago, Illinois, where he completed his foot-and-ankle fellowship training. Dr. Bitterman serves as chair of the Department of Orthopaedic Surgery at Huntington Hospital and is co-chair of the Research Committee for the Huntington Hospital Orthopaedic Surgery Residency program. His research interests include clinical outcomes after foot-and-ankle surgery, Achilles tendon pathology, connective tissue disorders, patient comprehension, infection control, and residency training. He has published on Marfan syndrome and is a member of the Professional Advisory Board of The Marfan Foundation.

Antonio Bulbena-Vilarrasa, M.D., Ph.D., M.Sc., is distinguished professor of psychiatry and chair of the Department of Psychiatry at the Universitat Autònoma de Barcelona. He has created and coordinated several networks of services, including general hospital, psychiatric hospital, community care, inpatient and outpatient adult and child psychiatry, mobile teams, and inpatient and outpatient addiction psychiatry, which has become the largest psychiatric network in Europe. Dr. Bulbena's main research focus is the interface between somatic and mental illnesses, especially between new somatic biomarkers and anxiety disorders and related conditions. In particular, he has studied the relationship between anxiety disorders and joint hypermobility syndrome (hypermobile-type Ehlers-Danlos), which he originally described in 1988. Recently, he developed a new model of anxiety disorders based on the relationship between the connective tissue and the autonomic nervous system, called the "neuroconnective phenotype." He is chair of the Psychiatric & Psychological Aspects Working Group of the International Consortium of Ehlers-Danlos Syndromes and Hypermobility Spectrum Disorders. Dr. Bulbena trained in top academic institutions in Spain and in the United Kingdom and has more than 200 publications in respected medical journals.

Pradeep Chopra, M.D., is assistant professor (clinical) at Brown Medical School and director of the Center for Complex Conditions, Rhode Island. He is board certified in pain medicine, and his area of interest is complex chronic pain conditions. Dr. Chopra is a recognized international expert on many of the complex pain conditions, including connective tissue disorders such as Ehlers-Danlos syndromes, Marfan syndrome, and complex regional pain syndrome. He has authored and coauthored multiple peer-reviewed journal articles and books on such conditions. Dr. Chopra's primary training is in anesthesia and critical care medicine, with a fellowship in pain medicine, all from Harvard Medical School. He is a member of the Pain Management Working Group of the International Consortium of Ehlers-Danlos Syndromes and Hypermobility Spectrum Disorders, and is the recipient of multiple awards from Harvard, as well as the Schwartz Center Compassionate Care Award.

Harry C. Dietz, III, M.D. (through July 2021), is Victor A. McKusick professor of medicine and genetics and an investigator at the Howard Hughes Medical Institute at the Johns Hopkins University School of Medicine. Recognized as a leading authority on Marfan syndrome and related connective tissue disorders, Dr. Dietz and his team have made critical contributions to the clinical and molecular characterization of many vascular connective tissue disorders, including Marfan, Loeys-Dietz, and Shprintzen-Goldberg syndromes. His group has pioneered therapeutic strategies for these and other conditions, including vascular Ehlers-Danlos syndrome. Dr. Dietz leads a multidisciplinary team focused on the clinical care of patients with connective tissue disorders and has a long history of service to patient advocacy groups, including the DEFY Foundation. Currently, he serves on the Professional Advisory Board of The Marfan Foundation and as chair of the Medical Advisory Council of the Loeys-Dietz Syndrome Foundation. He has received more than 50 national and international awards and honors, including the Antoine Marfan Award from the National Marfan Foundation and the Art of Listening Award from the Genetic Alliance. Dr. Dietz received his medical degree from the State University of New York Upstate School of Medicine and completed a pediatric residency and a cardiology fellowship at Johns Hopkins University School of Medicine before joining its faculty. He is a member of both the National Academy of Medicine and the National Academy of Sciences and previously served on the National Academies' Committee on Accelerating Rare Diseases Research and Orphan Product Development.

Clair A. Francomano, M.D., is professor and director of the Medical Genetics Residency in the Department of Medical and Molecular Genetics at Indiana University (IU) School of Medicine and serves as director of the Ehlers-Danlos Society Center for the Ehlers-Danlos Syndromes at IU Health. Her academic medical career has been dedicated to the clinical and molecular aspects of the hereditary disorders of connective tissue, including Marfan and Stickler syndromes, a variety of skeletal dysplasias, and the Ehlers-Danlos syndromes (EDS), which have been her primary focus during the past 15 years. Dr. Francomano has worked closely with the Ehlers-Danlos Society and the International Consortium on the Ehlers-Danlos Syndromes and Hypermobility Spectrum Disorders, currently chairing the Medical and Scientific Board for the Ehlers-Danlos Society and serving on the Steering Committee for the International Consortium. She is a member of the medical board of the Ehlers-Danlos Syndrome Research Foundation and is a member of the EDS Community Coalition. The Ehlers-Danlos Society awarded Dr. Francomano their Lifetime Achievement Award in 2019 for her contributions to persons living with EDS. Dr. Francomano has edited four books and published over 150 papers in the peer-reviewed biomedical literature.

Walter R. Frontera, M.D., Ph.D., F.R.C.P., is professor of physical medicine and rehabilitation and physiology at the University of Puerto Rico School of Medicine. He formerly served as inaugural chair and professor of physical medicine and rehabilitation at Harvard Medical School and Vanderbilt University School of Medicine. Dr. Frontera's main research interest is the mechanisms underlying muscle atrophy and weakness in the elderly, and the development of rehabilitative interventions for sarcopenia. He is editor in chief of the *American Journal of Physical Medicine and Rehabilitation* and the immediate past president of the International Society of Physical and Rehabilitation Medicine. Dr. Frontera received his medical degree from the University of Puerto Rico School of Medicine and a Ph.D. in applied anatomy and physiology from Boston University. He is a member of the National Academy of Medicine and has served on numerous National Academies' committees, including the Standing Committee of Medical and Vocational Experts for the Social Security Administration's Disability Programs, the Committee on the Use of Selected Assistive Products and Technologies in Eliminating or Reducing the Effects of Impairments, and the Planning Committee on Long-Term Health Effects Stemming from

COVID-19 and Implications for the Social Security Administration. Dr. Frontera is also a fellow of the Royal College of Physicians in London.

Petra M. Klinge, M.D., Ph.D., is director of the Pediatric Neurosurgery Division and director of the Research Center and Clinic for Cerebrospinal Fluid Disorders at the Neurosurgery Foundation, and professor in the Department of Neurosurgery at the Warren Alpert Medical School of Brown University. She specializes in the surgical treatment of patients with brain tumors, hydrocephalus, and Alzheimer's disease, as well as pediatric diseases and treatment of congenital diseases like Chiari and spinal malformations. Dr. Klinge is a member of the American Association of Neurosurgeons and the Congress of Neurological Surgeons. She is editor in chief of the Elsevier journal *Interdisciplinary Neurosurgery: Advanced Techniques and Case Management* and associate editor of *Clinical Neurology and Neurosurgery*. Dr. Klinge is a member of the executive committee of the Scientific Education & Advisory Board of the Bobby Jones Chiari & Syringomyelia Foundation and is a member and past president of the International Society for Hydrocephalus and Cerebrospinal Fluid Disorders. She serves on the Ehlers-Danlos Syndromes Community Coalition and the Neurology Working Group of the International Consortium of Ehlers-Danlos Syndromes and Hypermobility Spectrum Disorders. Dr. Klinge received her medical degree at the University of Kiel and completed her neurosurgical residency at Hannover Medical School in Germany. Since 2014, she has specialized in the diagnosis and treatment of neurological and neurosurgical spine and brain conditions associated with connective tissue disorders and conducts specific research to advance the science and recognition of the clinical pathology and provides educational presentations on these conditions.

Barbara L. Kornblau, J.D., O.T.R/L., F.A.O.T.A., C.C.M., C.D.M.S., C.P.E., is a professor in and program director of the Occupational Therapy Program for Idaho State University. She also serves as a consultant to the United Spinal Association, the Coalition for Disability Health Equity, and previously served as a consultant to the American Association on Health and Disability on disability access and disability employment and policy issues. Ms. Kornblau is past president of the American Occupational Therapy Association, a former Robert Wood Johnson Health Policy Fellow in the Offices of Senators Harkin and Rockefeller, an attorney, a Certified Case Manager, a Certified Disability Management Specialist, a Certified Pain Educator, and a person with a disability. She is recognized as an expert in disability policy, return to work issues, assistive technology, and reasonable accommodations under the Americans with Disabilities Act and the Rehabilitation Act. She received a J.D. from the University of Miami and an occupational therapy degree from the University of Wisconsin–Madison.

She previously served on two National Academies' committees for the Social Security Administration, including the Committee on Functional Assessment for Adults with Disabilities.

Deborah Krakow, M.D., is a professor in and chair of the Department of Obstetrics and Gynecology and professor of human genetics, pediatrics, and orthopaedic surgery at the David Geffen School of Medicine at the University of California, Los Angeles (UCLA). She obtained her medical degree from the Chicago Medical School and completed her residency in obstetrics and gynecology, and fellowships in maternal fetal medicine and medical genetics. Dr. Krakow has a 20-year career in caring for patients with and studying the molecular biology underlying connective tissue disorders, and she has published more than 100 articles on heritable disorders of the musculoskeletal system. She is codirector of the International Skeletal Dysplasia Registry and serves on the medical advisory boards of the Osteogenesis Imperfecta Foundation and Little People of America.

Cheryl Lynn Maier, M.D., Ph.D., is medical director of the Special Coagulation Laboratory and assistant professor in the Department of Pathology and Laboratory Medicine at Emory University School of Medicine. She completed her M.D. and Ph.D. at Yale School of Medicine, with a concentration in immunology, before completing a pathology residency and a clinical fellowship in transfusion medicine and coagulation at Emory. Dr. Maier also completed a 2-year postdoctoral research fellowship investigating the immune response to transfused blood products. More recently, she secured extramural funding from the National Heart, Lung, and Blood Institute with a K99/R00 career development award, studying platelet immunology. Dr. Maier's interest in heritable disorders of connective tissue (HDCT) relates to the oftentimes subtle yet potentially significant bleeding diatheses these patients experience. She is particularly interested in ways that defects in collagen and other tissues contribute to bleeding in patients with HDCT, as well as any associated consequences on innate and adaptive immune responses in these patients.

Anne L. Maitland, M.D., Ph.D., is assistant professor in the Department of Medicine, Division of Allergy and Clinical Immunology, at the Icahn School of Medicine at Mount Sinai and attending physician at the Mount Sinai South Nassau Chiari EDS Program. She is also medical director of Comprehensive Allergy & Asthma Care and of 3 Pillars Therapeutics. Dr. Maitland serves as chair of the American Academy of Allergy, Asthma, and Immunology (AAAAI) Mast Cell Activation Disorders Committee and of the Allergy & Immunology Working Group of the International Consortium of Ehlers-Danlos Syndromes and Hypermobility Spectrum Disorders. She serves as an expert consultant for facilitating the North America Allied Health Providers Extension for Community Healthcare Outcomes educational program for the Ehlers-Danlos Society. Dr. Maitland is a member of the Ehlers-Danlos Syndromes Community Coalition and of the medical board of the Ehlers-Danlos Syndrome Research Foundation. In addition, she is an active member of the AAAAI committee to meet the needs of the underserved, as well as of the National Medical Association Allergy & Immunology faculty. Dr. Maitland is active in local societies and the surrounding communities to increase awareness of immune-mediated disorders, including primary immune deficiency and mast cell disorders. She is a fellow of the American College of Allergy, Asthma and Immunology. Her clinical interests include efforts to improve the surveillance, diagnosis, and management of individuals affected by immediate and delayed disorders and those who are susceptible to severe or recurrent infections, as well as the diagnosis and treatment of mast cell disorders in the context of connective tissue disorders. Dr. Maitland previously served on speakers' bureaus and advisory committees for Regeneron, Genentech, and Sanofi.

Reed E. Pyeritz, M.D., Ph.D., recently retired as William Smilow Professor of Medicine and is emeritus professor of genetics at the Perelman School of Medicine at the University of Pennsylvania. His field of clinical service, research, and teaching was medical genetics, for which he was a member of the first class of professionals to receive certification by the American Board of Medical Genetics. From 1978 to the present, his clinical and research interests have focused on heritable disorders of connective tissue, particularly Marfan syndrome. Dr. Pyeritz was founder of the National Marfan Foundation (now The Marfan Foundation) in 1980 and served as chair of its Professional Advisory Board, of which he remains a member, for many years. He has published more than 300 research papers, reviews, and chapters on Marfan syndrome and related disorders, such as vascular Ehlers-Danlos syndrome. He is coeditor of *Principles and Practice of Medical Genetics and Genomics.*

Leslie N. Russek, Ph.D., P.T., D.P.T., O.C.S., is professor emeritus in the Physical Therapy Department at Clarkson University, where she taught musculoskeletal physical therapy, foundational sciences, and research methods. She has been researching and publishing in the area of hypermobile Ehlers-Danlos syndrome (hEDS) for more than 20 years. She has also published in the areas of fibromyalgia and chronic pain, including a textbook chapter on chronic pain. Dr. Russek is a member of the Allied Health Working Group of the International Consortium of Ehlers-Danlos Syndromes and Hypermobility Spectrum Disorders. She serves as an expert consultant for facilitating the North America Allied Health Providers

Extension for Community Healthcare Outcomes educational program for the Ehlers-Danlos Society. Dr. Russek continues to treat patients with hypermobility spectrum disorder (HSD) and hEDS part time and frequently provides lectures about HSD to patients and health care providers.

Eric Lowell Singman, M.D., Ph.D., is professor at the University of Maryland School of Medicine's Department of Ophthalmology and Visual Sciences. A board certified ophthalmologist, he has subspecialty fellowship training in neuro-ophthalmology. After his fellowship, Dr. Singman practiced neuro-ophthalmology for 14 years in Lancaster, Pennsylvania, and was an attending neuro-ophthalmologist at the Lancaster Rehabilitation Hospital, as well as at Sinai Hospital of Baltimore's Comprehensive Concussion Clinic. Previously, he was associate professor of ophthalmology at the Wilmer Eye Institute at the Johns Hopkins Hospital and division chief at the Program of All-Inclusive Care for the Elderly clinic. He founded and directed the Wilmer Clinic for Vision Concerns after Traumatic Brain Injury at Johns Hopkins. He also co-founded the Wilmer Genetic Eye Disease Center. Dr. Singman has served as a subject matter expert on brain injury at the Department of Defense (DoD) Vision Center of Excellence on multiple occasions and has chaired grant review committees for the DoD Vision Research Program. His clinical expertise includes diagnosis of visual dysfunction after brain injury, as well as the impact of Ehlers-Danlos syndromes (EDS) on vision. His research interests have focused on automation of the eye examination, using big data to explore the impact of brain injury on vision and the visual sequelae of hypermobile EDS. Dr. Singman also serves as a district medical adviser for Federal Occupational Health as well as the U.S. Marshall Service, particularly in the area of evaluating visual system disability claim reports for federal employees with work-related injuries.